Advances in Computational Intelligence for Health Informatics and Computer-Aided Diagnosis

This book provides a comprehensive overview of the intersection of computational intelligence, health informatics, and computer-aided diagnosis (CAD). The book explores and highlights the latest advancements, methodologies, applications, and tools in these fields.

Advances in Computational Intelligence for Health Informatics and Computer-Aided Diagnosis: Methods, Applications, and Tools covers a broad spectrum of computational intelligence approaches, from basic concepts to advanced methodologies. The focus on health informatics reflects the book's commitment to researching data integration, privacy issues, and interoperability issues that are crucial in today's healthcare landscape. The book's core is its in-depth examination of CAD systems, which encompasses numerous healthcare sectors and underlines the technological complexity involved in building accurate and efficient diagnostic tools. Some of the other key areas covered include: medical imaging analysis, disease identification and diagnosis, and drug research and development. It also provides case studies that demonstrate how computational intelligence methods are applied in real-world healthcare scenarios, giving readers a practical understanding of the subject matter. The authors then discuss future trends and directions in computational intelligence for health informatics.

The book is designed to serve as a guide for academics, professionals, and students who are curious about the challenges of integrating contemporary computational approaches into medical diagnostics and decision support.

Advances in Computational Intelligence for Health Informatics and Computer-Aided Diagnosis

Methods, Applications, and Tools

Edited by
A. Malini, Surbhi Bhatia Khan, S. Kayalvizhi, and Mohammed Saraee

CRC Press
Taylor & Francis Group
Boca Raton London New York

CRC Press is an imprint of the
Taylor & Francis Group, an **informa** business

Designed cover image: A. Malini

First edition published 2025
by CRC Press
6000 Broken Sound Parkway NW, Suite 300, Boca Raton, FL 33487-2742

and by CRC Press
4 Park Square, Milton Park, Abingdon, Oxon, OX14 4RN

CRC Press is an imprint of Taylor & Francis Group, LLC

ISBN: 978-1-032-77657-6 (hbk)
ISBN: 978-1-032-77658-3 (pbk)
ISBN: 978-1-003-48423-3 (ebk)

DOI: 10.1201/9781003484233

Typeset in Times
by Newgen Publishing UK

Contents

Preface....vii
About the Editors....ix
List of Contributors....xi

Chapter 1 Overview of Computational Intelligence for Health Informatics and Computer-Aided Diagnosis....1

S. Kayalvizhi, A. Malini, Surbhi Bhatia Khan, and Mohammed Saraee

Chapter 2 From Pixels to Prognosis: Machine Learning Approaches for Medical Imaging Diagnosis....11

T. Priyadarsini and Saranya J.

Chapter 3 Development of an Advanced Lung Cancer Diagnosis System: Using Image Processing and Machine Learning....22

S. Kayalvizhi, Kuraganti Harish, and Yakub Mathew

Chapter 4 Machine Learning Algorithms for Medical Diagnosis and Prognosis....31

P. Muthu, S. Latha, S. Hannah Pauline, R. Jansi, and Samiappan Dhanalakshmi

Chapter 5 Exploring Deep Learning Models in Medical Image Analysis for Human Disease Detection and Classification....53

Nithyakalyani Krishnan and P. Muthu

Chapter 6 Machine Learning Approach for Different Habitual Activity Versus Sleep Intermittent Stages from Time-Efficient Perspectives based on Facial Features....78

Krishnakumar K. and S. Latha

Chapter 7 A Survey of Interoperability and Security Challenges in the IoT Healthcare Environment....106

Parthiban S. and Saranya J.

Chapter 8 Automated Cardiovascular Disease Prediction Using Ant Colony Optimization with a Deep Learning Improved Neural Network 132

K. Sathya, R. Shanthi, J. Esther, C. Selvi, and M. Pandiyan

Chapter 9 Utilizing Explainable Artificial Intelligence for Parkinson's Disease Diagnosis through the Analysis of Spiral and Wave Drawings with Integrated Data Augmentation 156

S. Murugaveni, Harisudha Kuresan, N. Sri Sai Charan Reddy, Perala Manoj, and Gaddam Rohit

Chapter 10 Review of Medical Sensors for Healthcare Monitoring Systems Using Machine Learning Algorithms 171

M. K. Srilekha, S. Uma Maheswari, N. R. Shanker, and J. Gayathri

Chapter 11 Breast Cancer Classification Using Machine Learning: A Study 193

S. Muthumari, J. Suganthi, B. Nagarajan, and M. Mageshwari

Chapter 12 Secure Compressive Sensing in Medical Imaging Using Fractional-Order Hyperchaotic Systems 206

S. Kayalvizhi and S. Malarvizhi

Chapter 13 Early-Stage Lung Cancer Classification Using Spatial FusionNet 221

Meghna Vaddadi, Netaliya Ahmed, Nimmy B. Mathew, and A. Anilet Bala

Chapter 14 Practical Applications: Specific Diseases or Conditions Where AI Has Made a Significant Impact: A Review 243

Saranya J., Selvakumar V. S., Suganthi S., and Dinesh K.

Chapter 15 Medical Impact Assessment of Industrial Emissions: Predicting the Air Quality Index 261

Eshaan Abbas Jafri, Raj Tetarwal, Udhaya Kumar, and Kasthuri Bha J. K.

Index 279

Preface

The advent of computational intelligence has revolutionized many sectors, and healthcare is no exception. The integration of advanced computational methods and artificial intelligence (AI) into health informatics and computer-aided diagnosis has opened new frontiers in medical research and clinical practice. This book, titled "Advances in Computational Intelligence for Health Informatics and Computer-Aided Diagnosis: Methods, Applications, and Tools," seeks to provide an in-depth exploration of the latest advancements and their transformative impact on healthcare.

The chapters in this book are carefully curated to cover a broad spectrum of topics within this rapidly evolving field. We begin with an overview of computational intelligence in healthcare, establishing the foundation for understanding the diverse methods and applications discussed in subsequent chapters. The book delves into the application of machine learning for medical imaging diagnosis, presenting innovative approaches from pixels to prognosis.

We explore the development of an advanced lung cancer diagnosis system utilizing image processing and machine learning, followed by an examination of automated dementia detection through genetic algorithms and differential evaluation models. The potential of deep learning models in medical image analysis for human disease detection and classification is also discussed, showcasing cutting-edge research in this area.

Further, the book addresses machine learning approaches for analyzing habitual activities and sleep patterns using facial features, and the challenges of interoperability and security in Internet of Things (IoT)-based healthcare systems. The intelligent prediction of cardiovascular diseases using ant colony optimization and enhanced deep learning models is presented, highlighting the fusion of bio-inspired algorithms with AI.

The utilization of explainable AI for diagnosing Parkinson's disease through spiral and wave drawing analysis is another key topic, emphasizing the importance of transparency in AI systems. A review of medical sensors in healthcare monitoring systems and the role of machine learning algorithms offers insights into the growing field of wearable health technology.

Additionally, the book covers specific applications such as breast cancer classification using machine learning, secure compressive sensing in medical imaging, and early-stage lung cancer classification through improved data processing with Spatial FusionNet. The final chapters provide a comprehensive review of the practical applications of AI in diagnosing specific diseases or conditions and assess the medical impact of industrial emissions on air quality.

This compilation serves as a valuable resource for researchers, practitioners, and students interested in the intersection of computational intelligence and healthcare. By showcasing a diverse range of methods, applications, and tools, this book aims to inspire further innovation and collaboration in the pursuit of improved healthcare outcomes through advanced technology.

About the Editors

Dr A. Malini is an associate professor in the School of Computer Science and Engineering at Vellore Institute of Technology, Chennai, Tamil Nadu. She has 20+ years of teaching experience. She obtained her doctoral degree from Anna University, Chennai. She is a lifetime member of the Computer Society of India. She has published 50+ research articles in refereed journals and international/national conferences. She has contributed 20+ chapters to books. She has contributed to three edited books on artificial intelligence (AI) and machine learning. Dr Malini has contributed voluntarily as a reviewer for reputed international journals and session chair for international conferences. She acted as a mentor and won Smart India Hackathon 2022 held at NIT Assam. She holds two Indian design patents. Her research interests include software engineering, software testing, mobile application development, green computing, Internet of Things (IoT), AI, and machine learning.

Surbhi Bhatia Khan is currently working at the School of Science, Engineering and Environment at University of Salford, United Kingdom. She is listed in the top 2% researchers released by Stanford University, USA. She earned Project Management Professional Certification from the reputed Project Management Institute, USA. She also has an Adjunct Professor position at Chandigarh University, India. She has more than 13 years of academic and teaching experience in different universities. She has published 150+ papers in many reputed journals in high indexed outlets, with many best paper awards. Her areas of interest are sentiment analysis, deep learning/machine learning, and data science in healthcare.

S. Kayalvizhi is an accomplished academician and researcher, currently serving as an Assistant Professor (Senior Grade) in the Department of Electronics and Communication Engineering at SRM Institute of Science and Technology, Kattankulathur, Tamilnadu, India. She holds a Ph.D. in Compressive Sensing and Signal Processing from the SRM Institute of Science and Technology, awarded in 2021. With over 20 years of academic experience, has made significant contributions to the fields of signal processing, machine learning, and healthcare technologies. She has published 40+ papers in renowned international journals and conference proceedings, showcasing her expertise in areas such as deep learning, IoT-based healthcare systems, and AI-driven disease prediction models. She has contributed 10+ chapters to books.

Mo Saraee holds a chair in data science. His research focuses on data science, machine learning, data and text mining, natural language processing (NLP), big data, and medical informatics, addressing multi-disciplinary, cross-school topics with transformative impact and benefiting local communities, with a dedication to action through the real-world application of research, including developing and integrating innovative data mining approaches to improve human health, in collaboration with both Salford City Council and the NHS. His research has been published in leading journals, such as the *British Medical Journal*, *Knowledge-Based Systems*, and *Neurocomputing*. He is the Editor-in-Chief for the *International Journal of Web Research*.

Contributors

Eshaan Abbas Ja
Department of Electronics and Communication Engineering, Faculty of Engineering and Technology, SRM Institute of Science and Technology, Kattankulathur, Chengalpattu District, Tamil Nadu 603203, India

Netaliya Ahmed
Department of Electronics and Communication Engineering, SRM Institute of Science and Technology, Kattankulathur-603203, Chennai, Tamil Nadu, India

A. Anilet Bala
Department of Electronics and Communication Engineering, SRM Institute of Science and Technology, Kattankulathur 603203, Chennai, Tamil Nadu, India

Surbhi Bhatia Khan
School of Science, Engineering and Environment, University of Salford, Manchester, United Kingdom; University Centre for Research and Development, Chandigarh University, Mohali, Punjab, India; Division of Research and Development, Lovely Professional University, Phagwara, India

Samiappan Dhanalakshmi
Department of Electronics and Communication Engineering, Faculty of Engineering and Technology, SRM Institute of Science and Technology, Kattankulathur, Chengalpattu District, Tamil Nadu 603203, India

Dinesh K
Department of Electronics and Communication Engineering, Rajalakshmi Engineering College, Thandalam, Tamil Nadu 602 105, India

J. Esther
Department of Computer Applications, Tagore College of Arts and Science, Chennai, Tamil Nadu, India

J. Gayathri
Assistant Professor, Department of Electronics and Communication Engineering, Veltech Multitech Dr. RR & SR Engineering College, Avadi, Tamil Nadu, India

S. Hannah Pauline
Department of Electronics and Communication Engineering, Faculty of Engineering and Technology, SRM Institute of Science and Technology, Kattankulathur, Chengalpattu District, Tamil Nadu 603203, India

Kuraganti Harish
Department of Electronics and Communication Engineering, Faculty of Engineering and Technology, SRM Institute of Science and Technology, Kattankulathur, Chengalpattu District, Tamil Nadu 603203, India

R. Jansi
Department of Electronics and Communication Engineering, Faculty of Engineering and Technology, SRM Institute of Science and Technology, Kattankulathur, Chengalpattu District, Tamil Nadu 603203, India

Kasthuri Bha J. K.
Department of Electronics and Communication Engineering, Faculty of Engineering and Technology, SRM Institute of Science and Technology, Kattankulathur, Chengalpattu District, Tamil Nadu 603203, India

S. Kayalvizhi
Assistant Professor- Senior Grade, Department of Electronics and Communication Engineering, Faculty of Engineering and Technology, SRM Institute of Science and Technology, Kattankulathur, Chengalpattu District, Tamil Nadu 603203, India

Krishnakumar K
Department of Electronics and Communication Engineering, Faculty of Engineering and Technology, SRM Institute of Science and Technology, Kattankulathur, Chengalpattu District, Tamil Nadu 603203, India

Nithyakalyani Krishnan
Department of Biomedical Engineering, College of Engineering and Technology, Faculty of Engineering and Technology, SRM Institute of Science and Technology, Kattankulathur, Tamil Nadu 603203, India

Udhaya Kumar
Department of Electronics and Communication Engineering, Faculty of Engineering and Technology, SRM Institute of Science and Technology, Kattankulathur, Chengalpattu District, Tamil Nadu 603203, India

Harisudha Kuresan
Department of Electronics and Communication Engineering, Faculty of Engineering and Technology, SRM Institute of Science and Technology, Kattankulathur, Chengalpattu District, Tamil Nadu 603203, India

S. Latha
Department of Electronics and Communication Engineering, Faculty of Engineering and Technology, SRM Institute of Science and Technology, Kattankulathur, Chengalpattu District, Tamil Nadu 603203, India

M. Mageshwari
S.M.S College of Arts and Science, Sivakasi, Virudhunagar District, Tamil Nadu 626123, India

S. Malarvizhi
Professor, Department of Electronics and Communication Engineering, Faculty of Engineering and Technology, SRM Institute of Science and Technology, Kattankulathur, Chengalpattu District, Tamil Nadu 603203, India

A. Malini
School of Computer Science and Engineering, Vellore Institute of Technology, Chennai, Tamil Nadu, India

Perala Manoj
Department of Electronics and Communication Engineering, Faculty of Engineering and Technology, SRM Institute of Science and Technology, Kattankulathur, Chengalpattu District, Tamil Nadu 603203, India

Nimmy B. Mathew
Department of Electronics and Communication Engineering, SRM Institute of Science and Technology, Kattankulathur-603203, Chennai, Tamil Nadu, India

Yakub Mathew
Department of Electronics and Communication Engineering, Faculty of Engineering and Technology, SRM Institute of Science and Technology, Kattankulathur, Chengalpattu District, Tamil Nadu 603203, India

S. Murugaveni
Department of Electronics and Communication Engineering, Faculty of Engineering and Technology, SRM Institute of Science and Technology, Kattankulathur, Chengalpattu District, Tamil Nadu 603203, India

P. Muthu
Department of Biomedical Engineering, College of Engineering and Technology, Faculty of Engineering and Technology, SRM Institute of Science and Technology, Kattankulathur, Tamil Nadu 603203, India

S. Muthumari
Sri S. Ramasamy Naidu Memorial College, Sattur, Tamil Nadu, India

B. Nagarajan
SRM Institute of Science and Technology, Kattankulathur, Chengalpattu, Tamil Nadu, 603203, India

M. Pandiyan
Department of Computer Applications, Faculty of Science and Humanities, SRM Institute of Science and Technology, Kattankulathur, Chengalpattu, Tamil Nadu, 603203, India

Parthiban S
Assistant Professor, Department of Electronics and Communication Engineering, V.R.S. College of Engineering and Technology, Arasur – 607107, Villupuram, Tamil Nadu, India

T. Priyadarsini
Assistant Professor, Department of Electronics and Communication Engineering, V.R.S. College of Engineering and Technology, Arasur – 607107, Villupuram, Tamil Nadu, India

Gaddam Rohit
Department of Electronics and Communication Engineering, Faculty of Engineering and Technology, SRM Institute of Science and Technology, Kattankulathur, Chengalpattu District, Tamil Nadu 603203, India

Mohammed Saraee
School of Science, Engineering and Environment, University of Salford, Manchester, United Kingdom

Saranya J
Associate Professor, Department of Electronics and Communication Engineering, Rajalakshmi Engineering College, Thandalam – 602105, Tamil Nadu, India

K. Sathya
Department of Computer Applications, Faculty of Science and Humanities, SRM Institute of Science and Technology, Kattankulathur, Chengalpattu, Tamil Nadu, 603203, India

Selvakumar V. S
Professor, Department of Electronics and Communication Engineering, Rajalakshmi Engineering College, Thandalam, Tamil Nadu 602 105, India

C. Selvi
Department of Computer Applications, Vel Tech Ranga Sanku Arts College, Chennai, Tamil Nadu, India

N. R. Shanker
Professor, Department of Computer Science Engineering, Aalim Muhammed Salegh College of Engineering, Avadi, Tamil Nadu, India

R. Shanthi
Department of Computer Applications, Faculty of Science and Humanities, SRM Institute of Science and Technology, Kattankulathur, Chengalpattu, Tamil Nadu, 603203, India

N. Sri Sai Charan Reddy
Department of Electronics and Communication Engineering, Faculty of Engineering and Technology, SRM Institute of Science and Technology, Kattankulathur, Chengalpattu District, Tamil Nadu 603203, India

M. K. Srilekha
Assistant Professor, Department of Electronics and Communication Engineering, College of Engineering and Technology, SRM Institute of Science and Technology, Kattankulathur-603203, Tamil Nadu, India

J. Suganthi
Christ (Deemed to be) University, Bengaluru, India

Suganthi S
Professor, Department of Electronics and Communication Engineering, Rajalakshmi Engineering College, Thandalam, Tamil Nadu 602105, India

Raj Tetarwal
Department of Electronics and Communication Engineering, Faculty of Engineering and Technology, SRM Institute of Science and Technology, Kattankulathur, Chengalpattu District, Tamil Nadu 603203, India

S. Uma Maheswari
Assistant Professor, Department of Electronics and Communication Engineering, College of Engineering and Technology, SRM Institute of Science and Technology, Kattankulathur-603203, Tamil Nadu, India

Meghna Vaddadi
Department of Electronics and Communication Engineering, SRM Institute of Science and Technology, Kattankulathur-603203, Chennai, Tamil Nadu, India

1 Overview of Computational Intelligence for Health Informatics and Computer-Aided Diagnosis

S. Kayalvizhi, A. Malini, Surbhi Bhatia Khan, and Mohammed Saraee

1.1 INTRODUCTION

Health informatics is the interdisciplinary field that focuses on the acquisition, storage, retrieval, and use of healthcare information to support decision-making, improve patient care, and advance biomedical research [1]. It involves the application of information technology, data science, and computational methods to manage and analyze health-related data effectively.

Here's a breakdown of its significance:

Improving Patient Care: Health informatics makes it easier to manage patient records effectively and gives medical professionals rapid access to vital data. Better patient outcomes, decreased medical errors, and enhanced care coordination result from this.

Enhancing Healthcare Efficiency: Health informatics makes healthcare companies more productive and effective by automating repetitive work, optimizing resource allocation, and streamlining administrative processes.

Facilitating Research and Innovation: Researchers may access enormous volumes of healthcare data using health informatics, which can then be evaluated to find trends, patterns, and insights. Biomedical research is accelerated by this data-driven strategy, which results in novel findings, therapies, and medical advancements.

Supporting Public Health Initiatives: When it comes to tracking disease outbreaks, keeping an eye on population health trends, and developing focused

DOI: 10.1201/9781003484233-1

interventions to stop the spread of infectious diseases and other dangers to public health, health informatics is essential.

Empowering Patients and Consumers: Through patient portals, mobile health apps, and wearable devices, health informatics empowers individuals to take control of their health, engage in preventive care, and make informed decisions about their healthcare needs.

Overall, health informatics is essential for transforming healthcare delivery, promoting evidence-based practice, and driving continuous improvement in the quality, safety, and efficiency of healthcare services. The rest of the chapter is organized as follows: 2. Foundations of Computational Intelligence, 3. Overview of Various Computational Intelligence Methodologies, 4. Applications, 5. Challenges and Limitations, 6. Case Studies, 7. Conclusion.

1.2 FOUNDATIONS OF COMPUTATIONAL INTELLIGENCE

Computational intelligence (CI) encompasses a broad range of techniques inspired by natural intelligence, such as human reasoning and learning processes [2–6]. Some key concepts and techniques of CI are as follows:

1.2.1 Artificial Neural Networks (ANN)

- Neural networks (NNs) seen in animal brains serve as the model for ANNs.
- They are made up of layers of networked nodes, or neurons, that can learn from data through a process known as training.
- Pattern recognition, classification, regression, and function approximation are among the tasks that ANNs are utilized for.

ANNs serve as foundational tools in CI, significantly impacting the analysis of medical data. Within the realm of healthcare, ANNs are pivotal in various applications, including diagnostic systems, medical image analysis, predictive modeling, drug discovery, personalized medicine, and time series data analysis [7]. In diagnostic systems, ANNs leverage patient data, such as symptoms and test results, to assist clinicians in accurately identifying diseases, ranging from cancer to neurological disorders. Moreover, ANNs excel in medical image analysis tasks, such as tumor detection and segmentation, by processing magnetic resonance imaging (MRI) scans, X-rays, and histopathological slides with remarkable accuracy, facilitated by specialized architectures like convolutional NNs (CNNs). By using ANNs for predictive modeling, medical practitioners can maximize clinical decision-making by predicting patient outcomes, illness progression, and therapy responses based on past data. Furthermore, by evaluating chemical structures and forecasting compound actions, ANNs significantly contribute to drug discovery and development by accelerating the identification of promising therapeutic options. In personalized medicine, ANNs use unique patient data, such as genetic profiles and biomarkers, to customize treatment regimens that maximize benefits and minimize side effects. Moreover, ANNs play a critical role in the analysis of time series data from electronic health records (EHRs) and wearable devices, supporting the prediction of health outcomes, monitoring of chronic conditions, and early illness identification. Despite their efficacy, ensuring the interpretability and explainability of ANN models remains a challenge, necessitating ongoing research efforts to address these concerns. Ethical and regulatory considerations, such as data privacy and compliance with standards like the Healthcare Portability and Accountability Act (HIPAA) and General Data Protection Regulation (GDPR), are paramount in the ethical deployment of ANNs in medical data analysis, safeguarding patient privacy and confidentiality. Overall, ANNs represent a transformative force in CI for medical data, offering immense potential to revolutionize diagnosis, treatment, and patient care while demanding careful attention to ethical, regulatory, and interpretability aspects [8].

1.2.2 Evolutionary Computation (EC)

- Natural selection and biological evolution are the main sources of inspiration for EC algorithms.
- EC approaches include evolutionary tactics, genetic algorithms (GAs), and genetic programming.
- EC algorithms are applied to difficult problem solving, search and exploration tasks, and optimization challenges.

1.2.3 Fuzzy Logic

- A mathematical framework for handling ambiguity and imprecision is fuzzy logic.
- It extends classical binary logic by allowing degrees of truth between 0 and 1, rather than just true or false.
- Fuzzy logic is used in systems where precise mathematical modeling is difficult, such as control systems, decision-making processes, and expert systems.

1.2.4 Swarm Intelligence

- The cooperative behavior of various animal groups and social insect colonies serves as an inspiration for swarm intelligence systems.
- Ant colony optimization (ACO), particle swarm optimization (PSO), and bee colony optimization (BCO) are a few examples.
- Swarm intelligence algorithms are frequently applied in uncertain and dynamic situations for tasks involving search, optimization, and decision-making.

1.2.5 Probabilistic Reasoning

- Probabilistic reasoning techniques, such as Bayesian networks and probabilistic graphical models, are used to model uncertainty and make inferences from uncertain data.
- They are particularly useful for tasks such as diagnosis, prediction, decision-making under uncertainty, and risk assessment.

1.2.6 Hybrid Systems

- Hybrid systems combine multiple CI techniques or integrate CI with other computational approaches, such as traditional optimization methods or statistical techniques.
- Hybrid systems frequently seek to better address difficult problems by combining the advantages of many approaches.

These are just a few key concepts and techniques within the broad field of CI. Every strategy has advantages and disadvantages, and the best approach will rely on the particular requirements and issue domain. CI continues to evolve, with researchers exploring new methods and hybrid approaches to tackle increasingly complex real-world challenges.

1.3 OVERVIEW OF VARIOUS COMPUTATIONAL INTELLIGENCE METHODOLOGIES

1.3.1 Neural Networks (NN)

- NNs are computer architectures that draw inspiration from the composition and operation of the human brain.
- They are made up of interconnected nodes, or neurons, arranged in layers, which include an output layer, an input layer, and one or more hidden layers.
- In order for NNs to discover patterns and relationships from data, they are trained using techniques like backpropagation.
- They are employed in tasks including function approximation, regression, classification, and pattern recognition.

1.3.2 Genetic Algorithms (GA)

- GAs are optimization techniques that draw inspiration from the concepts of genetics and natural selection.
- They begin with the creation of a population of potential solutions, which are subsequently refined through the application of operators like crossover, selection, and mutation over the course of multiple generations.
- In a variety of fields, GAs are employed to identify the best or almost best answers to optimization and search issues.

1.3.3 Fuzzy Logic

- A mathematical framework for handling ambiguity and imprecision is fuzzy logic.
- It extends classical binary logic by allowing degrees of truth between 0 and 1, rather than just true or false.
- Fuzzy logic is particularly useful in systems where precise mathematical modeling is difficult, such as control systems, decision-making processes, and expert systems.

1.3.4 Expert Systems

- Expert systems are computer programs designed to mimic a human expert's decision- making process within a certain field.
- They are composed of an inference engine that uses the rules to solve problems or make decisions, and a knowledge base that holds domain-specific data and rules.
- Expert systems find application in a variety of domains, including engineering, finance, and medical, for activities including diagnosis, troubleshooting, and advising services.

Every one of these approaches has advantages and disadvantages, and the best approach will rely on the particular issue domain, the type of data, and the intended results.

In practice, researchers and practitioners often combine multiple methodologies or hybridize them to leverage their complementary strengths and address complex real-world problems more effectively [9].

1.4 APPLICATIONS

CI techniques have a wide range of applications in health informatics, contributing to various aspects of healthcare delivery, research, and management [10]. Here are some key applications:

1.4.1 Disease Diagnosis and Prognosis

- CI techniques, such as ANNs and support vector machines, are used for diagnosing diseases based on medical data such as symptoms, medical images, and patient history.
- They can also be employed for predicting disease progression and prognosis, aiding in treatment planning and patient management.

1.4.2 Medical Image Analysis

- Medical pictures such as X-rays, MRI scans, and histopathology images are analyzed using CI approaches, which include deep learning algorithms like CNNs.
- These methods help radiologists and pathologists with diagnosis and treatment planning by automating the processes of abnormality detection, segmentation, and classification.

1.4.3 Health Monitoring and Wearable Devices

- Continuous health monitoring is made possible by the integration of CI algorithms into wearable technology and remote monitoring systems.
- These algorithms analyze physiological data, including heart rate, blood pressure, and activity levels, to identify abnormalities, forecast health risks, and offer users individualized feedback and interventions.

1.4.4 Electronic Health Records (EHR)

- CI techniques are utilized for analyzing and mining electronic health records to extract valuable insights for clinical decision-making, population health management, and healthcare quality improvement.
- Natural language processing (NLP) algorithms are employed for extracting information from unstructured clinical notes and reports, enabling structured data analysis.

1.4.5 Drug Discovery and Development

- To find possible drug candidates, forecast drug-target interactions, and enhance drug qualities, CI approaches are utilized in drug discovery and development processes.
- Among the CI methods used in drug development are virtual screening, molecular docking, and quantitative structure-activity relationship (QSAR) modeling.

1.4.6 Healthcare Management and Decision Support

- Healthcare management systems and decision support tools use CI techniques to optimize resource allocation, boost workflow effectiveness, and improve patient outcomes.
- Predictive analytics and optimization algorithms are used for capacity planning, staff scheduling, and healthcare logistics management.

1.4.7 Personalized Medicine

- By assessing individual patient data to customize treatments and interventions based on the patient's distinct traits, genetic makeup, and reaction to therapy, CI methods enable customized medicine.
- They facilitate precision medicine initiatives by identifying biomarkers, predicting treatment outcomes, and optimizing treatment regimens.

These uses show how CI has a major impact on enhancing patient outcomes, advancing healthcare delivery, and spurring breakthroughs in health informatics. CI approaches will become more and more important as technology develops in order to revolutionize healthcare and deal with the many issues that the healthcare sector is confronting.

1.5 CHALLENGES AND LIMITATIONS

While CI techniques offer significant benefits and opportunities in health informatics, they also face **several challenges and limitations**. Here are some key ones:

1.5.1 Data Quality and Quantity

- CI techniques require large amounts of high-quality data for training robust models. However, healthcare data often suffer from issues such as incompleteness, inconsistency, and inaccuracies.
- Limited availability of labeled data for supervised learning tasks can hinder the development and performance of CI models, particularly in medical imaging and rare disease contexts.

1.5.2 Interpretability and Transparency

- Many CI models, especially deep learning models, are thought of as "black boxes," which makes it difficult to decipher their judgments and comprehend the underlying logic.
- Lack of interpretability and transparency can impede trust and acceptance among healthcare professionals, regulators, and patients, limiting the adoption of CI solutions in clinical practice.

1.5.3 Ethical and Privacy Concerns

- Healthcare data are sensitive and subject to strict privacy regulations (e.g., HIPAA in the United States and GDPR in the European Union). CI techniques raise concerns about data security, patient privacy, and confidentiality.
- Unauthorized access, data breaches, and misuse of healthcare data pose ethical risks and legal liabilities, necessitating robust security measures and privacy-preserving techniques.

1.5.4 Integration with Existing Healthcare Systems

- It can be difficult to integrate CI technologies into current healthcare workflows and systems because of compatibility problems, aversion to change, and interoperability challenges.
- To reach their full potential and guarantee that healthcare professionals can use them, CI apps must smoothly interface with clinical decision support systems, EHRs, and other healthcare IT infrastructure.

1.5.5 Validation and Reproducibility

- Validating the performance and generalizability of CI models in healthcare settings is essential but often challenging due to the heterogeneity of patient populations, variations in data sources, and lack of standardized evaluation protocols.
- Reproducing research findings and benchmarking CI algorithms across different datasets and institutions are crucial for establishing their reliability, scalability, and clinical utility.

1.5.6 Resource Constraints

- Deep learning is one of the more computationally demanding CI techniques, requiring a significant amount of computer resources (e.g., GPUs and high-performance computing equipment).
- Limited access to computational resources, expertise, and funding can be barriers to developing and deploying CI solutions, especially in resource-constrained healthcare settings and underserved communities.

Addressing these challenges and limitations requires interdisciplinary collaboration among researchers, clinicians, policymakers, and industry stakeholders. Strategies such as data sharing initiatives, transparent model development practices, regulatory frameworks, and ethical guidelines can help mitigate risks and promote responsible use of CI in health informatics.

1.6 CASE STUDIES

Certainly! Here are a few **case studies** showcasing the application of CI in health informatics:

1.6.1 Diagnosis and Prognosis of Breast Cancer

- Researchers at a medical institution developed a CI-based system for diagnosing and predicting the prognosis of breast cancer.
- Using a combination of ANNs and GAs, the system analyzed mammography images and patient data to classify tumors, predict tumor characteristics, and estimate patient survival rates.
- The system demonstrated high accuracy in diagnosing breast cancer subtypes and predicting patient outcomes, providing valuable decision support for oncologists and improving patient management strategies.

1.6.2 Medical Image Analysis for Brain Tumor Detection

- A group of scientists used CNNs, a deep learning approach, to automatically identify brain cancers in MRI data.
- The CNN model learnt to recognize and separate tumor regions from healthy brain tissue by training on a sizable dataset of tagged MRI images. In terms of brain tumor detection, the developed system performed on par with human radiologists, saving a great deal of time and effort in the diagnosis and treatment planning processes.

1.6.3 Personalized Medicine in Diabetes Management

- A healthcare organization implemented a personalized medicine approach for managing diabetes using CI techniques.

- Machine learning algorithms were used to evaluate patient data, including medical history, genetic information, lifestyle characteristics, and glucose monitoring data, in order to customize treatment regimens for each patient.
- The system generated personalized recommendations for medication dosage, dietary interventions, and lifestyle modifications based on the patient's unique characteristics and responses to therapy, leading to improved glycemic control and patient outcomes.

1.6.4 Drug Discovery Using Virtual Screening

- Pharmaceutical researchers virtually screened possible medication options for a given condition using CI techniques including GAs and molecular docking.
- By simulating the interaction between drug molecules and target proteins, the researchers identified promising lead compounds with high binding affinity and favorable pharmacological properties.
- The process of finding new drugs was sped up and expenses related to experimental screening and testing were decreased by the quick identification and improvement of promising drug candidates made possible by virtual screening.

These case studies illustrate the diverse applications of CI in health informatics, spanning disease diagnosis, medical imaging, personalized medicine, and drug discovery. Healthcare companies can improve patient care, expedite clinical workflows, and spur innovation in healthcare delivery by utilizing sophisticated computational approaches.

1.7 CONCLUSION

In summary, CI has become a potent and adaptable instrument in the field of health informatics, providing creative answers to a variety of medical problems. In order to improve patient outcomes, enhance clinical decision-making, and spur medical innovation, CI enables the analysis, interpretation, and utilization of enormous amounts of healthcare data through the application of techniques like ANNs, GAs, fuzzy logic, and expert systems.

There are numerous and significant uses of CI in health informatics. Personalized medicine, drug development, medical image analysis, health monitoring, disease diagnosis, and prognosis are just a few of the areas where CI approaches are revolutionizing healthcare research, management, and delivery. Healthcare organizations can get important insights from complicated healthcare data by utilizing machine learning, data mining, and optimization algorithms. This can result in more precise diagnoses, more successful treatments, and improved patient care.

However, the adoption of CI in health informatics is not without challenges and limitations. Issues such as data quality and quantity, interpretability and transparency, ethical and privacy concerns, integration with existing healthcare systems, validation and reproducibility, and resource constraints pose significant obstacles to the widespread deployment and acceptance of CI solutions in clinical practice. Researchers, physicians, legislators, and industry stakeholders must work together to build robust, dependable, and ethical CI applications that adhere to the strictest safety, efficacy, and ethical guidelines in order to tackle these difficulties.

Despite these challenges, the potential of CI in health informatics remains immense. With continued research, innovation, and interdisciplinary collaboration, CI promises to revolutionize healthcare delivery, accelerate medical discoveries, and empower individuals to lead healthier lives. By leveraging the capabilities of CI, we can build a future where healthcare is more personalized, precise, and accessible to all.

REFERENCES

1. Aggarwal, C. C. (Ed.). (2016). *Healthcare Data Analytics*. Chapman and Hall/CRC.
2. Bellazzi, R., & Zupan, B. (Eds.). (2008). *Artificial Intelligence in Medicine* (Vol. 48). Springer Science & Business Media.
3. Dua, S., & Acharya, U. R. (2019). Applications of artificial intelligence and deep learning in cardiovascular imaging. *Journal of Medical Systems*, 43(2), 40.
4. Gandomi, A. H., & Haider, M. (2015). Beyond the hype: Big data concepts, methods, and analytics. *International Journal of Information Management*, 35(2), 137–144.
5. Kotsiantis, S. B., Zaharakis, I., & Pintelas, P. E. (2006). Machine learning: A review of classification and combining techniques. *Artificial Intelligence Review*, 26(3), 159–190.
6. Lecun, Y., Bengio, Y., & Hinton, G. (2015). Deep learning. *Nature*, 521(7553), 436–444.
7. Lisboa, P. J. (Ed.). (2013). *Artificial Intelligence in Medicine*. Springer Science & Business Media.
8. Luo, W., Phung, D., Tran, T., Gupta, S., Rana, S., Karmakar, C., ... & Berk, M. (2016). Guidelines for developing and reporting machine learning predictive models in biomedical research: A multidisciplinary view. *Journal of Medical Internet Research*, 18(12), e323.
9. Mamoshina, P., Vieira, A., Putin, E., & Zhavoronkov, A. (2016). Applications of deep learning in biomedicine. *Molecular Pharmaceutics*, 13(5), 1445–1454.
10. Topol, E. J. (2019). High-performance medicine: The convergence of human and artificial intelligence. *Nature Medicine*, 25(1), 44–56.

2 From Pixels to Prognosis

Machine Learning Approaches for Medical Imaging Diagnosis

T. Priyadarsini and Saranya J.

2.1 INTRODUCTION

Modern technology and medical diagnostics working together has created new opportunities in the rapidly evolving field of healthcare. With the help of artificial intelligence (AI), primarily machine learning (ML) and medical imaging, this chapter opens up a revolutionary new era for improved diagnosis. The confluence of these two fields holds great promise for altering our perception and understanding of medical imaging pictures. As one employs ML algorithms to interpret diagnostic images, a new era of medical diagnosis will be ushered in, and this study guides us through many of the details that occur. Beyond technicalities, though, our adventure continues. Examining the complex terrain of using ML into medical diagnostics, we address ethical issues and obstacles. The objective of this chapter is to present the opportunities while also providing a balanced viewpoint on the moral ramifications and real-world constraints in the healthcare industry. Come explore with us the cutting-edge research, practical applications, and cooperative projects that are propelling the smooth assimilation of ML into standard medical procedures. We want you to understand how ML can revolutionize diagnostic procedures by the end of this chapter, and to see a future in healthcare where technology and medicine work together to improve people's lives all around the world.

In tumor analysis, ML plays a critical role in early detection through image analysis, accurate tumor region segmentation, pathology analysis support, treatment outcome prediction, tumor progression prediction[1], understanding genomic data for targeted therapies, and drug discovery support. Improved patient outcomes, personalized medication, and a deeper understanding of cancer pathways are all benefited by these ML applications in cancer research and treatment. ML finds application in drug development, radiomics, personalized treatment planning, and the integration of diverse medical datasets, among other areas of cancer research and therapy. By analyzing massive datasets, ML expedites the drug discovery process. It also customizes treatment regimens according to the unique characteristics of each patient, extracts useful information from medical imaging to forecast treatment response, and adjusts to new data for ongoing learning in the ever-evolving field

DOI: 10.1201/9781003484233-2

of cancer research. Through the integration of various data sources, ML improves decision-making processes, which in turn leads to better patient outcomes, more precise diagnoses, and a deeper comprehension of cancer biology. Ultimately, this aids in the development of more efficient and individualized cancer care plans.

2.2 OVERVIEW OF TUMOR DIAGNOSIS

Cancer is a serious worldwide health concern that is typified by the body's aberrant cells growing and spreading out of control[2]. Researchers are working on developing better diagnostic and therapeutic approaches for various cancer kinds, such as lung, prostate, and breast cancers, in order to enhance patient outcomes and life expectancy[3]. For more effective therapy and higher survival rates, early tumor detection is essential. In order to enable more successful therapeutic interventions, early diagnostic approaches concentrate on recognizing tumors at their earliest stages. Early tumor diagnosis is greatly aided by a variety of imaging modalities, including endoscopy, ultrasonography, X-rays, and magnetic resonance imaging (MRI), and positron emission tomography (PET) scans, in addition to tumor-related biomarkers[3,4].

2.2.1 Advancement of Technologies for Tumor Diagnosis

The field of medical diagnostics is dynamic, and the introduction of tumor diagnostic technology has changed the way humans feel about and approach cancer diagnosis. Beginning with its early conceptualization and ending with the modern age of precision medicine, this chapter examines deeply the development of these technologies[2]. In order to begin our journey, let's take a look at the key turning points that made tumor detection technology possible. This section highlights the first steps that paved the way for the revolution in cancer diagnostics, from the development of early biomarker identification to the introduction of imaging tools. Technologies for imaging are essential to the diagnosis of tumors. This section describes the evolution of radiography from classic radiography to the complex modern modalities like computed tomography (CT), PET, and MRI[5,6]. Our capacity to see and identify tumors with previously uncommon precision has been greatly enhanced by the advancement of imaging. Tumor diagnostics has been redefined by the combination of genetic and molecular methods. Here, we examine the revolutionary advancements in transcriptomics, proteomics, and genomes that have made it possible to comprehend the molecular signatures connected to various tumor types at a deeper level. Next-generation sequencing and liquid biopsies have created new opportunities for non-invasive, tailored diagnostic techniques.

The field of tumor diagnostics has expanded into new areas in recent years due to the synergy between AI and this technology. In order to help find patterns[7] and anomalies that the human eye might miss, this section explores how ML algorithms examine large datasets. AI combined with tumor diagnostics offers enormous promise for targeted treatment plans and early detection (Table 2.1).

TABLE 2.1
Evaluation of different imaging methods Wang et al[2]

Technique	Imaging time	Penetration depth	Resolution	Invasiveness	Radiation
Endoscopy	Real time	Surface	Camera dependent	True	Nil
US	Real time	Not deep	Limited	Nil	Nil
CT	Short period	Depth	High	Nil	True
MRI	Short period	Unlimited	Field dependent	Nil	Nil
PET	Short period	Depth	1 mm to 2 mm	Nil	true

2.3 ANALYSIS OF TUMOR DETECTION

2.3.1 Deep Learning Overview[8]

Deep neural networks are neural networks that have several hidden layers. They are highly knowledgeable about learning hierarchical functions from data. A supervised learning algorithm is used to train neural networks. It adjusts the weights of the connections based on the error in the output compared to the actual target[9]. It measures the difference between the expected output and the real target. The aim is to reduce this loss during training[10]. Optimization algorithms, like gradient descent, are techniques used to adjust weights efficiently during training[8]. Convolutional neural networks (CNNs) are designed specifically to process input that resembles a grid, such as images and videos[11]. It maintains a hidden state that captures information about previous inputs, allowing it to handle sequential dependencies. Random forest is an ensemble learning technique that can be deployed at places that require higher level prediction accuracy by combining many decision trees[12].

2.3.2 Datasets

The website address of the dataset is www.kaggle.com. Three types of brain tumors are included: meningiomas (708 images), gliomas (1426 images), and pituitary tumors (930 images), totaling 3064 T1-weighted contrast enhanced pictures from more than 200 patients. Three planes were used to collect all the images from more than 200 patients: axial (994 images), sagittal (1025 images), and coronal (1045 images). Non-deep learning and deep learning techniques are used, binary classification is applied (gliomas and meninges), and multiclass classification is also applied (pituitary, gliomas, and meninges tumor). Sentiment analysis is a very effective technique for extracting stated emotions from unstructured texts by converting the data into an organized manner[13]. In order to increase accuracy and sensitivity, we concentrate on reducing type one false positive rate (FPR) and type two false negative rate (FNR) mistakes[14].

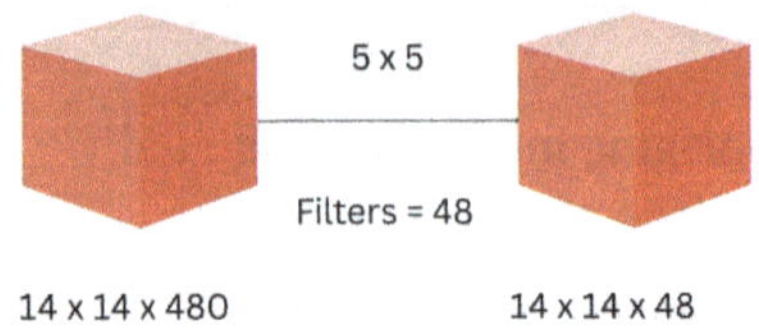

FIGURE 2.1 5 × 5 convolution with 48 filters.

2.3.3 Convolutional Neural Networks (CNNs)

One of the primary features of CNN methods for extracting information from images is feature extraction. CNNs are therefore more suited to additional image analysis[1].

- We use multiple layers to train the CNN networks[15].
- By utilizing the various layers, the feature space is enhanced.
- Edges, colors, and other first-order properties are acquired from the initial layers.
- Higher-order features that are linked to the input image data are trained using later layers.
- The last layer provides its features to the categorization layer[16].

By employing the transfer learning technique, the CNN networks are trained on pre-trained networks rather than starting from scratch. The network's depth is increased by the new inception module. Compensation for the deeper network is done by optimizing the network, which lowers the total computational cost and permits a sizable quality boost[17]. This method involves using the additional 1 × 1 convolutional layers with the rectified linear activation function.

1 × 1 convolution: The architecture of the Inception employs 1 × 1 convolution. The architecture's weights and biases are decreased in number by using these convolutions. We can increase the depth of the architecture by decreasing the parameters.
Here is an illustration of 1 × 1 convolution:

For instance, if we wish to conduct 5 × 5 convolution with 48 filters without utilizing an intermediary 1 × 1 convolution: Convolution with filters is shown in Figure 2.1.

Total number of operations: (14 × 48 × 14) × (5 × 5 × 480) = 112.9 Mega

With 1 × 1 convolution: Convolution with convolution is shown in Figure 2.2.

(16 × 14 × 14) × (480 × 1 × 1) + (14 × 48 × 14) x (5 × 16 × 5) = 1.5 M + 3.8 M = 5.3 M, which is much smaller than 112.9M.

2.3.4 Training Network

An equal-sized input image is needed to train the CNN, but the image sizes in the brain tumor dataset vary. To make the new images the same size as the input images, we utilize the resize function in the MATLAB toolbox. The CNN GoogLeNet pretrained architecture is shown in Figure 2.3.

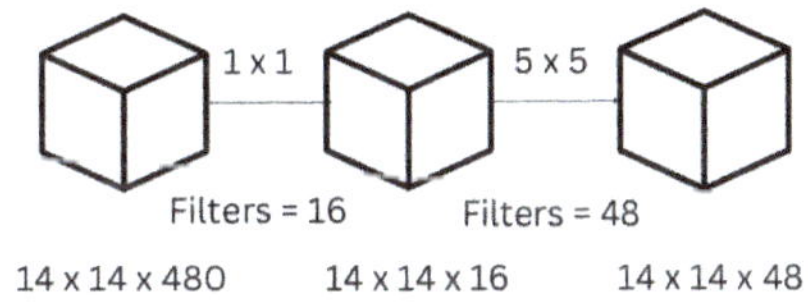

FIGURE 2.2 5 × 5 convolution with 1 × 1 convolution.

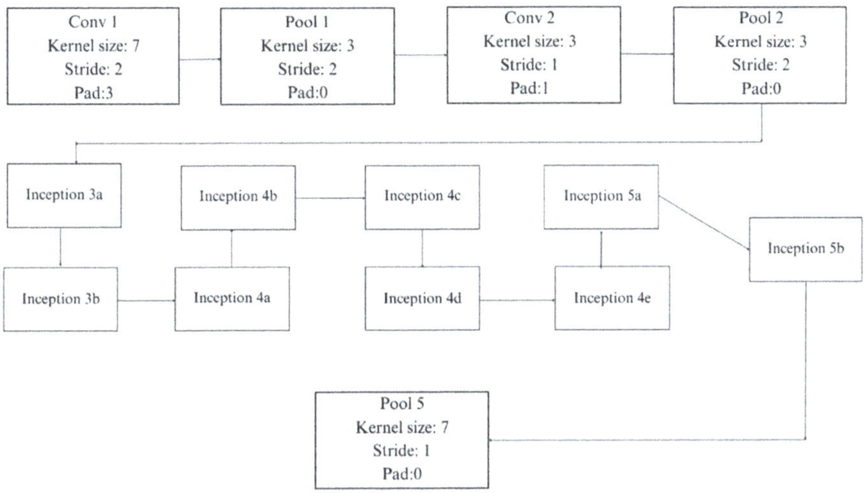

FIGURE 2.3 Convolutional neural network (CNN) GoogLeNet pretrained architecture[39].

2.3.5 Transfer Learning

In this method, new dataset models are initialized using the pre-trained models. More than 14 million images are used to train the ImageNet dataset for the classification layer. The later layers use a smaller dataset to fine-tune the model; the earlier layers provide a broader range of options. When we have limited data, using transfer learning becomes a dependable choice because we don't need to train a CNN from scratch[7]. We can determine which layer needs to be retrained based on the characteristics of the dataset.

By using a transfer learning approach, we use GoogLeNet and ResNet101 hyperparameters for optimization in this work. Applying the ImageNet dataset, which includes more than 1 million photos[5], GoogLeNet and ResNet101 are trained. There are 1000 established classifications, and each of the photos belongs to one of them. ReNet101 and optimized GoogLeNet are used to train the training dataset. After fine-tuning the network, we extract features from the last Average Pool layer and apply a sigma activation function. The final Pool layer[18] is made up of 1024 output nodes. Because there are three classes in the dataset used in this study, the final three layers of GoogLeNet and ResNet101 are modified to accomplish the purpose. The fully connected layers of GoogLeNet and ResNet101 are substituted in all cases by a different completely connected layer with an output of size three. Next, the softmax and cross-entropy layers are removed. They are swapped out for new, identically named layers in order to mix in with the recently connected layer. For fully linked layers, the number of neurons is set to three in order to categorize the three different types of tumors. Instead of using softmax, we evaluate the performance of this suggested model on GoogLeNet and ResNet101 using support vector machine and *K*-nearest neighbor (KNN) classifiers.

2.3.6 GoogLeNet

The convolutional, GoogLeNet, and FC layers of the transfer learning approach are effectively used to accomplish the tasks. Fixed input photos are preferred when using completely linked layers, however images of any size can be supported without any issues. How to perform transfer learning with CNN techniques and information layers is detailed in references 6 and 8. Since there is a continuing demand for precise and computationally efficient models, the correctness of the technique and approach has a considerable influence on the medical industry[19].

2.3.7 ResNet101

The 50-layer residual network (ResNet) design is a modified version of the ResNet101 architecture[6,20], which is named after the 101 layers of the residual network. ResNets

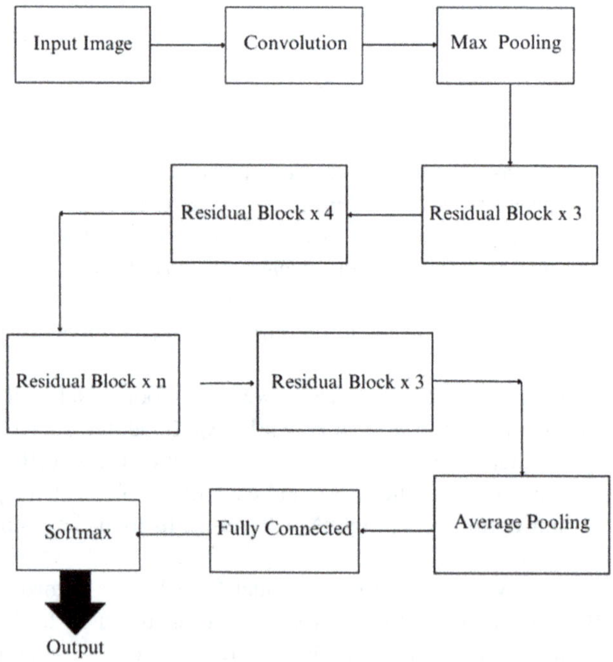

FIGURE 2.4 Residual network general architecture[39].

have been used to solve several computer vision and related problems. A variety of uses for ImageNet exist for ResNet, one of the most sophisticated large-scale CNN designs (i.e., object identification and recognition, different categorization objectives). In a CNN, there are often several layers that are trained to carry out different jobs and are connected to one another in a specific way.

ResNet connections, which keep gradients from vanishing to zero after the chain rule is applied, are the foundation of the design and its implementation[21]. The ResNet general architecture is shown in Figure 2.4. ResNet101 consists of 33 filters (blocks) and 104 convolutional layers, one block for each layer. Of the 33 levels, 19 make direct use of the output from earlier layers; this is referred to as a residual link.

In order to acquire an input from other levels, the summing operator at the conclusion of each layer uses the remaining connections as its first operand. The preceding block's output feeds into the next four layers, which use it as an input for the convolutional layer with a stride of one and a filter size of 1 × 1. After the normalization processes are finished, the output is moved using this normalization layer to the summing operator at the block's output. Each block's depth can change based on how dense it is[10]. The overall design in Figure 2.4 shows the reflection of ResNet101.

2.4 BASED ON THE PARAMETERS OF THE PERFORMANCE METRICS

To identify different forms of brain tumors, we calculate sensitivity, specificity, overall accuracy, and the area under the receiver operating curve.

2.4.1 Sensitivity

To determine the proportion of people who, among those who genuinely have the condition, test positive for it:

Sensitivity = (Summation of True Positive/Summation of Condition Positive)

2.4.2 Specificity

To measure the percentage of non-disease cases:

Specificity = (Summation of True Negative/Summation of Condition Negative)

Based on an individual test result, negativity is considered.

2.4.3 Positive Predictive Value (PPV)

It helps evaluate dependability of a test in identifying true positive cases:

Positive Predictive Value = (Summation of True Positive/Summation of Predicted Condition Positive)

2.4.4 Negative Predictive Value (NPV)

It helps evaluate the dependability of a test in correctly identifying true negative cases:

Negative Predictive Value = (Summation of True Negative/Summation of Predicted Condition Negative)

2.4.5 Total Accuracy

The percentage of accurate predictions that are both positive and negative among all cases analyzed is known as accuracy. In terms of mathematics, the overall accuracy is calculated as follows:

Total Accuracy = (Summation of True Positive + Summation of True Negative)/(Summation of Predicted Condition Positive + Summation of Predicted Condition Negative)

2.5 BRAIN METASTASES

Since cerebral metastases are commonly estimated to occur in 8–14 persons per 100,000, appropriate therapy for secondary central nervous system cancers is crucial from a therapeutic standpoint. Brain metastases, the most frequent intracranial malignancy[22,23], will eventually affect 20 to 40% of cancer patients. Furthermore, as the prevalence of brain metastases rises, managing intracranial metastases becomes increasingly crucial. This can be largely attributed to improved diagnostic imaging quality and utilization. Better systemic treatments are also managing metastatic illness, but because of the blood-brain barrier[24], they are less successful intracranially.

Patients with brain metastases frequently experience seizures, particularly as their disease burden increases[25]. The most frequent cancers that result in cerebral metastases are colorectal (1.8%), kidney (6.5%), lung (20%), and melanoma (6.9%). Patients with brain metastases have reported seizure rates that vary greatly depending on histology[23,25,26–29]from 13 to 48%. Research shows that 67%[25,30] of patients who have cerebral metastases from malignancy are particularly at higher risk of experiencing seizures[31]. Their propensity to be hemorrhagic and cortical may be connected to this. Compared to 16–33% of breast cancer patients and 21% of individuals with gastrointestinal malignancy[20,25,29,32,33], 29–48% of lung cancer patients experience seizures.

Although there are no randomized controlled trials (RCTs) to guide the choice of antiepileptic drugs (AED) for individuals with brain metastases, non-enzyme-inducing antiepileptic drugs (EIAEDs) are recommended and lower extremity venous (LEV) study has been shown to be effective in treating intracranial tumors[34,35]. Seventy-seven percent of patients with brain metastases who received LEV monotherapy experienced at least a 50% decrease in seizure frequency. Three modern antiepileptic medications—levetiracetam, oxcarbazepine, and topiramate—were used in 38 patients with brain metastases. We found that all these drugs were highly effective in reducing the frequency of seizures[25,36]. Certain specialists advise a slow taper and discontinuation of AEDs three to six months after surgery[37] for individuals with brain metastases who are seizure-free and whose malignancies have been effectively treated with radiation therapy[38].

2.6 CONCLUSION

ResNet101, a CNN, fared better in multiclass classification using characteristics extracted from a fully linked layer in deep learning and input into a support vector machine and KNN than when it used a softmax approach with transfer learning. In addition, deep learning outperformed typical handmade characteristics created using supervised ML techniques in terms of predictive performance for classifying binary data. To enhance the clinical results for brain cancer patients, the suggested strategy may be helpful in diagnosis, prognosis, and therapy planning. Further research can incorporate other deep learning algorithms, a larger dataset, additional clinical factors, and different kinds of brain tumors.

REFERENCES

1. Englot, D. J., Chang, E. F., & Vecht, C. J. (2016). Epilepsy and brain tumors. *Handbook of Clinical Neurology*, 134, 267–285.
2. Wang, H., Yang, S., Chen, L., Li, Y., He, P., Wang, G., Dong, H., Ma, P., & Ding, G. (2024). Tumor diagnosis using carbon-based quantum dots: Detection based on the hallmarks of cancer. *Bioactive Materials*, 33, 174–222.
3. Pruitt, A. A. (2015). Medical management of patients with brain tumors. *Continuum (Minneapolis, Minn.)*, 21(2 Neuro-oncology), 314–331.
4. Pol, R., & Balague, N. From microscopic to macroscopic sports injuries, Applying the complex dynamic systems approach to sports medicine: A narrative review. *British Journal of Sports Medicine*, 53, 1214–1220.
5. Krizhevsky, A., Sutskever, I., & Hinton, G. E. (2017). ImageNet classification with deep convolutional neural networks. *Communications of the ACM*, 60, 84–90.
6. Hoai An Le Thi, Hoai Minh Le, and Tao Pham Dinh (2019). Automatic identification of intracranial hemorrhage on CT/MRI image using meta-architectures improved from region-based CNN. In *World Congress on Global Optimization* (pp. 740–750). Springer.
7. Szegedy, C., Liu, W., Jia, Y., Sermanet, P., Reed, S., Anguelov, D., ... & Rabinovich, A. (2015). Going deeper with convolutions. *IEEE Conference on Computer Vision and Pattern Recognition (CVPR)* (pp. 1–9). IEEE Computer Society.
8. Ferentinos, K. P. (2018). Deep learning models for plant disease detection and diagnosis. *Computers and Electronics in Agriculture*, 145, 311–318.
9. Iqbal, S., Siddiqui, G. F., Rehman, A., Hussain, L., Saba, T., Tariq, U., & Abbasi, A. A. (2021). Prostate cancer detection using deep learning and traditional techniques. *IEEE Access*, 9, 27085–27100.
10. Ahmet, F. Y. D. (2019). Early detection of skin cancer using deep learning architectures: Resnet-101 and Inception-v3. In *2019 Medical Technologies Congress (TIPTEKNO)* (pp. 1–4). IEEE.
11. Schneider, S., Taylor, G. W., & Kremer, S. C. (2018). Deep learning object detection methods for ecological camera trap data. *15th Conference on Computer and Robot Vision (CRV)* (pp. 321–328). IEEE.

12. Nagaesvara, E. B. R., Aadhithya, M., Malini A. (2023). *An Analysis of Machine Learning Techniques for Forest Cover Type Classification. IEEE 6th International Conference on Contemporary Computing and Informatics* (Vol. 6, pp. 489–494), Curran Associates, Inc.
13. Chakraborty, K., Bhatia, S., Bhattacharyya, S., Platos, J., Bag, R., & Hassanien, A. E. (2020). Sentiment analysis of COVID-19 tweets by deep learning classifiers—A study to show how popularity is affecting accuracy in social media. *Applied Soft Computing Journal*, 97, 106754.
14. Safdar, S., Rizwan, M., Gadekallu, Reddy, T., Javed, A. R., Imam Rahmani, M. K., Jawad, K., & Bhatia, S. (2022). Bio-imaging-based machine learning algorithm for breast cancer detection. *Diagnostics*, 12(5), 1134. https://doi.org/10.3390/diagnostics12051134
15. Chen, T., Xu, R., He, Y., & Wang, X. (2017). Improving sentiment analysis via sentence type classification using BiLSTM-CRF and CNN. *Expert Systems with Applications*, 72, 221–230.
16. Sun, C., Shrivastava, A., Singh, S., & Gupta, A. (2011). Revisiting unreasonable effectiveness of data in deep learning era. *Paper Presented at: Proceedings of the IEEE International Conference on Computer Vision* (pp. 843–852). IEEE.
17. www.geeksforgeeks.org/understanding-googlenet-model-cnn-architecture/ [Accessed 6th March 2024].
18. Abbasi, A. A., Hussain, L., Awan, I. A., Abbasi, I., Majid, A., Nadeem, M. S. A., & Chaudhary, Q. A. (2020). Detecting prostate cancer using deep learning convolution neural network with transfer learning approach. *Cognitive Neuro-Dynamics*, 14, 523–533.
19. Sriram, G. K., Karunasagar, A., Sudharsan, R., & Malini, A. (2023). Deep learning approaches for Pneumonia classification in healthcare. *3rd International Conference on Innovative Practices in Technology and Management, ICIPTM 2023, Curran Associates, Inc.*
20. Khan, M., Khan, M. A., Ahmed, F., Mittal, M., Goyal, L. M., Hemanth, D. J., & Satapathy, S. C. (2019) Gastrointestinal diseases segmentation and classification based on duo-deep architectures. *Pattern Recognition Letters*, 131, 193–204.
21. He, K., Zhang, X., Ren, S., & Sun, J. (2016). Deep residual learning for image recognition. (Institute of Electrical and Electronics Engineers) *IEEE Conference on Computer Vision and Pattern Recognition.*
22. Perucca, E. (2013). Optimizing antiepileptic drug treatment in tumoral epilepsy. *Epilepsia*, 54(Suppl 9), 97–104.
23. Maschio, M., Dinapoli, L., Zarabia, A., & Jandolo, B. (2006). Issues related to the pharmacological management of patients with brain tumors and epilepsy. *Functional Neurology*, 21(1), 15–19.
24. Rahman, Z., Wong, C. H., Dexter, M., Olsson, G., Wong, M., Gebsky, V., ... & Bleasel, A. B. (2015). Epilepsy in patients with primary brain tumors: The impact on mood, cognition, and HRQOL. *Epilepsy & Behavior*, 48, 88–95.
25. Maschio, M., Dinapoli, L., Gomellini, S., Ferraresi, V., Sperati, F., Vidiri, A., ... & Jandolo, B. (2010). Antiepileptics in brain metastases: Safety, efficacy and impact on life expectancy. *Journal of Neuro-Oncology*, 98(1), 109–116.
26. Vecht, C. J., & Wilms, E. B. (2010). Seizures in low- and high-grade gliomas: Current management and future outlook. *Expert Review of Anticancer Therapy*, 10(5), 663–669.

27. Van Breemen, M. S. M., Wilms, E. B., & Vecht, C. J. (2007). Epilepsy in patients with brain tumors: Epidemiology, mechanisms, and management. *The Lancet Neurology*, 6(5), 421–430.
28. Vecht, C. J., Kerkhof, M., & Duran-Pena, A. (2014). Seizure prognosis in brain tumors: New insights and evidence-based management. *The Oncologist*, 19(7), 751–759.
29. Avila, E. K., & Graber, J. (2010). Seizures and epilepsy in cancer patients. *Current Neurology and Neuroscience Reports*, 10(1), 60–67.
30. Klein, M., Engelberts, N. H. J., van der Ploeg, H. M., Kasteleijn-Nolst Trenité, D. G., Aaronson, N. K., Taphoorn, M. J., ... & Heimans, J. J.. (2003). Epilepsy in low-grade gliomas: The impact on cognitive function and quality of life. *Annals of Neurology*, 54(4), 514–520.
31. Tremont-Lukats, I. W., Ratilal, B. O., Armstrong, T., & Gilbert, M. R. (2008). Antiepileptic drugs for preventing seizures in people with brain tumor. *Cochrane Database of Systematic Reviews*, 2, CD004424.
32. Happold, C., Gorlia, T., Chinot, O., Gilbert, M. R., Nabors, L. B., Wick, W., ... & Weller, M. (2016). Does valproic acid or levetiracetam improve survival in glioblastoma? A pooled analysis of prospective clinical trials in newly diagnosed glioblastoma. *Journal of Clinical Oncology*, 34(7), 731–739.
33. Lwu, S., Hamilton, M. G., Forsyth, P. A., Cairncross, J. G., & Parney, I. F. (2010). Use of peri-operative anti-epileptic drugs in patients with newly diagnosed high grade malignant glioma: A single center experience. *Journal of Neuro-Oncology*, 96, 403–408.
34. Ruda, R., & Soffietti, R. (2015). What is new in the management of epilepsy in gliomas?. *Current Treatment Options in Neurology*, 17(6), 351.
35. Froscher, W., Kirchstein, T., & Rosche, J. (2014). Anticonvulsant therapy in brain-tumor related epilepsy. *Journal of Epileptology*, 82(14), 678–690.
36. Wu, A. S., Trinh, V. T., Suki, D., Graham, S., Forman, A., Weinberg, J. S., ... & Lang, F. F. (2013). A prospective randomized trial of perioperative seizure prophylaxis in patients with intraparenchymal brain tumors. *Journal of Neurosurgery*, 118(4), 873–883.
37. Arvold, N. D., Pinnell, B. A., Mahadevan, A., Connelly, S., Silverman, R., Weiss, S. E., ... & Alexander, B. M. (2016). Steroid and anticonvulsant prophylaxis for stereotactic radiosurgery: Large variation in physician recommendations. *Practical Radiation Oncology*, 6(4), 89–96.
38. Vecht, C., Royer-Perron, L., Houillier, C., & Huberfeld, G. (2017). Seizures and anticonvulsants in brain tumours: Frequency, mechanisms and anti-epileptic management. *Current Pharmaceutical Design*, 23(42), 6464–6487.
39. Anjum, S., Hussain, L., Ali, M., Alkinani, M. H., Aziz, W., Gheller, S., Abbasi, A. A., Marchal, A. R., Suresh, H., & Duong, T. Q. (2021). Detecting brain tumors using deep learning convolutional neural network with transfer learning approach. *International Journal of Imaging Systems and Technology*, 1–17, volume 31.

3 Development of an Advanced Lung Cancer Diagnosis System

Using Image Processing and Machine Learning

S. Kayalvizhi, Kuraganti Harish, and Yakub Mathew

3.1 INTRODUCTION

Medical imaging is essential for diagnosing diseases like lung cancer, but accurately interpreting complex images can be challenging. Deep learning methodologies, like convolutional neural networks, have been applied for the analysis of medical images, enhancing diagnostic precision [1]. In particular, the Inception v3 architecture is famous for its effectiveness in image classification tasks. However, Inception v3 may not always provide the best features for specific diagnostic tasks. Researchers have combined Inception v3 with traditional machine learning techniques, such as Extreme Gradient Boosting (XGBoost), to overcome this limitation and improve predictive performance. The resulting Inception v3+XGBoost model has shown promise in predicting lung cancer from computed tomography (CT) images. Building an effective predictive model requires careful preprocessing of input data. In the case of lung cancer detection from CT images, preprocessing techniques like Z-score normalization, contrast limited adaptive histogram equalization (CLAHE), and *K*-means clustering, are utilized to elevate the caliber and significance of the task at hand. Z-score normalization standardizes the intensity values of CT images to mitigate variations in image intensity across different scans. CLAHE enhances the contrast and visibility of subtle features within the CT images. *K*-means clustering isolates the regions of interest for analysis, reducing the computational complexity of the model and improving its ability to focus on relevant image regions. By integrating these preprocessing techniques with the Inception v3+XGBoost model, researchers aim to develop a robust and accurate tool for the early detection and diagnosis of lung cancer from CT images. This interdisciplinary approach harnesses the strengths of both deep learning and traditional machine learning, paving the way for more effective medical image analysis and improved patient outcomes.

DOI: 10.1201/9781003484233-3

3.2 LITERATURE SURVEY

In [2], researchers proposed a new approach for categorizing various types of lung cancer from whole-slide pathology images using deep learning. The method eliminates the need for manual annotations, making the workflow more efficient and speeding up the classification process, ultimately facilitating prompt and accurate diagnosis. Another study addressed the challenge of classifying lung cancer histologically from CT images using deep learning algorithms. This approach offers a non-invasive and efficient method of histological classification, allowing clinicians to make informed treatment decisions based on CT imaging alone.

In [3], researchers explored machine learning techniques for extracting radiomic biomarkers from imaging data, which can help personalize cancer care by quantifying subtle imaging features capturing valuable information about tumor phenotype, microenvironment, and response to treatment. The fourth study introduced a new approach to enhance the prediction of lung cancer from CT images by using an adaptive hierarchical heuristic mathematical model with the assistance of deep learning. The proposed approach achieves better predictive performance by combining traditional mathematical modeling techniques with deep learning features and adapts to variations in image characteristics, optimizing prediction accuracy across different patient populations and imaging protocols.

Finally, in [4], researchers focused on diagnosing breast cancer from mammography images. The researchers introduced a finely tuned VGG16 model called BreastNet18, designed to classify breast lesions accurately. They conducted extensive ablation studies to analyze the individual network components' contribution to diagnostic performance, which offered insights into model architecture optimization. BreastNet18 demonstrates high accuracy in distinguishing between benign and malignant lesions, making it a reliable tool for early detection and risk stratification in breast cancer screening programs.

These studies demonstrate the potential of machine learning combined deep learning techniques to improve cancer diagnosis and treatment. They offer innovative and efficient methods for categorizing cancer types, classifying histological subtypes, extracting radiomic biomarkers, predicting cancer from imaging data, and diagnosing breast cancer [5,6]. These approaches have the potential to enhance current clinical practices and improve patient outcomes.

3.3 PROPOSED METHODOLOGY

3.3.1 Data Preprocessing

3.3.1.1 Z-Score Normalization

Algorithm

1. Compute the average and the variation from the average for every characteristic present in the dataset. For each data point x in the dataset:
   - Subtract the mean (μ) of the feature from x.

- Divide the result by the standard deviation (σ) of the feature.
- This gives you Z for that data point: $Z = \frac{x - \mu}{\sigma}$.

3.3.1.2 CLAHE

Algorithm

1. **Divide the Image into Tiles**: The input image is divided into non-overlapping tiles or patches.
2. **Compute Histograms**: Compute the histogram for each tile.
3. **Apply Histogram Equalization**: Perform histogram equalization on each tile, redistributing pixel intensities to enhance local contrast.
4. **Clipping**: Clip the histogram at a specified level to prevent noise over-amplification, typically by limiting the contrast enhancement.
5. **Interpolation**: Combine the equalized tiles to form the final enhanced image. This may involve techniques like bilinear interpolation to smooth transitions between tiles.

3.3.1.3 *K*-Means Clustering

Algorithm

1. The first step of the algorithm randomly chooses *K* initial cluster centroids from the data points.
2. In the second step, the algorithm calculates the distance of each data point to each centroid and assigns the data point to the cluster with the closest centroid.
3. In the third step, the algorithm updates to determine the central point of each cluster. We calculate the average of all the data points that have been assigned to that particular cluster.
4. The second and third steps are repeated until convergence is achieved. This means that the process of the algorithm comes to a halt either when the centroids show negligible changes or when the maximum number of iterations is completed.
5. Finally, in the last step, the act of dividing data points into *K* clusters is determined by certain standards, with the final centroids representing each cluster's center.

3.3.1.4 Inception v3 Model

Algorithm

1. The Inception v3 model was designed for image classification. It starts by taking input images of a fixed size, generally 244 × 244 × 3 pixels.
2. The model then uses convolutional layers that extract low-level features from the input images. These layers use small filters to capture local patterns.
3. The core of the Inception v3 model consists of multiple Inception modules stacked on top of each other. Each module contains parallel branches with

different convolutional operations, which allows the network to capture features at different scales.

4. Max pooling layers are included between convolutional layers to downsample feature maps. The pooling layers reduce spatial dimensions and computational complexity while preserving important features.
5. Toward the end of the network, global average pooling is applied to reduce the spatial dimensions of the feature maps. This is followed by fully connected layers that perform classification based on the extracted features.
6. The ultimate layer of the network is a layer that utilizes the softmax function that computes the probability distribution over the output classes. This enables the Inception v3 model to predict the class labels of input images.
7. Inception v3 is trained using backpropagation and gradient descent to minimize a loss function, such as categorical cross-entropy.
8. Transfer learning is often employed in Inception v3, where the model is pretrained on a large dataset like ImageNet and fine-tuned on a specific task with a smaller dataset.
9. During inference, the model outputs the predicted class probabilities for the input image.

3.3.2 Feature Extraction

Algorithm

1. **Input Parameters**: The function **extract_features** takes two parameters:
   - **Model**: The pre-trained Inception v3 model is used to extract features.
   - **Generator**: The data generator provides batches of input images and their corresponding labels.
2. **Feature Extraction Loop**: The function iterates over the batches generated by the input **generator**. For each batch:
   - It extracts features using the **model.** The **Predict** method, which applies the pre-trained Inception v3 model to the input image batch, produces a batch of feature vectors.
   - It appends the extracted features and corresponding labels to separate lists.
3. **Concatenating Features and Labels**: After iterating through all batches, the function concatenates the extracted features and labels into two arrays using **np.vstack**.
4. **Returning Features and Labels**: Finally, the function returns the concatenated features and labels as NumPy arrays.

3.3.3 XGBoost Model

Algorithm

1. Initialization: The model is initialized with an initial prediction, usually the mean of the target variable. Additionally, several parameters, such as the maximum tree depth, learning rate, and regularization terms, are set at this stage.

2. Gradient Calculation: Once the initialization is done, the gradient of the loss function is computed concerning the model's prediction. Common loss functions, such as the squared error for regression and logistic loss for classification, are used to compute the gradient.
3. Tree Building: A decision tree is built to minimize the negative gradient of the loss function. XGBoost uses a regularized form of tree boosting to control model complexity and prevent overfitting. Each tree is built sequentially to correct the residuals of the previous trees.
4. Leaf Weight Calculation: The optimal weights for the ultimate layer of the network constitutes a layer that utilizes the softmax function. This calculation involves computing the similarity scores between each instance and the leaf nodes.
5. Update Model Prediction: The model's prediction is updated by adding the predictions of the new tree, weighted by a shrinkage parameter (learning rate). This step ensures that the model learns incrementally and avoids overfitting.
6. Regularization: To control model complexity and improve generalization performance, regularization techniques such as shrinkage (learning rate) and tree pruning are applied.
7. Iteration: Steps 2–6 are repeated The given process continues until it reaches a specific stopping point, which could be a maximum limit or any other criterion that has been set, such as number of trees or observing no significant improvement in the validation error.
8. Prediction: Finally, during inference, the target variable is predicted for new instances by aggregating the predictions of all the trees in the ensemble.

3.4 PERFORMANCE EVALUATION

Multiple models for detecting lung cancer, which are based on Inception v3 and XGBoost, have been thoroughly evaluated to determine how well they can precisely identify cancerous lesions from CT images. The models use various preprocessing techniques, such as *K*-means clustering for image segmentation, Z-score normalization, and CLAHE. The goal of the evaluation is to assess the ability of these models to accurately detect lung cancer.

Experimental Setup: A diverse dataset is used to train and evaluate a model for detecting cancerous regions in lung CT images. The dataset is preprocessed with a *K*-means clustering technique for image segmentation to identify areas of interest. Z-score normalization is applied to standardize the intensity of pixels, and CLAHE is used to enhance contrast, ensuring that the images are consistent and of improved quality.

Model Training and Validation: A model called Inception v3 is used to process a dataset, extracting important features that are then fed into XGBoost classifiers. The model's hyperparameters are optimized through cross-validation, and steps are taken to address class imbalance to ensure proper model training. The models are then

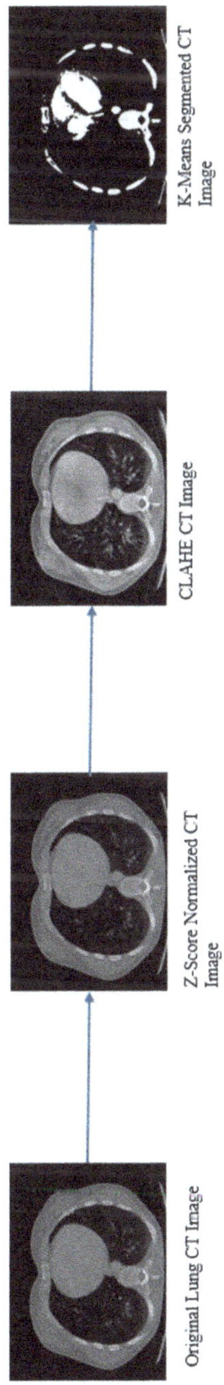

FIGURE 3.1 Preprocessing technique flow diagram.

evaluated on a separate validation set using common metrics such as accuracy, sensitivity, specificity, and AUC-ROC.

Results: Two models, Inception v3+XGBoost, were evaluated for their ability to detect lung cancer lesions. They showed similar performance but with slight variations in different evaluation metrics. The Inception v3+XGBoost model was found to be more effective in discriminating between cancerous and non-cancerous regions, as it exhibited higher accuracy and AUC-ROC values.

Discussion: Inception v3, for instance, is equipped with advanced convolutional layers and inception modules that are highly effective in identifying complex patterns and features that are significant in detecting lung cancer.

Conclusion: The study compared the effectiveness of different techniques in detecting lung cancer from CT images. The combination of Inception v3 and XGBoost showed better results in terms of sensitivity and specificity compared to other methods. The study emphasized the significance of utilizing multiple deep learning architectures and preprocessing techniques to develop reliable and precise computer-aided diagnosis (CAD) systems for lung cancer detection. These findings have important implications for enhancing patient outcomes and clinical decision-making in the field of oncology (Figures 3.1 to 3.4) (Table 3.1).

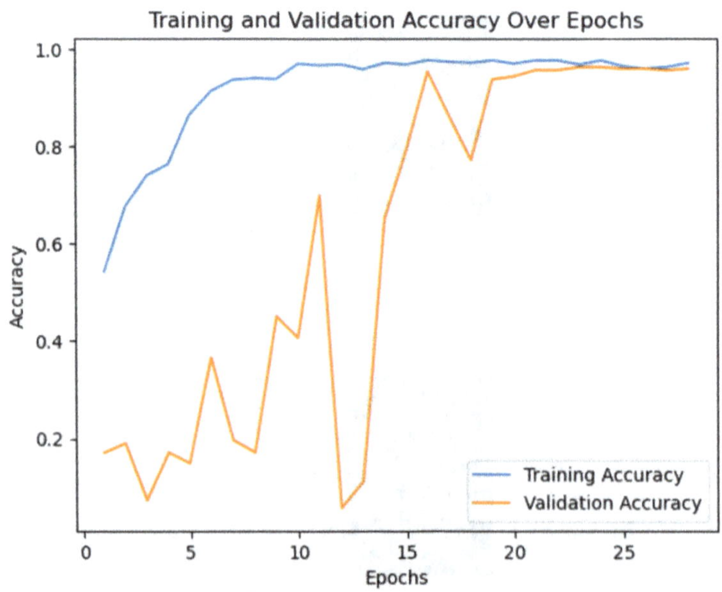

FIGURE 3.2 OUTPUT 1: Validation and training accuracy over epochs for the Inception v3 model.

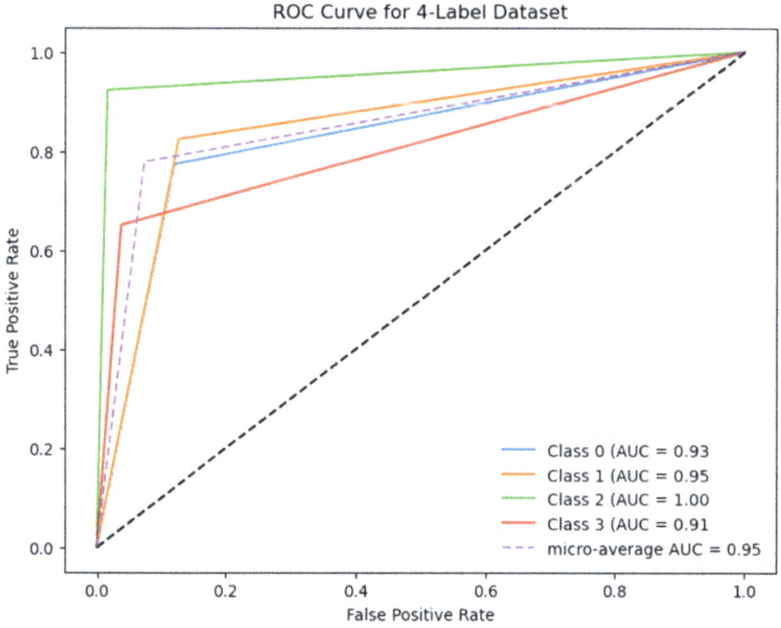

FIGURE 3.3 OUTPUT 2: ROC curve of the four classes of data from the Inception v3+XGBoost model.

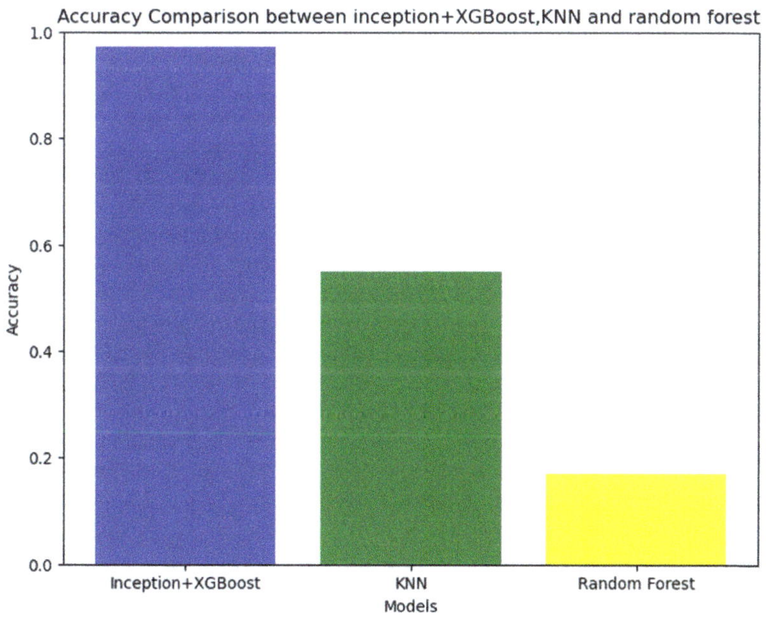

FIGURE 3.4 OUTPUT 7: Comparison of the accuracy of different models.

TABLE 3.1
Model accuracy, loss, validation accuracy, and validation loss

Model	Accuracy	Loss	Validation accuracy	Validation loss
Inception v3+XGBoost	97%	0.0913	96.1%	0.9587

3.5 CONCLUSION

The combination of advanced deep learning models, such as Inception v3, with XGBoost for detecting lung cancer using CT images, has shown promising results. By using preprocessing techniques, such as Z-score normalization, CLAHE, and *K*-means clustering, the models were able to extract features effectively and improve the accuracy of detection. The experimental results demonstrate that the Inception v3 model combined with XGBoost achieved a higher accuracy of 95%. Overall, integrating deep learning models with traditional machine learning algorithms presents a robust approach for accurate and efficient lung cancer detection from CT images. Further research and optimization of preprocessing techniques and model architectures could potentially enhance the performance and applicability of these methods in clinical settings. Ultimately, this could aid in early detection and improved prognosis for patients with lung cancer.

REFERENCES

1. C. Parmar et al., "Machine Learning Methods for Quantitative Radiomic Biomarkers," in *Science Report,* vol. 5, p. 13087, 2015, doi: 10.1038/srep13087
2. J. Pati, "Gene Expression Analysis for Early Lung Cancer Prediction Using Machine Learning Techniques: An Eco-Genomics Approach," in *IEEE Access*, vol. 7, pp. 4232–4238, 2019, doi: 10.1109/ACCESS.2018.2886604
3. R. Siegel, D. Naishadham and A. Jemal, "Cancer Statistics, 2013," in *CA Cancer Journal of Clinical*, vol. 63, pp. 11–30, 2013.
4. Yu, K.-H. et al., "Predicting Non-Small Cell Lung Cancer Prognosis by Fully Automated Microscopic Pathology Image Features," in *Nature Communication*, vol. 7, p. 12474, 2016, doi: 10.1038/ncomms12474
5. H. Yu, Z. Zhou and Q. Wang, "Deep Learning Assisted Predict of Lung Cancer on Computed Tomography Images Using the Adaptive Hierarchical Heuristic Mathematical Model," in *IEEE Access*, vol. 8, pp. 86400–86410, 2020, doi: 10.1109/ACCESS.2020.2992645
6. Z. Li et al., "Deep Learning Methods for Lung Cancer Segmentation in Whole-Slide Histopathology Images—The ACDC@LungHP Challenge 2019," in *IEEE Journal of Biomedical and Health Informatics*, vol. 25, no. 2, pp. 429–440, Feb. 2021, doi: 10.1109/JBHI.2020.3039741

4 Machine Learning Algorithms for Medical Diagnosis and Prognosis

P. Muthu, S. Latha, S. Hannah Pauline, R. Jansi, and Samiappan Dhanalakshmi

4.1 INTRODUCTION

One of the primary causes of dementia, Alzheimer's disease, can have detrimental effects on a person's daily life if it is not identified and treated early. The Mini-Mental State Examination (MMSE) Predictor aids in the diagnosis of dementia. Organization, planning, communication, memory, problem solving, thinking, motor capabilities, and coordination are among the cognitive impairments brought on by dementia in an individual. The types of progressive dementia include vascular, Alzheimer's, fronto-temporal, Lewy body, Creutzfeldt–Jakob, Wernicke–Korsakoff, Huntington's, normal pressure, and mixed hydrocephalus dementia. The reasons for dementia occurrence are aging, family history, traumatic heart health, and brain wound. Currently there is no permanent cure for dementia. Alzheimer's treatment is in the clinical trial stage. The World Health Organization devised action plans for the health response to dementia from 2017 to 2025, giving it high priority. Figure 4.1 shows the dementia types.

Rishad et al. reviewed machine learning and neuroimaging techniques for diagnosing dementia [1]. Deep learning with multimodal image analysis has proven to give promising results for dementia detection. The clinical diagnosis of dementia is performed by neuro-imaging methods like magnetic resonance imaging (MRI), single photon emission computed tomography (SPECT), computed tomography (CT), or positron emission tomography (PET). The processes' neuroimages are split into training and test data. Relevant features are extracted, selected, and optimized. Dementia classification, prediction, and differentiation machine learning or deep learning models are performed. The following performance metrics are used to evaluate computer-aided dementia diagnosis: missing value confiscation, accuracy, precision, sensitivity, and confusion matrix [2]. The types of dementia, causing memory loss to adverse conditions, are given in Figure 4.1.

Electronic big data available for dementia are high-dimensional and sparse [3]. Gavin et al. proposed an entropy regularization with ensemble deep neural network (ECNN) for feature analysis in the dementia dataset. Ten indicators of dementia were studied, with hypertension being the significant feature. The model provided an

DOI: 10.1201/9781003484233-4

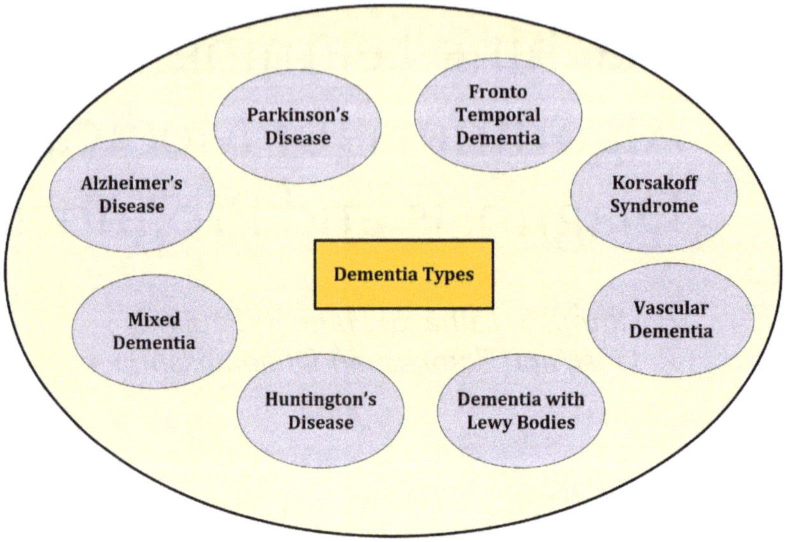

FIGURE 4.1 Types of dementia.

accuracy of 75.5%. ECNN is a deep neural network (DNN) method with two hidden layers containing 50 and 30 neurons. Low variance principal components were removed, which also led to data loss in the feature space. A disconnection occurred between dimensionality reduction and estimation. Feature selection while in the training phase and feedback helped to overcome both problems. The features may be either disconnected, partially connected, or fully connected to the model. The last two connection types were the favorable ones for removing redundant features. The highly ranked features for the ECNN model were hypertension, tablets, prefilled syringe, increased blood glucose, social groups, nightmares, and third-party encounters [4].

Delirium, which may occur in dementia patients, and their psychomotor behaviors were studied with machine learning models by Chang et al. [5,6]. Learning from examples of the module 2 algorithm achieved the best prediction results in identifying psychomotor the habits of delirium-affected individuals. The classifications were based on dementia level, educational qualification, dehydration, sleep issues, gender, Foley catheter, and haloperidol in hyperactive and hypoactive dementia [7].

The daily activities of dementia-affected individuals can't be monitored continuously. Using signal processing and machine learning can identify issues in appliance usage by affected persons [8, 9]. The random forest (RF) and support vector machine (SVM) algorithms have been modeled using the data. The RF algorithm outperformed the other methods with 96.34% specificity and 96.34% sensitivity. Changes in routine and behavior pattern have been analyzed by the approach. There are four types of devices: on/off devices, multi-state or finite-state devices, continuous variable devices, and long-period active devices. Seasonal changes influencing dementia patients have not been identified [10, 11].

Males with inflammatory bowel disease (IBD) and Crohn's disease (CD) had a higher threat of dementia compared to females in the long run. Niamh et al. developed many classification workflows and imputation based on computational expense and diagnostic classification performance to overcome many missing data problems in the test and training sets [12]. Missing data may lead to diagnosis delay and changes in predictions of the disease. In a minimized feature set, applying iterative imputation in the training data has proved to be computationally effective. Predictive Mean Matching (PMM) with Multivariate Imputation via Chained Equations (MICE) has been used for data imputation. The coefficients are obtained by linearly regressing the obtained data in columns, creating a new list using random data from the posterior predictive distribution, predicting closer missing values, and randomly assigning missing values. The process is repeated ten times to achieve the imputed dataset. After imputation, classification is performed and performance is analyzed.

Fubao et al. proposed a multi-class deep learning approach for dementia-based classification with an informed questionnaire [13, 14]. The DNN gave an accuracy of 88% for detecting normal, mild, and very mild cognitive dementia, and moderate and severe dementia. Fifty features were selected from the neuropsychological tests to form the questionnaire. SVM, multilayer perceptron (MLP), Naive Bayes, AdaBoost, RC-Forest, LogitBoost, and RF algorithms were also used for classification. Gavin et al. proposed entropy regularization with DNNs to identify significant features and to provide predictive results of patient hospitalization with dementia [15]. They tried reducing the feature set and obtained a maximum efficiency of 75.9%. Initially low variant principal components were removed. Information entropy had a peak value of 0.5. Entropy regularization brought the first layer of the neural network toward [0,1]. Feedback on the selected features is given to input each time and direct feature reduction is performed. The features may be disconnected, partially connected, or fully connected to improve prediction performance.

The opportunities, challenges, and issues of using machine learning for dementia research was studied by Gavin et al. [16]. The study was performed for the neuroimaging, speech analysis, and cognitive assessment of dementia patients. The authors strongly recommended an automatic diagnostic method since radiologist checks are time consuming, concentrate on certain brain areas only, and depend on the medical professional. For dementia assessments, both linear and nonlinear computations with feature extracted data are frequently used in the literature. Chao et al. combined machine learning methods with electroencephalography (EEG) signals [17]. They used the directed transfer function to find the interregional directed connectivity. They classified the EEG signal using linear discriminant analysis (LDA), backpropagation, and SVM in order to identify dementia. After Fisher selection, SVM classification yielded accuracy, specificity, and sensitivity of 86.11%, 85.71%, and 86.67%, respectively

Rodrigo et al. [18] proposed evolutionary computation (EC)-based MRI analysis for the diagnosis of Alzheimer's disease. There were three categories: mild cognitive, Alzheimer's disease, and cognitive normal. The process of evaluating slice grouping included choosing slice features, standardizing data, using principal component analysis (PCA) to reduce dimensions, class balance, and assessing the correctness of training and testing.

Machine learning algorithms are used to classify data from the dementia dataset. EC approaches are used for feature reduction and selection, and the results are compared before and after EC application. Section 4.2 of this chapter presents the methodology, Section 4.3 presents the results and discussion, and Section 4.4 wraps up the chapter.

4.2 METHODOLOGY

The dataset, classification techniques (classification and regression tree (CART), naive Bayes, logistic regression, and SVM), and EC approaches (genetic algorithm (GA) and differential evolution (DE)) are all covered in detail in this section. The findings and discussion cover machine learning techniques both with and without feature reduction using EC techniques.

Metrics for categorization performance are used to gauge performance. Figure 4.2 shows the block diagram for the suggested categorization model.

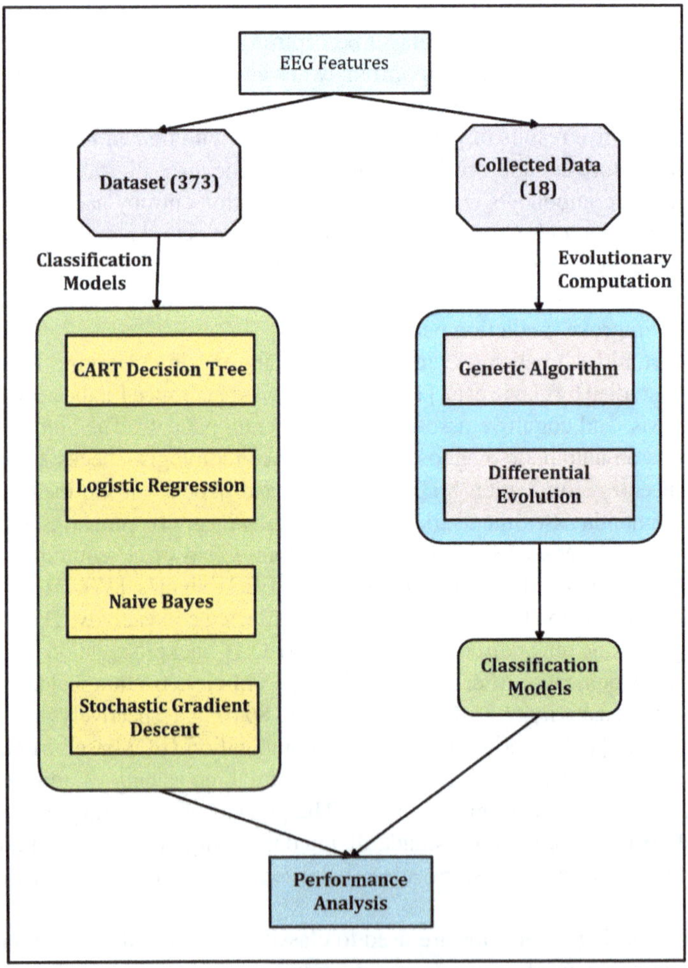

FIGURE 4.2 Overview of the proposed classification model.

4.2.1 Dataset

Battineni's "Dementia Prediction Dataset" from Kaggle was used for applying the proposed method of EC with Machine Learning (ECML). The dataset consisted of dementia MRI data from 186 individuals aged between 60 and 96. Each person was scanned multiple times to get a total of 336 data: 190 data were for individuals without dementia and 146 were for individuals with dementia [19].

The SRM Medical College Hospital and Research Center in Kattankulathur, Tamil Nadu, India, granted ethical permission for the collection of dementia data. At the SRM Medical College Hospital and Research Center in Kattankulathur, Chennai, India, eight data were gathered from patients with dementia and ten from people without dementia.

4.2.2 Dementia Analysis

EEG is a modality that helps to acquire electrical signal electrodes kept near the individual's scalp. The amplitude and frequency of the signal depends on the person's current mental state. For a dementia patient, slow wave activity increases, the alpha frequency reduces, and beta frequencies and the posterior dominant rhythm reduce in the EEG signal [20]. Visual EEG evaluation has been proven to be the best quantitative analysis for dementia classification. A reduction in beta and increase in theta is the identification mark for early stages of dementia. Quantitative EEG (QEEG) includes time-frequency study along with time and frequency analysis, which evaluates individuals' cognitive functions.

The following personal information was included in the dementia dataset that we collected and the data that we collected. The following factors were taken into consideration: the individual's sex, left or right handedness, age, socio-economic status (SES), degree of education, MMSE, clinical diagnosis rating (CDR), average whole brain volume (aWBV), approximated total intracranial volume (aTIV), and Atlas scaling component (ASC). The first five features provide personal details about the person, which helps in learning about our study population. The remaining five features may be considered for the classification and analysis of dementia.

MMSE is a questionnaire-based evaluation method used to identify the cognitive status of the individual. The value ranges from 0 to 30, with lower values indicating the presence of cognitive impairments. The severity, functional, behavioral and cognitive status of the person can be found by the CDR parameter. The value ranges from 0 to 1, with 0 indicating an individual without dementia and 1 indicating an individual with dementia. When dura is not identifiable, Total Intercranial Volume (TIV) provides the predicted capacity of the cranial cavity defined by the cerebral contour or supratentorial dura matter [21]. aTIV is a covariate, measured in mm^3. Whole Brain Volume (WBV) is the native WBV and aWBV is the normalized one, measured in mg. Matching the person with the atlas target is done using the volume scaling factor Atlas scaling factor (ASF). The brain MRI data points metric is subjected to affine transformation and its determinant is obtained.

Dementia affected refers to an individual with significant dementia and non-dementia confirms that the individual does not have dementia. Converted refers to the person who is converted to significant dementia after the initial valuations.

4.2.3 Machine Learning Technique Classification

The purpose of the chapter is to use machine learning models with and without EC to categorize an individual as dementia affected or non-dementia individual. Using the available dementia EEG dataset, logistic regression, CART decision tree, Naive Bayes, and gradient descent algorithms were run. Testing was done using the data we obtained from the SRM Medical College Hospital in Chennai following training.

4.2.3.1 CART Decision Tree

Gini impurity is used by the decision tree algorithm CART to divide the tree into nodes. At each node point, the best split is obtained. The given input needs to be split based on the best split point. The process is continued until either the stopping criteria is met or there is no possibility of further splitting. The sum of the squared probabilities of every class is stored in the Gini index. Skewed categorial and numerical variables can be handled with the CART structure effectively. The structure is unmodified, even when the root square value or log values are replaced in the variable. Beginning with the root node, tree building is performed. Partitioning is stopped at any level when all data samples are in similar classes. A less complex tree is structured by tree pruning [22]. The modified Gini index is given by

$$Gini(DS) = 1 - \sum_{j} n^2(j) \tag{1}$$

The normalized weight of the classes with the j class that approaches the point is denoted by $n(j)$. The total for every node is computed.

4.2.3.2 Logistic Regression

Logistic regression models the probability of the discrete output from the available input variable. The approach is used since the target is categorial. The linear combination of weighted predicting variables with sigmoid activation is used in logistic regression classification [23, 24]. The probability with repression and activation, called the odds ratio, can be found using the following equation:

$$\log\left(\frac{q}{1-q}\right) = \sum_{j=1}^{m} w_j x_j + c \tag{2}$$

where c is the bias term, w_j is the jth feature's coefficient, q is the probability of having dementia, and x is the feature set. The product of the scaling factor and absolute values sum, called the regularization factor, is added to the total cost to overcome the overfitting problem. The hyperplane decision boundary between the two classes needs to be flexible and nonlinear in covariates.

4.2.3.3 Naive Bayes

Naive Bayes is a probability-based classifier with independent assumptions between the features. Each feature individually contributes to classification. Accuracy increases with kernel density estimation for kernel smoothing. The likelihood table is generated using features from the frequency table [25]. The posterior probability is estimated using the Bayes theorem. Bayes with feature selection is given by

$$c(F) = \arg \max_{\alpha C} P(c) \prod_{j=1}^{m} P(a_j \mid c) \tag{3}$$

The selective parameter for test occurrence F is a_j, and the number of selective parameters is m. The total probability over all the components of the mixture is the likelihood. Since it may receive two votes and become more relevant than the other features, the connected features are eliminated.

4.2.3.4 Gradient Descent Algorithm

Gradient descent is an optimization algorithm that reduces the cost function. In stochastic gradient descent, data are chosen randomly in a batch instead of working on all the data. The frequency updates are computationally expensive, which may lead to noisy gradients and an increase in the error rate. The initial results and their errors are found first. With the current learning rate, at every iteration, the modified biases and weights are computed. If the computed error is greater than the current error by a threshold value, the previous error values are retained. The process is continued with a reduced learning rate. For the ith iteration, random sample y^t, parameters θ, learning rate α, and gradient b, the update is given by

$$\theta_i = \theta_{i-1} - \alpha b_i \tag{4}$$

Using the gradient descent approach requires careful adjustment of the learning rate, as well as a lowering of the learning rate during the training phase [26]. Changes in the parameter training result from the current gradient being derived from the directions of the past and present gradients.

4.2.4 Evolutionary Computation (EC) Algorithms

EC is a population dependent stochastic optimization approach to arrive at the global optimal solution. The initial population is randomly created with an algorithm. The size of the population needs to be maintained throughout. A fitness function evaluates how close individuals are to the optimum. The individual with the maximum fitness value is the chosen one. The EC cycle is represented in Figure 4.3.

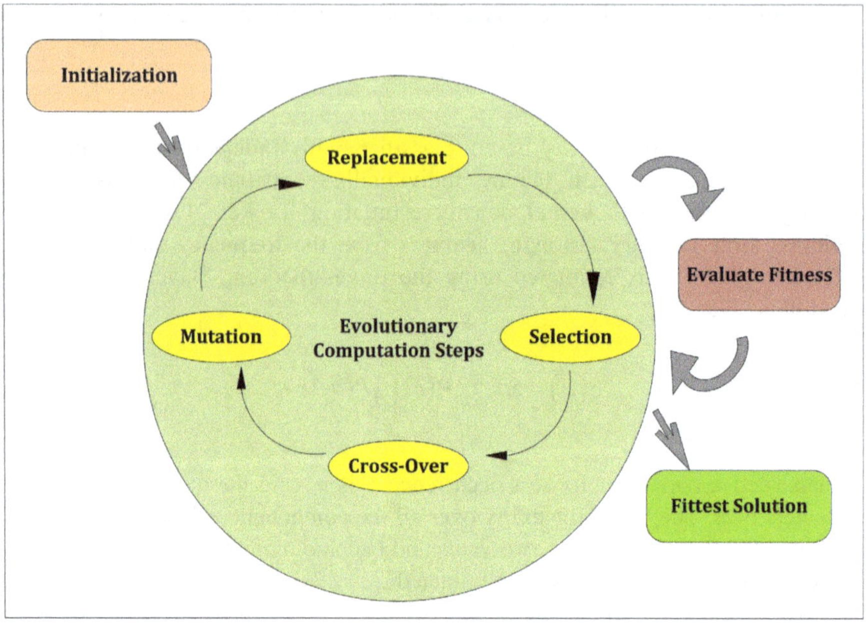

FIGURE 4.3 Evolutionary computation cycle.

GA and DE EC approaches are used to optimize the dementia database. The algorithms change the ways in which individuals are represented.

4.2.4.1 Genetic Algorithm

GA is used to optimize decision trees and other machine learning algorithms that require a genetic depiction of the solution domain and a fitness function to appraise the solution domain. All possible solutions of the problem are referred to as the population. Other parameters of GA include allele, chromosomes, genes, genetic operators, fitness function, and selection.

The steps the algorithm follows are initialization, fitness assignment, selection, reproduction, and termination. The advantages of GA include its parallel capability operation and solution to problems, and it does not need derivative information.

For each chromosome, the fitness values are computed. The initial population for *n* chromosomes is generated. Based on the crossover probability, the crossover operation is applied on selected pairs. Based on the mutation probability, mutation is applied in the offspring. The newly created population replaces the old population. This iterative process leads to the best solution [27, 28]. The process of GA is given in Figure 4.4.

Boltzmann selection is applied to the dementia database, which is dependent on sampling techniques and entropy. The premature convergence problem that exists in the dataset may be solved by the Boltzmann selection process. The procedure is enhanced with elitism selection in order to reduce the likelihood of knowledge loss. By using precedence preserving crossover, the discrete solution as it is presented in

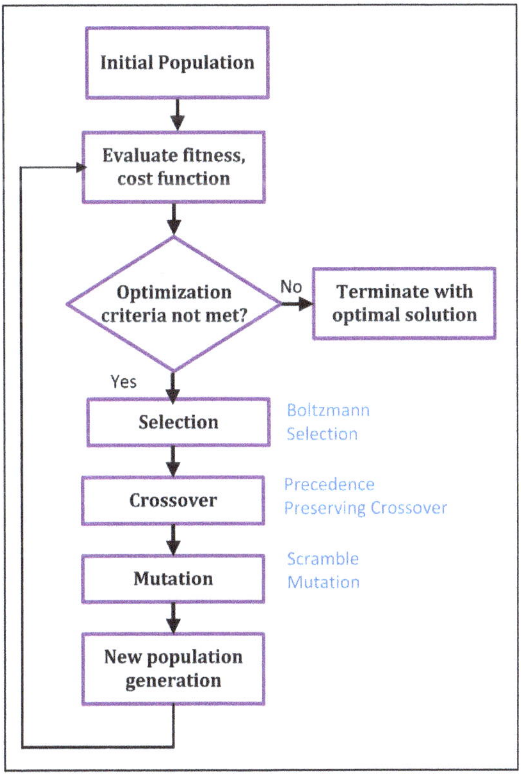

FIGURE 4.4 Genetic algorithm process.

the base data is kept organized (PPX). When choosing among candidates from both parents, PPX is helpful. Scramble mutation is applied to identify if the generated fitness is enhanced, and if the generated fitness values are in the correct range and in order.

4.2.4.2 Differential Evolution

General-purpose optimization known as DE unravels design and non-design optimization attempts. It is the most important global numerical optimization algorithm in the evolutionary algorithm family. The differential mutation operator is the fundamental element of DE. The parents in the mutation operator are randomly chosen from the current population. The appropriate species typically have sufficient information, which increases their chances of being used to lead other species. Any real, vector-valued function can be quickly and effectively optimized using simple vector functions and random draws. DE lacks continuity and differentiability features, which are necessary in a number of common optimization methods [29, 30].

The model is metaheuristic and depends on evolutionary biology concepts. Genetic indications of available results for the real-valued fitness functions are available for the consequent generations. The individual gene's mutation and crossover produce the analysis.

DE can quickly and accurately use both approximate and exact optimal designs to evaluate some or all of the parameters in linear and nonlinear models. DE is also capable of successfully deciphering other complicated design challenges, including high-dimensional ones.

Let us consider the following scenario: We want to minimize a real-valued function h:RN→R with N number of parameters, devoid of generality, by achieving x^*∈RV such that $h(x^*) \leq h(x)$ for all x∈RV. Within the search space of potential solutions, the boundaries of each N parameter define the fitness function's landscape.

4.3 RESULTS AND DISCUSSION

Logistic regression, naive Bayes, CART, and stochastic gradient descent algorithm are the four machine learning techniques that are used to classify dementia data in order to determine if the data are classed as dementia affected or not. We optimize the dataset using the EC techniques GA and DE. Next, classification techniques are used, and performance analysis is done both with and without the use of EC.

4.3.1 Performance Metrics

Statistical performance measures including parametric and non-parametric ones are required to identify the optimal classification algorithm for the available dementia dataset. This will aid in applying the best algorithms for practical use. For an imbalanced dataset, a greater number of performance measures are necessary, which aids in suitable model selection. The classification as dementia affected or non-dementia is a binary classification problem.

An individual with dementia is appropriately categorized as such and assigned the designation True Positive (TP). A True Negative (TN) is a person who is appropriately identified as not having dementia. It is a False Positive (FP) to predict that an individual has dementia when the reality is that the individual does not. False Negative (FN) refers to a prediction that an individual has dementia but the actual individual does not. The confusion matrix used to analyze classification performance is formed by these data. The ratio of accurate estimations to total estimates is known as accuracy:

$$Accuracy = \frac{TN + TP}{FP + FN + TP + TN} \tag{5}$$

Precision is the proportion of precise positive identifications among the actual constructive identifications:

$$Precision = \frac{TP}{TP + FP} \tag{6}$$

Recall or sensitivity specifies the proportion of correct predictions:

$$Recall = \frac{TP}{TP + FN} \tag{7}$$

The harmonic mean of precision and recall is provided by the F-score. The correctness of the exam is provided:

$$F\text{-}Score = 2 * \frac{Precision * Recall}{Precision + Recall} \tag{8}$$

Specificity predicts the true negatives of all the available categories:

$$Specificity = \frac{TN}{TN + FP} \tag{9}$$

The ability of a classifier to recognize the proper classes is measured by the area under the curve (AUC). The receiver operator characteristics (ROC) are summarized:

$$AUC = 0.5 * \left(\frac{TP}{TP + FN} + \frac{TN}{FP + TN} \right) \tag{10}$$

4.3.2 Feature Distribution

The feature distribution for dementia affected and non-dementia for aWBV, CDR, aTIV, MMSE, and ASC are plotted in Figure 4.5 (a–e). The values are normalized to remove data redundancy.

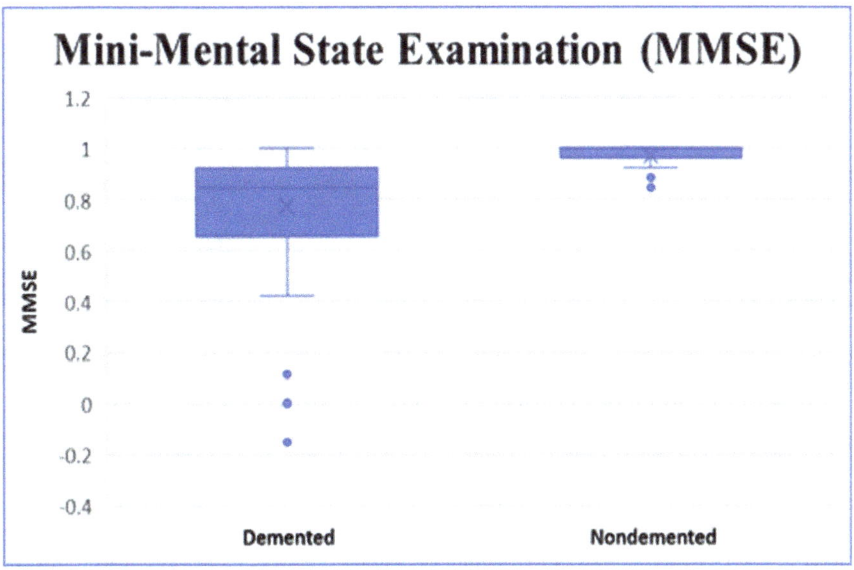

FIGURE 4.5 Feature distribution for (a) MMSE, (b) CDR, (c) aTIV, (d) aWBV, (e) ASF.

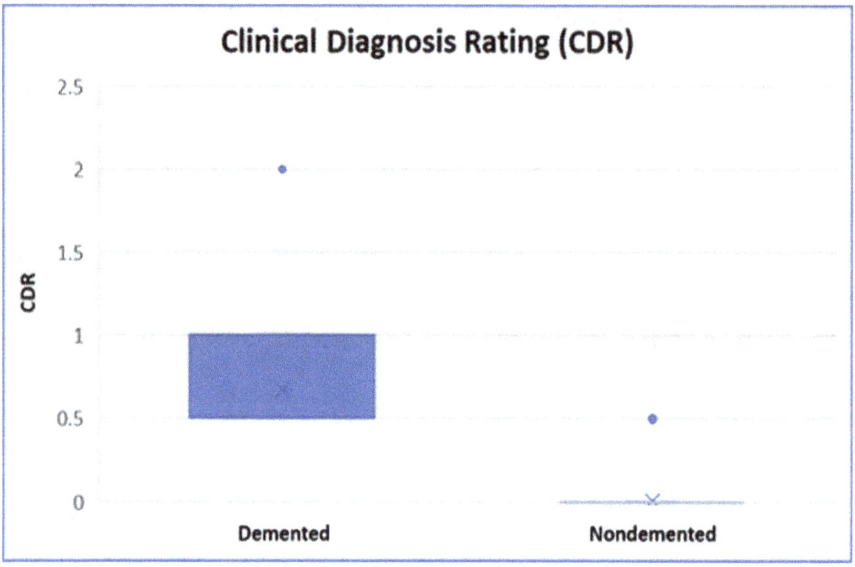

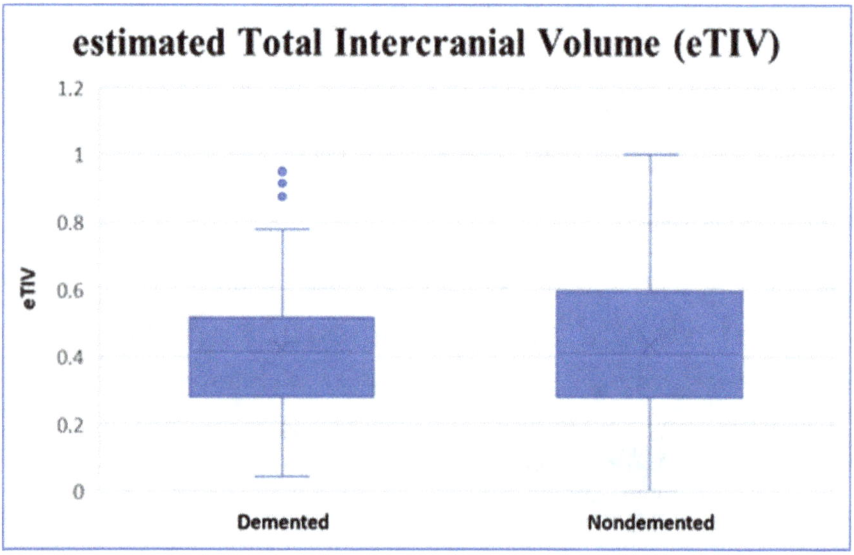

FIGURE 4.5 (Continued)

The box and whisker plots indicate that the dementia database features used for the classification as dementia affected and non-dementia varied significantly for both classes.

4.3.3 ML with and without EC

The ML algorithms' performance for the dementia dataset, logistic regression, naive Bayes, CART decision tree, and stochastic gradient descent are used [31]. Before using EC techniques, Table 4.1 expands the confusion matrix for the ML methods.

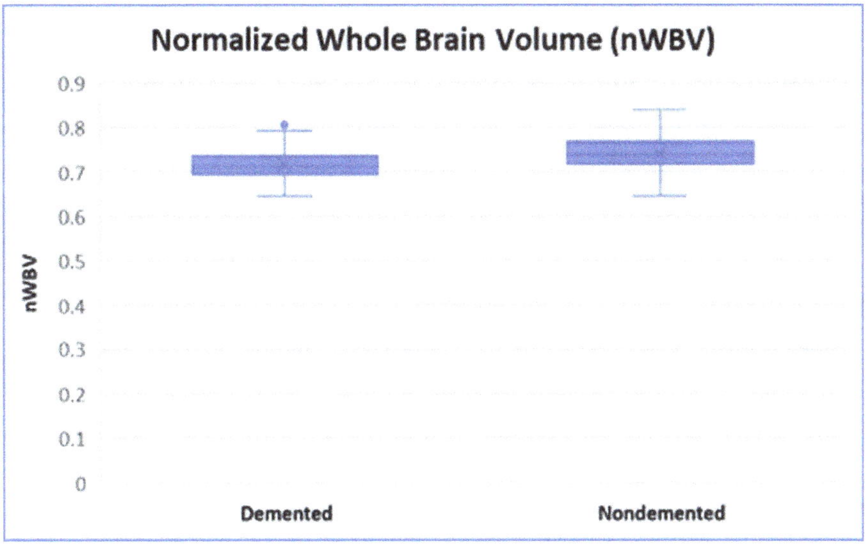

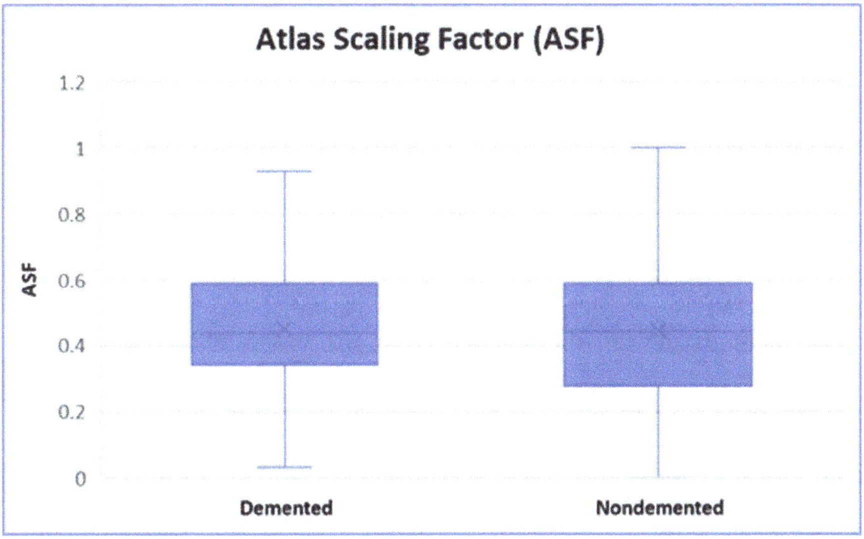

FIGURE 4.5 (Continued)

Predicted Values

The performance evaluation metrics for the classification algorithms used in the dementia classification are provided in Table 4.2.

Logistic Regression provides the best results among the applied machine learning algorithms for the dementia dataset. The confusion matrix for the ML algorithms following feature optimization using GA is shown in Table 4.3.

TABLE 4.1
Confusion matrix for the ML algorithms functional in the dementia dataset

Predicted Values	Actual Values							
	CART decision tree		Logistic regression		Naive Bayes		Stochastic gradient descent	
n = 336	Positive (1)	Negative (0)	Positive (1)	Negative (0)	Positive (1)	Negative (0)	Positive (1)	Negative (0)
Positive (1)	122	24	137	9	126	20	129	17
Negative (0)	36	154	8	182	21	169	19	171

TABLE 4.2
Performance measures of the ML systems functional in the dementia dataset

Classification model	Accuracy (%)	Precision (%)	Recall (%)	Specificity (%)	F-score (%)	AUC (%)
CART decision tree	82.14	83.56	77.21	86.51	80.25	81.86
Logistic regression	**94.94**	**93.83**	**94.48**	**95.28**	**94.15**	**94.88**
Naive Bayes	87.79	86.30	85.71	89.41	86.00	87.56
Stochastic gradient descent	89.28	88.35	87.16	90.95	87.75	89.05

TABLE 4.3
Confusion matrix for the ML algorithms after feature optimization by GA EC

Predicted Values	Actual Values							
	CART decision tree		Logistic regression		Naive Bayes		Stochastic gradient descent	
n = 336	Positive (1)	Negative (0)	Positive (1)	Negative (0)	Positive (1)	Negative (0)	Positive (1)	Negative (0)
Positive (1)	126	20	141	5	129	17	132	14
Negative (0)	30	160	5	185	17	173	15	175

Predicted Values

This is the data for the 336 data from the database, out of which 146 were dementia affected and 190 were non-dementia. Table 4.4 gives the performance of the ML algorithms after applying GA.

Table 4.4 also proves that logistic regression is the suitable approach for dementia classification. It shows significant improvement over applying the ML algorithms

TABLE 4.4
Performance measures of the ML models for the dementia data after feature optimization by GA

Classification model	Accuracy (%)	Precision (%)	Recall (%)	Specificity (%)	F-score (%)	AUC (%)
CART decision tree	85.11	86.30	90.76	88.88	88.47	89.82
Logistic regression	**97.02**	**96.57**	**96.57**	**97.36**	**96.57**	**96.96**
Naive Bayes	89.88	88.35	88.35	91.05	88.35	89.7
Stochastic gradient descent	91.36	90.41	89.79	92.59	90.09	91.19

TABLE 4.5
Confusion matrix for the ML algorithms after feature optimization by DE EC

Predicted Values	Actual Values: CART decision tree		Logistic regression		Naive Bayes		Stochastic gradient descent	
n = 336	Positive (1)	Negative (0)	Positive (1)	Negative (0)	Positive (1)	Negative (0)	Positive (1)	Negative (0)
Positive (1)	128	18	144	2	133	13	136	10
Negative (0)	26	164	3	187	14	176	12	178

TABLE 4.6
Performance measures of the ML models for the dementia dataset after feature optimization by DE

Classification model	Accuracy (%)	Precision (%)	Recall (%)	Specificity (%)	F-score (%)	AUC (%)
CART decision tree	86.90	87.67	83.11	90.10	85.32	86.60
Logistic regression	**98.51**	**98.63**	**97.95**	**98.94**	**98.28**	**98.44**
Naive Bayes	91.96	91.09	90.47	93.12	90.77	91.79
Stochastic gradient descent	93.45	93.15	91.89	94.68	92.51	91.19

directly on the dataset in terms of performance measures. After the features are optimized using the DE EC technique, Table 4.5 presents the confusion matrix of the machine learning algorithms.

Predicted Values

Table 4.6 gives the performance of the ML algorithms with DE EC.

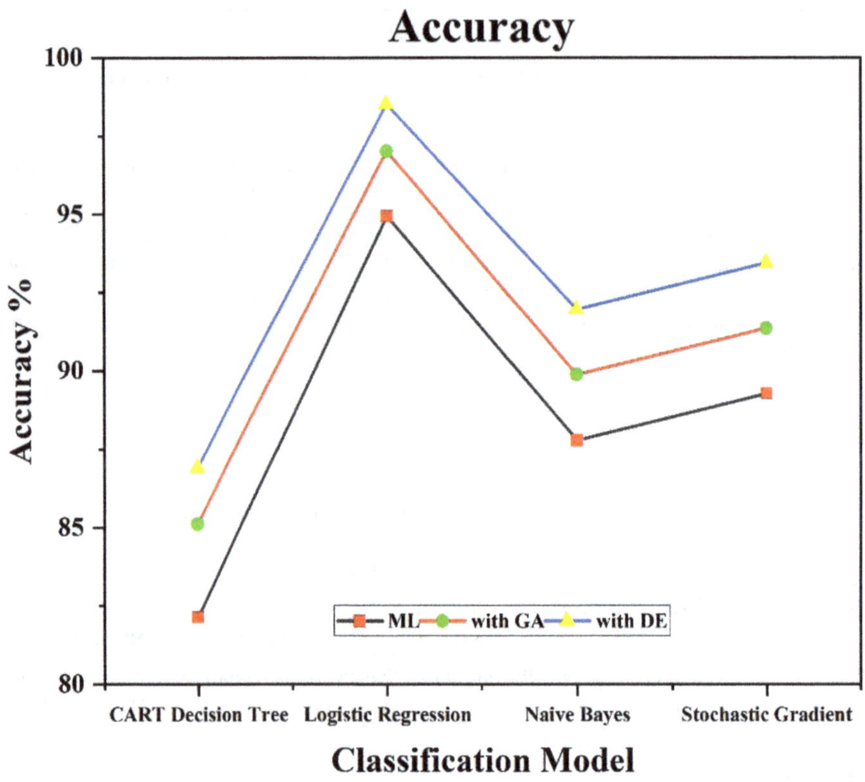

FIGURE 4.6 Classification performance measures: (a) accuracy, (b) precision, (c) recall, (d) specificity, (e) F-score, (f) area under the curve.

Again, this proves that logistic regression with DE EC remarkably improved performance over the rest of the algorithms. Figure 4.6 (a)–(f) provides the graphical representation for the performances of the ML algorithms with and without EC models.

The curves prove that, given the efficiency of logistic regression with DE optimization, it is the optimal classification model for dementia classification.

4.4 CONCLUSION

Three hundred and thirty-six data from the dementia dataset were classified by the ML models logistic regression, naive Bayes, CART, and stochastic gradient descent. Initially features were studied for their significance between dementia affected and non-dementia data. Logistic regression provided an accuracy of 94.94%, which is the highest recorded performance. EC algorithms GA and DE were applied to the models to optimize the feature set, so that classification performance improved. DE with logistic regression recorded the highest accuracy of 98.51%. The precision, recall, and specificity recorded for DE with logistic regression were 98.63%, 97.95%, and 98.94% respectively.

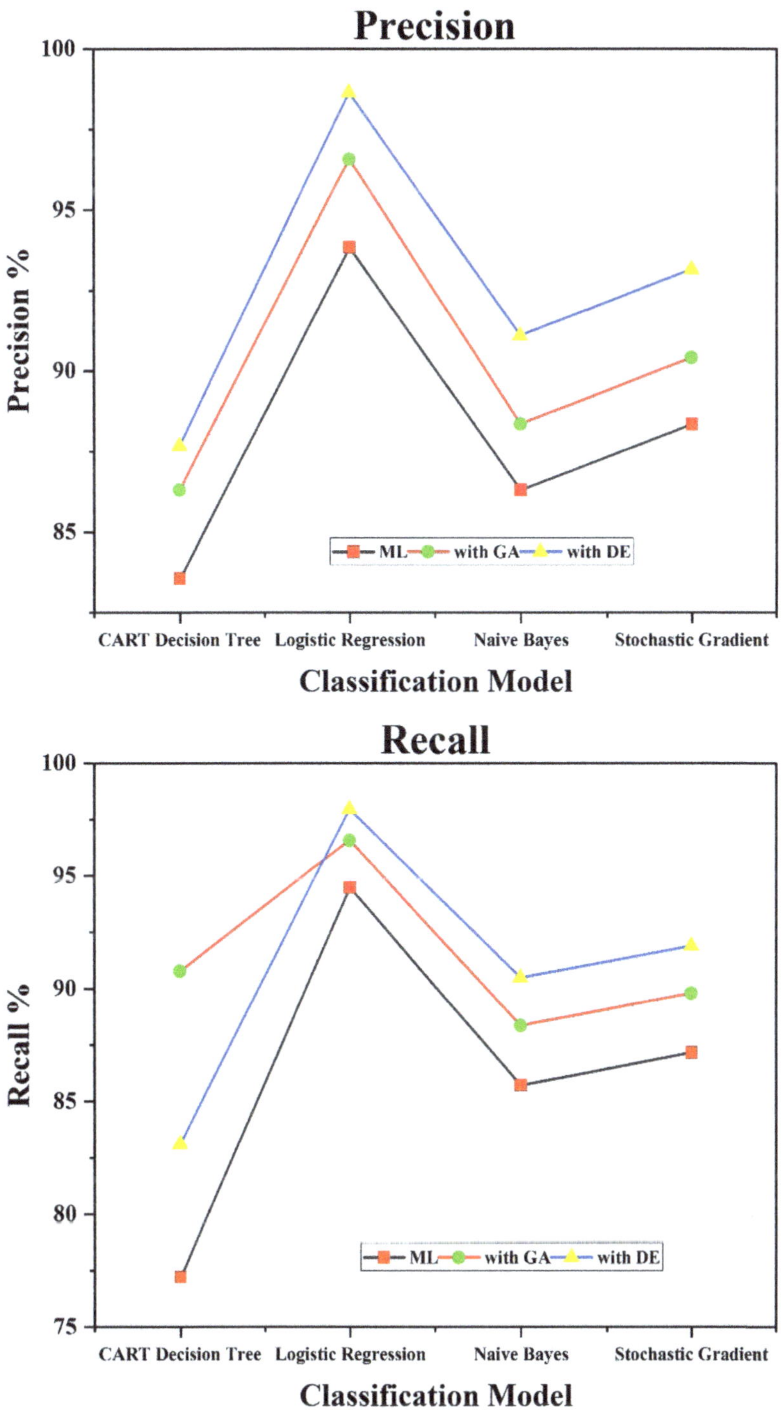

FIGURE 4.6 (Continued)

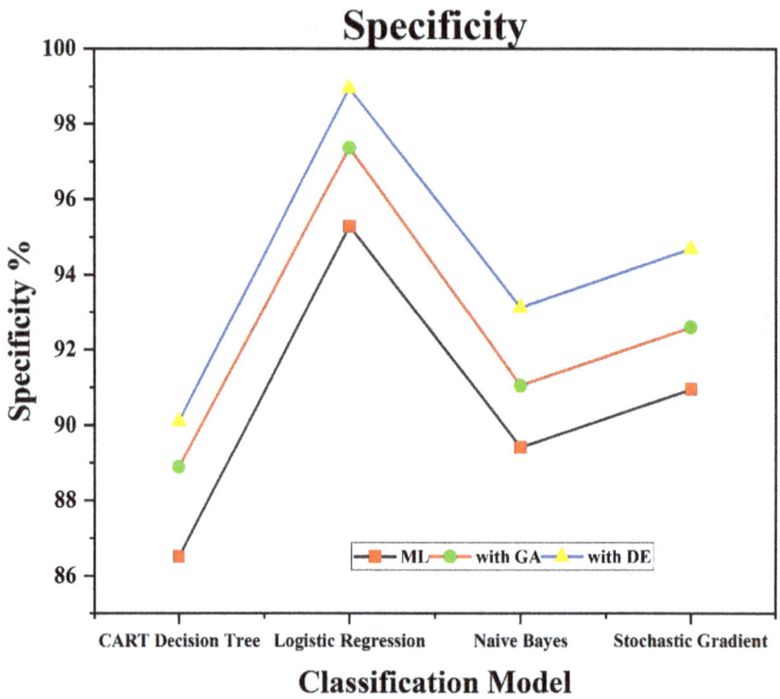

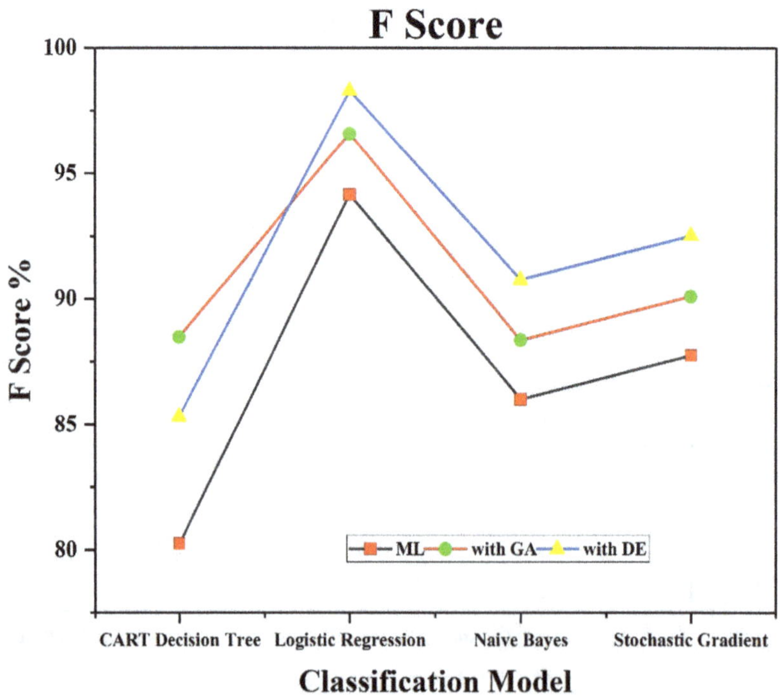

FIGURE 4.6 (Continued)

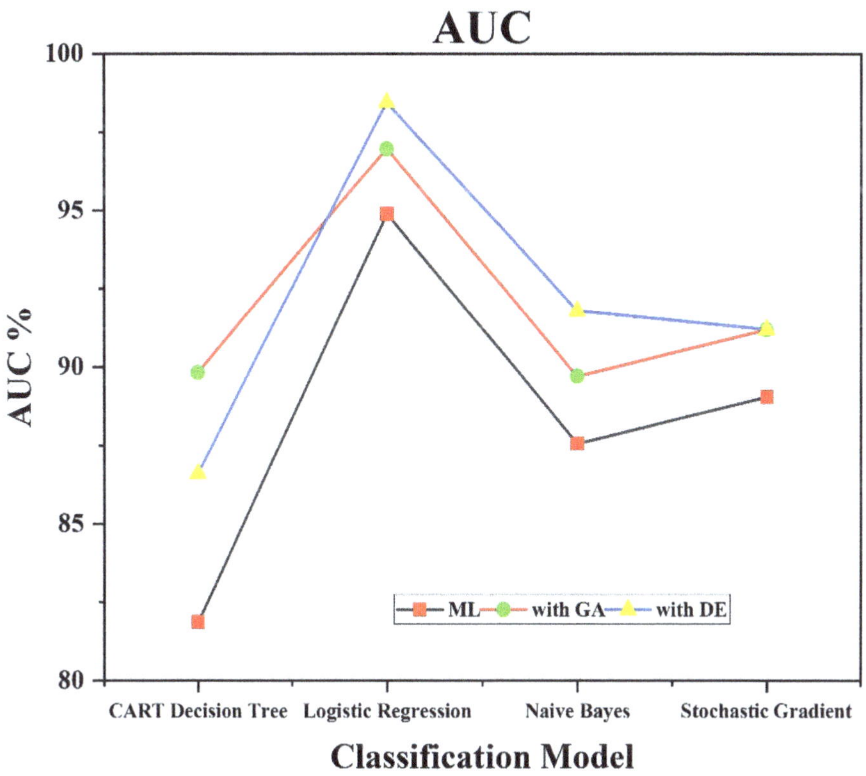

FIGURE 4.6 (Continued)

4.5 ETHICS STATEMENT

SRM Medical College Hospital and Research Centre in India provided ethical clearances. SRMIEC-ST0922-197 is the Ethics Clearance Number. For the purpose of participating in this study, the patients/participants gave their written informed consent.

REFERENCES

[1] M. R. Ahmed, Y. Zhang, Z. Feng, B. Lo, O. T. Inan and H. Liao, "Neuroimaging and Machine Learning for Dementia Diagnosis: Recent Advancements and Future Prospects," in *IEEE Review Biomedical Engineering*, vol. 12, pp. 19–33, 2019, doi: 10.1109/RBME.2018.2886237

[2] A. F. J. Geraets and A. K. Leist, "Sex/Gender and Socioeconomic Differences in Modifiable Risk Factors for Dementia," in *Science Report,* vol. 13, p. 80, 2023, doi: 10.1038/s41598-022-27368-4

[3] G. Tsang, S. -M. Zhou and X. Xie, "Modeling Large Sparse Data for Feature Selection: Hospital Admission Predictions of the Dementia Patients Using Primary Care Electronic Health Records," in *IEEE Journal of Translational Engineering*

in Health and Medicine, vol. 9, pp. 1–13, 2021, Art no. 3000113, doi: 10.1109/JTEHM.2020.3040236

[4] C. P. C. Kwok et al. "Dementia and Risk of Visual Impairment in Chinese Older Adults," in *Science Report*, vol. 12, pp. 18033, 2022, doi: 10.1038/s41598-022-22785-x

[5] C. -S. Son, W. -S. Kang, J. -H. Lee and K. J. Moon, "Machine Learning to Identify Psychomotor Behaviors of Delirium for Patients in Long-Term Care Facility," in *IEEE Journal of Biomedical and Health Informatics*, vol. 26, no. 4, pp. 1802–1814, April 2022, doi: 10.1109/JBHI.2021.3116967

[6] J. W. Błaszczyk, "Pathogenesis of Dementia," in *International Journal of Molecular Sciences,* vol. 24, no. 1, p. 543, doi: 10.3390/ijms24010543

[7] K. Nishikawa, K. Akihiro, R. Hirakawa, H. Kawano, Y. Nakatoh, "Machine Learning Model for Discrimination of Mild Dementia Patients Using Acoustic Features," in *Cognitive Robotics*, vol. 2, pp. 21–29, 2022, ISSN 2667-2413, doi: 10.1016/j.cogr.2021.12.003

[8] C. Chalmers, P. Fergus, C. A. C. Montanez, S. Sikdar, F. Ball and B. Kendall, "Detecting Activities of Daily Living and Routine Behaviours in Dementia Patients Living Alone Using Smart Meter Load Disaggregation," in *IEEE Transactions on Emerging Topics in Computing*, vol. 10, no. 1, pp. 157–169, 1 Jan.-March 2022, doi: 10.1109/TETC.2020.2993177

[9] Y. X., Teoh, K. W. Lai, J. Usman, S. L. Goh, H. Mohafez, K. Hasikin, P. Qian, Y. Jiang, Y. Zhang and S. Dhanalakshmi, "Discovering Knee Osteoarthritis Imaging Features for Diagnosis and Prognosis: Review of Manual Imaging Grading and Machine Learning Approaches," in *Journal of Healthcare Engineering*, vol. 2022, pp. 1 -9, 2022.

[10] G. Bivona, M. Iemmolo, L. Agnello, B. L. Sasso, C. M. Gambino, R. V. Giglio, C. Scazzone, G. Ghersi and M. Ciaccio, "Microglial Activation and Priming in Alzheimer's Disease: State of the Art and Future Perspectives," in *International Journal of Molecular Sciences*, vol. 24, no. 1, p. 884, 2023, doi: 10.3390/ijms24010884

[11] S.-Y. Chien, S. –F. Chao, Y. Kang, C. Hsu, M.-H. Yu and C.-T. Ku, "Understanding Predictive Factors of Dementia for Older Adults: A Machine Learning Approach for Modeling Dementia Influencers, in *International Journal of Human-Computer Studies*, vol. 165, p. 102834, 2022, ISSN 1071-5819, doi: 10.1016/j.ijhcs.2022.102834

[12] N. McCombe et al., "Practical Strategies for Extreme Missing Data Imputation in Dementia Diagnosis," in *IEEE Journal of Biomedical and Health Informatics*, vol. 26, no. 2, pp. 818–827, Feb. 2022, doi: 10.1109/JBHI.2021.3098511

[13] F. Zhu et al., "Analyze Informant-Based Questionnaire for The Early Diagnosis of Senile Dementia Using Deep Learning," in *IEEE Journal of Translational Engineering in Health and Medicine*, vol. 8, pp. 1–6, 2020, Art no. 2200106, doi: 10.1109/JTEHM.2019.2959331

[14] P. S. Q. Yeoh et al., "Emergence of Deep Learning in Knee Osteoarthritis Diagnosis," in *Computational Intelligence and Neuroscience*, vol. 2021, 2021.

[15] G. Tsang, S. -M. Zhou and X. Xie, "Modeling Large Sparse Data for Feature Selection: Hospital Admission Predictions of the Dementia Patients Using Primary Care Electronic Health Records," in *IEEE Journal of Translational Engineering in Health and Medicine*, vol. 9, pp. 1–13, 2021, Art no. 3000113, doi: 10.1109/JTEHM.2020.3040236

[16] G. Tsang, X. Xie and S. -M. Zhou, "Harnessing the Power of Machine Learning in Dementia Informatics Research: Issues, Opportunities, and Challenges," in *IEEE*

Reviews in Biomedical Engineering, vol. 13, pp. 113–129, 2020, doi: 10.1109/RBME.2019.2904488

[17] C. Wang, J. Xu, S. Zhao and W. Lou, "Identification of Early Vascular Dementia Patients With EEG Signal," in *IEEE Access*, vol. 7, pp. 68618–68627, 2019, doi: 10.1109/ACCESS.2019.2918251

[18] R. G. de Souza et al., "Computer-Aided Diagnosis of Alzheimer's Disease by MRI Analysis and Evolutionary Computing," in *Research Biomedical Engineering*, vol. 37, pp. 455–483, 2021, doi: 10.1007/s42600-021-00160-5

[19] G. Battineni, F. Amenta and N. Chintalapudi, "Data for: Machine Learning in Medicine: Classification and Prediction of Dementia by Support Vector Machines (SVM)", in *Mendeley Data*, vol. V1, 2019, doi: 10.17632/tsy6rbc5d4.1

[20] P. Durongbhan et al., "A Dementia Classification Framework Using Frequency and Time-Frequency Features Based on EEG Signals," in *IEEE Transactions on Neural Systems and Rehabilitation Engineering*, vol. 27, no. 5, pp. 826–835, May 2019, doi: 10.1109/TNSRE.2019.2909100

[21] S. Sargolzaei et al., "A Practical Guideline for Intracranial Volume Estimation in Patients with Alzheimer's Disease," in *BMC Bioinformatics*, vol. 16, no. Suppl 7, p. S8, 2015, doi: 10.1186/1471-2105-16-S7-S8. Epub 2015 Apr 23. PMID: 25953026; PMCID: PMC4423585.

[22] M. Seera and C. P. Lim, "Online Motor Fault Detection and Diagnosis Using a Hybrid FMM-CART Model," in *IEEE Transactions on Neural Networks and Learning Systems*, vol. 25, no. 4, pp. 806–812, Apr. 2014, doi: 10.1109/TNNLS.2013.2280280

[23] N. Steinauer, K. Zhang, C. Guo and J. Zhang, "Computational Modeling of Gene-Specific Transcriptional Repression, Activation and Chromatin Interactions in Leukemogenesis by LASSO-Regularized Logistic Regression," in *IEEE/ACM Transactions on Computational Biology and Bioinformatics*, vol. 18, no. 6, pp. 2109–2122, 1 Nov.-Dec. 2021, doi: 10.1109/TCBB.2021.3078128

[24] S. Latha, P. Muthu, K. W. Lai, A. Khalil and S. Dhanalakshmi. "Performance Analysis of Machine Learning and Deep Learning Architectures on Early Stroke Detection Using Carotid Artery Ultrasound Images," in *Frontiers in Aging Neuroscience*, vol. 13, p. 828214, 27 Jan. 2022, doi: 10.3389/fnagi.2021.828214. PMID: 35153728; PMCID: PMC8830903.

[25] X. Fang, "Inference-Based Naïve Bayes: Turning Naïve Bayes Cost-Sensitive," in *IEEE Transactions on Knowledge and Data Engineering*, vol. 25, no. 10, pp. 2302–2313, Oct. 2013, doi: 10.1109/TKDE.2012.196

[26] A. Byerly and T. Kalganova, "Homogeneous Vector Capsules Enable Adaptive Gradient Descent in Convolutional Neural Networks," in *IEEE Access*, vol. 9, pp. 48519–48530, 2021, doi: 10.1109/ACCESS.2021.3066842.

[27] S. Katoch, S. S. Chauhan and V. Kumar, "A Review on Genetic Algorithm: Past, present, and future," in *Multimedia Tools Applications*, vol. 80, pp. 8091–8126, 2021, doi: 10.1007/s11042-020-10139-6

[28] S. Latha, D. Samiappan, P. Muthu and R. Kumar. "Fully Automated Integrated Segmentation of Carotid Artery Ultrasound Images Using DBSCAN and Affinity Propagation," in *Journal of Medical and Biological Engineering*, vol. 41, no. 2, pp. 260–271, 2021.

[29] R. Storn and K. Price, "Differential Evolution-A Simple and Efficient Heuristic for Global Optimization Over Continuous Spaces," *Journal of Global Optimization*, vol. 11, pp. 341–359, 1997.

[30] Z. Stokes, A. Mandal and W. K. Wong, "Using Differential Evolution to Design Optimal Experiments," *Chemometr Intelligent Lab System,* vol. 199, p. 103955, 15 Apr. 2020.

[31] S. Latha and D. Samiappan, "Despeckling of Carotid Artery Ultrasound Images with a Calculus Approach," *Current Medical Imaging*, vol. 15, no. 4, pp. 414–426, 2019.

5 Exploring Deep Learning Models in Medical Image Analysis for Human Disease Detection and Classification

Nithyakalyani Krishnan and P. Muthu

5.1 INTRODUCTION

Deep learning (DL) is a novel research field that endeavors to bring machine learning (ML) closer to the human mind. To learn the target distribution, DL approaches necessitate an immense quantity of data. They have the potential to identify patterns of specific medical conditions at a faster pace than a clinician [1]. A wide range of artificial intelligence (AI)-based algorithms can be integrated into the DL platform to improve data analysis, diagnosis, and the simplification of complex data analysis [2]. There are various steps involved in each DL model, as depicted in Figure 5.1. To build a successful DL model, the first and most significant step is to define the network and architecture. Depending on the task to be completed, certain types of architecture are preferred. In DL, the compilation step involves configuring the model in order to complete the fitting/training process. Several of the important components of the evaluation procedure are defined during compilation. Fitting the model to the training dataset is the subsequent logical step after establishing the general architecture and constructing the model. A fit function is employed to train the model over a predetermined number of epochs.

The assessment of DL models is an essential phase in determining whether the expected results have been accomplished. During the pre-processing stage, the test data are split into multiple groups. It is crucial to consider the predictions on those groups when evaluating the efficiency of the model. The deployment phase is the last step in the model construction process. Although this is an optional step, deploying the model allows it to have great scope.

DOI: 10.1201/9781003484233-5

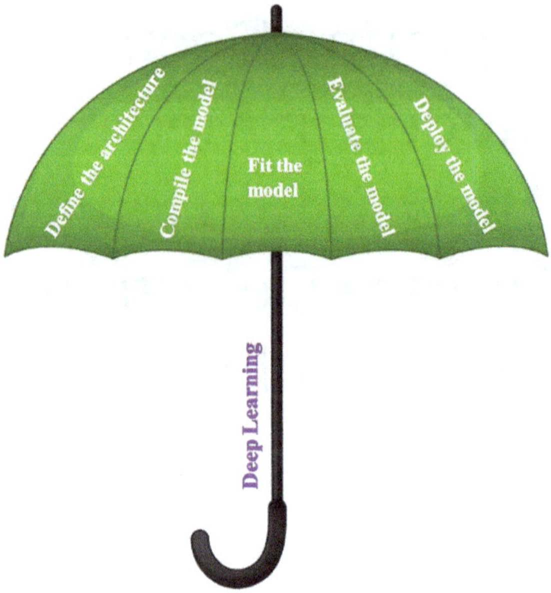

FIGURE 5.1 Illustration of the steps involved in a DL model.

5.2 DEEP LEARNING APPLICATIONS IN THE MEDICAL FIELD

5.2.1 Brain Image Analysis

Brain imaging techniques can be used to detect swelling and hemorrhage, and identify the effects of a stroke. Abnormal cell growth causes tumors in the brain. A brain tumor is a potentially lethal medical condition that, if not treated, can result in death [3]. As a result, estimating the size of the tumor early is critical for optimal treatment planning. Tumors are one of the most lethal malignancies in people of any age, and grading them is difficult for radiologists in health monitoring and automated diagnosis [4]. In an automated method for the detection of brain tumors, Hollon et al. integrated deep convolutional neural networks (DCNNs) and stimulated Raman histology (SRH) [5]. Computer-aided diagnosis (CAD) for medical applications presents a challenging task for brain tumor classification. Deepak et al. investigated a study on a three-class classification issue to differentiate between three forms of brain cancer: gliomas, meningiomas, and pituitary tumors. For feature recognition in images, deep transfer learning and a GoogLeNet that had already been trained were used. The features obtained were then categorized using verified classifier models [6]. Arshia et al. employed three convolutional neural network (CNN) architectures, namely AlexNet, GoogLeNet, and VGGNet, to categorize brain tumors [7]. Jyostna et al. introduced a more generalizable deep neural network (DNN) architecture for classifying tumors. Inception Net v2 and Xception networks were used to extract local feature representations, which were vectorized with proposed pooling-based techniques. In order to differentiate between tumor and non-tumor regions in the

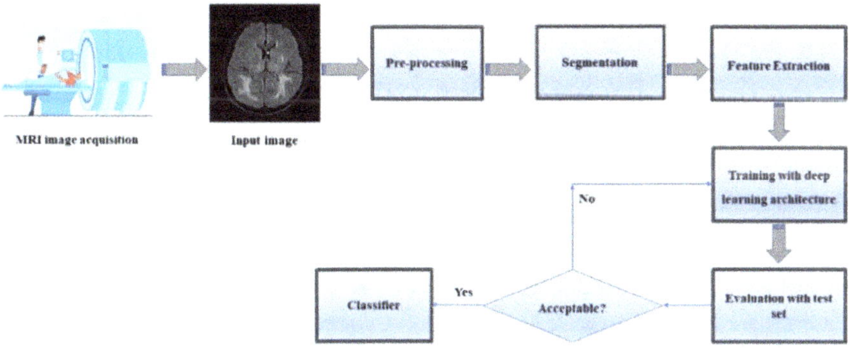

FIGURE 5.2 Generalized block diagram of brain disease detection based on MRI images using a DL model.

images, the approach is to prioritize the analysis of tumor areas while minimizing the focus on non-tumor areas [8].

Computed tomography (CT) and magnetic resonance imaging (MRI) are the predominant imaging modalities employed for the detection of brain abnormalities. Doctors prefer MRI due to the greater detail that can be observed [9]. The precise segmentation of the structures of interest is necessary for the quantitative analysis of brain MRI. The most widely used brain MRI segmentation techniques are DL-based, and it is becoming increasingly apparent that DL architectures outperform existing ML methods due to their capacity to learn and specialize over enormous amounts of data [10]. DL models are used to diagnose brain tumors by using MRI images as a result of the growth of AI. Based on MRI images, Figure 5.2 illustrates how DL techniques can be used to diagnose brain diseases. According to Gokay et al., CNN is used to segment brain tumors within three-dimensional (3D) brain tumor segmentation image sets. In semantic segmentation, MRI brain images are labeled according to their class. DL networks identify every pixel in an image for semantic segmentation [11]. Table 5.1 summarizes the datatype, detection modality, dataset, and network architecture that was used by previous researchers for brain image analysis. Figure 5.3 represents the block diagram of a brain tumor classification system.

5.2.2 Breast Cancer Detection

Breast cancer is a medical complication for which asymptomatic women undergo routine examinations to detect cancer before it becomes clinically apparent [10]. DL models such as CNN can be used to evaluate thermograms obtained by thermography. Breast thermograms can be automatically classified as normal or abnormal using CNNs. Roslidar et al. investigated the characteristics of breast thermograms and the differences between thermographic patterns in normal and malignant cases [14]. Breast cancer classification using sequential steps in image processing is shown in Figure 5.4. In a research study based on breast cancer detection, the Xception and Inception v3 models in combination attained mean accuracy of 97.5% among

TABLE 5.1
Summary of the datatype, detection modality, dataset, and network architecture employed for brain image analysis

Author	Datatype	Modality	Dataset	Network architecture	Results
Arshia et al. [7]	Brain MRI slices	MRI	Figshare	AlexNet, GoogLeNet and VGGNet	Among the three architectures involved in the study, the VGG16 model achieved the highest accuracy of 98.6% in terms of detection and classification.
Jyostna et al. [8]	Brain MRI images	MRI	Figshare and BraTS 2018	Xception and Inception ResNet v2 (IRV2)	This model attained a classification accuracy of 93.69%, surpassing the performance of the previous models.
Zeynettin et al. [10]	Brain MRI images	MRI	ImageNet	AlexNet	An extensive analysis was carried out to compare nine different classification algorithms for the segmentation of ischemic stroke lesions. The findings demonstrated that the combination of cascaded CNN and random decision forest approaches surpassed all other methods in terms of performance.
Gokay et al. [11]	Brain MRI images	MRI	BraTS	DCNN	Semantic segmentation method was implemented and their results were executed by a DL network for tumor prediction. The mean prediction ratio was 91.71 and mean IoU was 86.94.
Lu Li et al. [12]	Brain CT images	CT	Single comprehensive stroke center dataset and a benchmark dataset	U-Net	The U-Net model achieved performance with the highest location accuracy of 98.5% for detection and a Dice score of 0.8033.

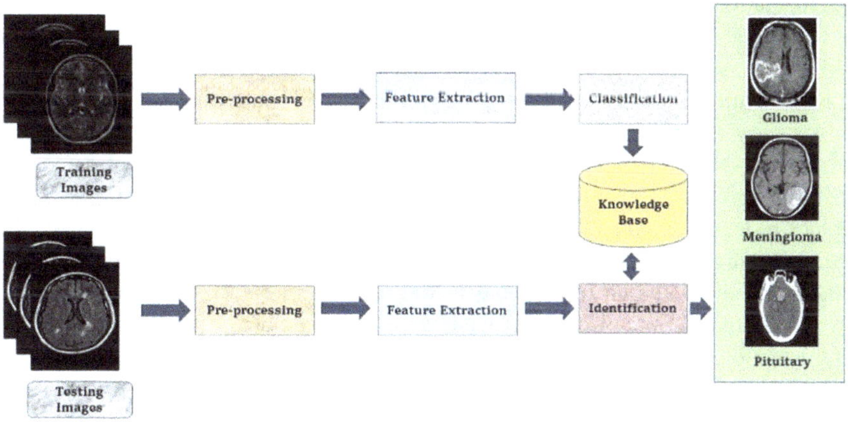

FIGURE 5.3 Representation of a brain tumor classification system.

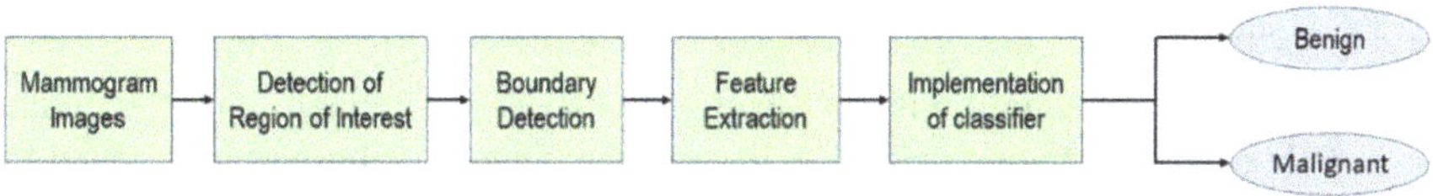

FIGURE 5.4 Block diagram for the classification of breast cancer in mammogram images.

multiple combinations of ensemble architectures using various pre-trained models. Based on the BreakHis dataset, several performance measures showed that the models outperformed existing advanced methods [15]. Umit et al. demonstrated that the diagnosis of breast cancer can be accomplished through the implementation of bidirectional long short-term memory (Bi-LSTM) and fully convolutional networks (FCN). FCN is implemented as an encoder to extract high-level features. The flattened layer is used to feed the FCN output to Bi-LSTM, which is then transformed into a one-dimensional sequence [16]. A DL approach was devised by Li Shen et al. that accurately identified cancer on screening mammograms. The approach was conducted using an end-to-end training dataset that included either full clinical annotation or partial clinical annotation [17]. VGG16 and AlexNet models were examined, with AlexNet being implemented for fine-tuning and the acquired features being classified using support vector machines (SVMs). In order to assess performance, a comprehensive series of tests was implemented on a histopathologic breast cancer dataset. The evaluation revealed that transfer learning outperformed SVM classification and deep feature extraction [18].

SanaUllah et al. developed a framework for the classification of breast cancer using cytology images and DL. Three distinct DL architectures, namely ResNet, VGGNet, and GoogLeNet, have been explored [19]. Yasin et al. investigated different methods, solutions, and data analysis methods for the automated detection of BC using histopathological images by implementing DCNN [20]. William et al. demonstrated the implementation of DL to identify cancer in cancer patients, surpassing five out of five full-time breast imaging specialists, with an average improvement in sensitivity of 14% [21]. An ensemble-based learning model was implemented by Abishek et al. for classification purposes. The proposed stacked ensemble obtained a classification accuracy rate of 98.08%, demonstrating the approach benefits, despite the fact that three CNNs were employed for training [22]. In recent years, object detection, speech recognition, and image recognition have all been greatly improved by the graphics processing unit (GPU) and DL. Researchers have found that CNNs are the most promising DL model for cancer diagnosis [23]. Meha et al. conducted an investigation into the potential of artificial neural networks (ANN), multi-layer perceptron neural organization (MLP), and CNN to differentiate breast malignancies for the early detection of breast cancer. The objective was to ascertain which technique is more effective for the analysis of breast cell malignancies [24]. Table 5.2 represents a brief summary of existing studies conducted on breast cancer detection and classification, and Table 5.3 represents the image dataset, segmentation, and classification techniques used by different researchers and their performance results based on DL.

5.2.3 Cardiovascular Imaging

DL-based image segmentation is now well-established as a reliable image segmentation method. A robust approach for main vascular segmentation was introduced by Su Yang et al. through the use of DL models with FCN. X-ray coronary angiography may reliably detect and segment major vessels using DL networks. The methodology for prediction could be implemented in real time with minimal image pre-processing [30]. Chest radiography (CXR) is a frequently employed thoracic imaging technique that is used to diagnose, treat, and identify a diverse array of cardiothoracic diseases. Nabulsi et al. developed a DL system (DLS) that differentiates between normal and abnormal CXRs by utilizing data that comprised a diverse array of CXR abnormalities [31]. The DL model was initially trained to identify anomalies in chest X-ray images using the ResNet-101 CNN architecture by Mohd et al., and subsequently retrained to identify characteristics from one million X-ray images [32]. Fabian et al. created nnU-Net, a DL technique for segmentation that can adapt its configuration dependent on the specific task. This includes modifying pre-processing, network design, training, and post-processing [33]. The aortic diameter was used to diagnose an ascending thoracic aortic aneurysm (ATAA). Using U-Net, ENet, and ERFNet approaches, the sustainability and effectiveness of DL for the automatic segmentation of ATAAs were evaluated. Clinically, DL for autonomous vascular segmentation can assist with patient treatment based on their individual risk profiles, as well as ATAA diagnosis [34]. Xiuquan et al. created an innovative comprehensive DL framework to simultaneously segment and visualize the left atrium [35]. The automatic segmentation of coronary arteries is essential in evaluating patients with coronary heart disease using coronary CT angiography (CCTA) images. Fangzheng et al. proposed a novel framework for segmenting CCTA images, which combines DL with digital image processing techniques [36].

TABLE 5.2
Summary of studies conducted with breast imaging

Author	Year	Modality	Region of interest	Inference
Jun Bai et al. [13]	2021	Digital breast tomosynthesis (DBT)	Breast	The automated detection of breast cancer was done using DBT. Utilizing DBT, it was possible to classify benign and malignant lesions.
Li Shen et al. [17]	2019	X-ray	Breast	Using automatic DL training methods, high accuracy was achieved on heterogeneous mammography platforms. These findings improved clinical tools, reducing false positives and false negatives in screening mammography.
Erkan et al. [18]	2018	Histopathological images	Breast	Transfer learning and deep feature extraction were evaluated for the purpose of detecting breast cancer using histopathological images.
Umit et al. [16]	2019	Histopathological images	Breast	An FCN and Bi-LSTM-based CNN model was recommended as a means of enhancing the efficacy of breast cancer diagnosis.
SanaUllah et al. [19]	2019	Cytology images	Breast	Based on deep transfer learning, a novel framework was suggested. Three potential CNN architectures were employed to derive features from breast cytology images. The proposed framework achieved an accuracy of 97.52%, while the GoogLeNet, VGGNet, and ResNet architectures achieved an average classification accuracy of 93.5%, 94.15%, and 94.35%, respectively.
Yasin et al. [20]	2020	Histopathological images	Breast	A robust transfer learning architecture was developed combining a fully connected classifier and previously trained DenseNet121 and ResNet-50 models. The suggested system was able to achieve up to 98% accuracy in multiclass classification and up to 100% accuracy in binary classification.

TABLE 5.3
Representation of the dataset, segmentation technique, and classification model used in different studies, along with their results

Author	Image dataset	Segmentation technique	Classification model	Results
Jitendra et al. [15]	BreakHis	Not specified	Xception, Inception v3, ResNetXt101, Inception ResNet v2 and DenseNet121	Xception, Inception v3, ResNetXt101, Inception ResNet v2, and DenseNet121 attained accuracies of 92.17%, 91.75%, 90.43%, 90.45%, and 89.13%. It was inferred that Xception and Inception v3 achieved the highest accuracy compared to Inception ResNet v2.
Umit et al. [16]	BreakHis and CIFAR-10	Not specified	FCN and Bi-LSTM	The AlexNet model was employed to evaluate the efficacy of breast cancer detection. The proposed approach performed better than all the training folds.
Maqsood et al. [25]	STARE, DRIVE, MESSIDOR, and DIARETDB1	Otsu thresholding	Not Specified	The Otsu thresholding segmentation method achieved accuracies of 95.45%, 97.88%, 99.20%, and 97.86% on different datasets.
Gaurav et al. [26]	APTOS	Not specified	DRISTI	The DRISTI model achieved an overall validation accuracy of 82% and a testing accuracy of 75.8% for five-class classification, and a validation accuracy of 96.2% and a testing accuracy of 95.5% for two-class classification.
Amita et al. [27]	Not specified	Gaussian mixture model (GMM)	DNN	The DNN classifier yielded the highest accuracy of 99.38% during the automated detection procedure, with minimal validation loss.

TABLE 5.3 (Continued)
Representation of the dataset, segmentation technique, and classification model used in different studies, along with their results

Author	Image dataset	Segmentation technique	Classification model	Results
Mingyu et al. [28]	Genomic Data Commons	Not specified	Inception v3	Inception v3 model was evaluated and achieved 96% accuracy.
Ramar et al. [29]	IITD-II Ear and AMI ear dataset	Not specified	DCNN	The DCNN model achieved a recognition rate of 97.36% and 96.99% for the applied two different datasets.

5.2.4 Eye Disease Detection

The most common cause of significant vision impairment is age-related macular degeneration (AMD). To identify individuals with AMD according to their disease condition, several classification schemes have been developed. Color fundus images were pre-processed in the first phase. They were then utilized to train several CNNs independently in the second step. A random forest algorithm was trained in the third phase to create an ensemble model based on the outcomes of the single CNNs [37]. DL was used to differentiate between healthy and pathological retinal fundus images and performance was additionally enhanced by using approaches for optimization, contrast amplification, and fine-tuning [38].

5.2.5 Skin Disease Detection

Michal et al. introduced a prototype to assess the proficiency of algorithms designed for lesion recognition and segmentation. Detection systems involving DL and traditional methods such as local brightness distribution and correlation were examined. The detection sensitivity and precision for the fusion of algorithms were 0.95 and 0.94, respectively. It was confirmed that the parameters analyzed were extremely accurate, especially for lesions over 3 mm in diameter which are the most likely to be malignant in nature [39]. Fawaz et al. devised a framework that combined DL and ML methods. In dermoscopic images, the active contour approach was applied for lesion segmentation. The textural properties of skin lesions were extracted using a hybrid feature extraction approach, namely utilizing the local binary pattern (LBP) and gray level co-occurrence matrix (GLCM). An ANN algorithm was used to process the features obtained. For accurate skin disease classification in the second system, CNN was applied and pre-trained from AlexNet and ResNet-50. According to the results of the studies, the suggested approach beat cutting-edge algorithms on the HP2 and ISIC 2018 datasets. Compared to the CNN model, the ANN model was the most accurate for PH2 (97.50%) and ISIC 2018 (98.35%) [40]. Marriam et al. created an automated system for early-stage skin melanoma segmentation using faster region-based recurrent CNN (RCNN) and fuzzy *k*-means clustering (FKM). Prior to utilizing the faster-RCNN for constructing a fixed-length feature vector, the images in the dataset required pre-processing to remove any noise and address illumination problems [41].

Ameri et al. developed a DCNN model for the purpose of detecting skin cancer using images of skin lesions to classify them into benign and malignant groups. The pre-trained model used was AlexNet and a transfer learning technique was employed. In this approach, raw images are taken as input and useful properties are extracted from them to enable automatic identification. Sensitivity and specificity can be modified by the user by altering the confidence threshold. The results indicated that DL has significant potential for the detection of both melanoma and non-melanoma skin cancer. The utilization of this technique by dermatologists can facilitate the diagnosis of skin cancer [42]. A fusion of the GrabCut method and adaptive neuro-fuzzy classifier (ANFC) model was developed and the pre-processing step was carried out using an inpainting approach and top hat filter. The filtered images were then segmented using the GrabCut method. A DL-based Inception model was then used to carry out the feature extraction process and finally classified into several classes using an ANFC technique [43].

5.2.6 Detection of Spinal Conditions

The implementation of DL techniques has become a recent advanced technique used for the detection of spinal disorders with MRI images. Figure 5.5 describes the workflow of a CNN-based DL technique employed for the detection of spinal conditions. Zamir et al. created and validated a DL technique to assess cervical spinal cord compression using MRI data. To build a DCNN and test it on the holdout dataset, they

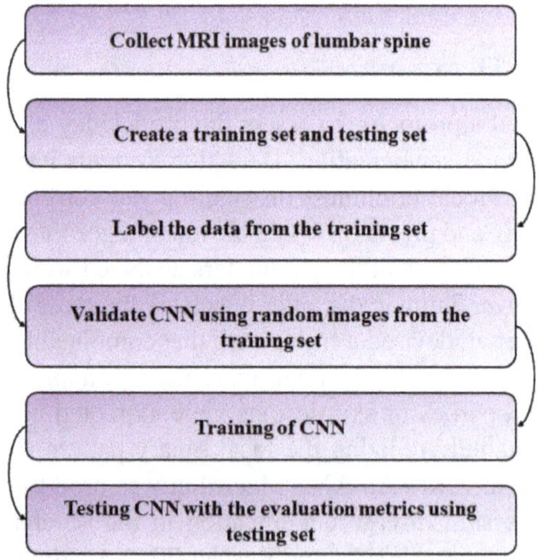

FIGURE 5.5 Representation of the workflow used for training and testing a CNN employed for the detection of spinal disorders.

used images from the training/validation dataset. With this model, cervical spine MRI image interpretation may be done more quickly and objectively [44]. Muscle fat infiltration (MFI) was reported in a variety of cervical spine conditions. It was difficult to identify an axial lumbar disc herniation because of limitations such as a complex background, noise, and blurry images. The most significant tasks in computer-assisted herniation diagnosis are disc segmentation and localization. Wafa et al. established a DCNN-based automatic system. This network analyzed the input MRI at different scales of context before combining the high-level features to improve the capacity of the system to locate the discs in the lumbar spine. The herniation was localized and detailed using the U-Net architecture [45]. MFI quantification necessitates time-consuming manual segmentation approaches that are rater-dependent. Seven cervical spine muscle groups were segmented using a CNN model trained in 100,000 iterations and the trained CNN model accuracy and reliability were assessed using an independent testing dataset [46].

5.2.7 Detection of Liver Diseases

Manually identifying cancer tissue is challenging and time-consuming. In order to make sure that patients are detected and treated effectively, CAD has been employed in the decision-making process. An investigation by Koichiro et al. examined the feasibility of classifying liver fibrosis stages using dynamic contrast-enhanced CT images and observed that DL models based on enhanced CT images contained a moderate level of accuracy for staging liver fibrosis [47]. Schmauch et al. proposed an DL algorithm that simultaneously detects and analyzes focal liver lesions (FLL). Three tasks were assessed, including lesion detection, malignancy determination, and lesion classification [48]. Figure 5.6 illustrates the different stages of liver disease leading to cirrhosis. Charlie et al. utilized multi-phasic MRI to create and verify a CNN-based DLS for identifying common liver pathologies. The DLS was proven to have 92% accuracy, 92% sensitivity, and 98% specificity. On average, the computation time for each lesion was 5.6 milliseconds [49]. By using segmented surfaces, Xi Fang et al. constructed a DL-based method for liver segmentation to help guide needle placement for finding and treating liver cancers. This segmentation method had a dice score of 96.1%. A set of images taken for the treatment of liver tumors was then merged using the surface-based image fusion technique [50].

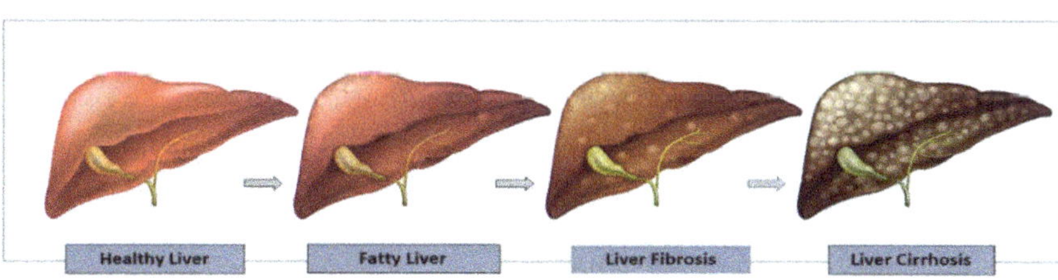

FIGURE 5.6 Diagrammatic representation illustrating the progression of different liver diseases.

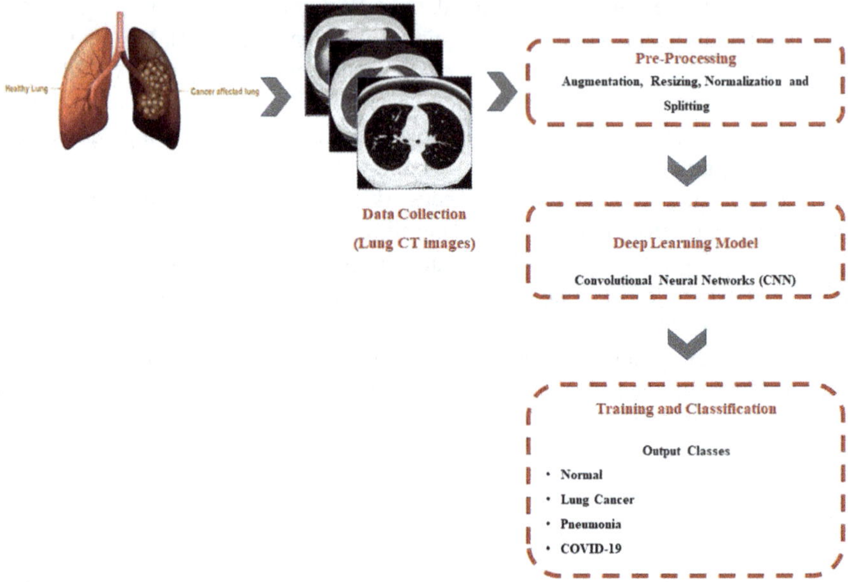

FIGURE 5.7 Process flow of a multi-class classification DL model based on CT lung images.

5.2.8 Lung Cancer Detection

Lung cancer must be diagnosed as early as feasible in order to improve patient survival rates. Using CT scans, the level of cancer and the location of tumors were determined. Figure 5.7 illustrates the process flow of a multi-class classification model based on CT lung images using DL. Linear discriminant analysis (LDA) and optimal DNNs (ODNNs) were used to analyze the lung CT data. A modified gravitational search algorithm was used to train the ODNN. This classifier achieved 95.26% sensitivity, 96.2% specificity, and 96.2% accuracy [51]. Malignant nodules can be classified using DL and the Early Lung Cancer Diagnosis using AI and Big Data (LUCINDA) study used lung nodules seen on thoracic CT scans to validate lung cancer prediction CNN (LCP-CNN) software [52]. According to Shreyesh et al., three popular DL architectures were compared, that is, ANN, CNN, and RNN, whereas traditional ML models were ignored. In both classification and regression, DL models outperformed traditional ML models [53]. Normal, viral pneumonia, and COVID-19 chest X-ray images are illustrated in Figure 5.8. A brief review of journals with their application and inference is summarized in Table 5.4.

5.2.9 Obesity Prediction

Obesity in children is a severe public health issue. The intervention procedure can be more effective in preventing and controlling childhood obesity if children who are at an elevated risk of acquiring the condition are identified early. Existing childhood

TABLE 5.4
A brief review of applications and inference from the various referred journals

Author	Application	Inference
Hollon et al. [5]	Brain tumor detection	The use of CNN for diagnosing SRH pictures was found to be more effective than the pathologist-based interpretation of conventional histologic images, with an overall accuracy of 94.6% compared to 93.9%.
Deepak et al. [6]	Brain tumor classification	Brain MRI scans were classified using a multi-class SVM with an error-correcting output code (ECOC) model. This model achieved a mean classification accuracy of 98%, surpassing all other methods.
Hyunkwang et al. [54]	Detection and classification of acute intra-cranial haemorrhage	The classifier achieved a performance of 98% sensitivity and 95% specificity for 200 cases, and 92% sensitivity and 95% specificity for 196 cases.
Umit at al. [15]	Breast cancer detection	For breast cancer detection, a pre-trained AlexNet model was employed. The Adam optimizer, an adaptive learning rate optimization technique, was used for training the model.
Sang et al. [55]	Glaucoma detection	The AUC of DCNN was approximately 0.1 higher in glaucoma-confirmed eyes than in glaucoma-suspected eyes. The AUC was diminished by 0.1 to 0.2 as a result of the inclusion of low-quality images in the analysis, which influenced the discriminative ability.
Rubina et al. [38]	Detection of diabetic eye diseases	ImageNet used the top two pre-trained CNN models. Several performance-improving approaches were used, including contrast amplification, optimization, and fine-tuning.
Gaurav et al. [26]	Diagnosis of diabetic retinopathy	The five-class training and validation accuracies were 99.21% and 75.50% for large datasets. On augmented APTOS, the accuracies for two-class training and validation were 99.96% and 97.05%. Cross-dataset and mixed dataset testing were implemented to demonstrate the efficacy of DRISTI.
Mohamed et al. [43]	Skin lesion segmentation and classification	GrabCut algorithm and ANFC model were utilized for segmentation.
Amita et al. [27]	Liver cancer detection	Using a DNN classifier over 200 epochs, this method obtained 99.38% accuracy and a 98.18% Jaccard index with a minimal validation loss of 0.062.

(continued)

TABLE 5.4 (Continued)
A brief review of applications and inference from the various referred journals

Author	Application	Inference
Koichiro et al. [47]	Liver fibrosis stages classification	There was a substantial association between the fibrosis score obtained from DL based on CT images (FDLCT score) and the stage of liver fibrosis.
Schmauch et al. [48]	Focal liver lesions diagnosis	For FLL detection and FLL characterisation, the models achieved mean AUC values of 0.93 and 0.91.
Xi Fang et al. [50]	Liver segmentation	The liver segmentation outcomes showed that the segmentation method developed was extremely accurate, with a Dice score of 96.1%.

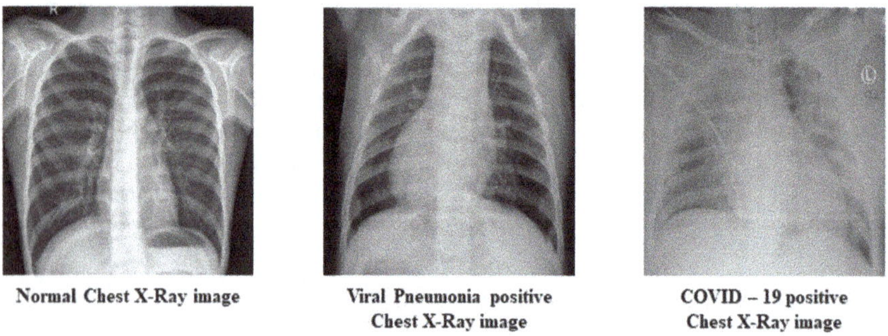

FIGURE 5.8 Representation of different X-ray classification in diagnosing diseases.

obesity prediction mostly relies on classic regression approaches based on a few hand-picked parameters and does not bring longitudinal patterns into account. DL methods, however, allow high-dimensional longitudinal datasets to be analyzed. An algorithm was developed by Mehak et al. to predict future obesity patterns from general information on a child's medical history. In order to build a new model for predicting child obesity patterns using electronic health records (EHR) data, a long short-term memory (LSTM) network and separate feed-forward network were utilized to simulate dynamic and static variables in the data [56]. Rashmi et al. evaluated skin temperature variations in several body locations, that is, the neck, forearm, abdomen, and calves, and also compared three study groups: normal, overweight, and obese. The abdomen and neck portions of the thermograms collected from the four study regions showed the highest temperature variations. Thermal imaging was employed to determine overweight and obesity using a modified pre-trained DL model based on a CNN [57].

5.2.10 Prediction and Classification of Lower Extremity Conditions

The ability of CNNs to detect anomalies in radiographs of the lower extremities was investigated in a study. Pre-training, dataset size, and model architecture were also investigated in order to make recommendations for future DL studies on limb radiographs. Maya et al. collected 93,455 lower extremity radiographs from various regions of the body in a large dataset and classified each one as normal or pathological. A 161-layer pre-trained CNN was able to complete the task of classifying abnormalities with area under the receiver operating characteristic (ROC) curve (AUC) of 0.880, sensitivity of 71.4%, and specificity of 96.1% [58]. Quilin et al. used a CNN DLS for investigating the motion recognition intention of lower limb prosthesis. A CNN model was created in an attempt to reconstruct the motion pattern. DL algorithms can improve the control performance of an intelligent lower limb prosthesis and enable it to operate in a range of motion modes by automatically recognizing and extracting features [59].

5.2.11 Detection of COVID-19

In most cases, CXR and CT imaging techniques have been used to diagnose the extremely infectious coronavirus disease-2019 (COVID-19). However, due to time constraints and significant risks of human error, diagnosing the infection by radiography was extremely difficult. A more automated and accurate method of detecting COVID-19 has been developed with the use of AI algorithms [60]. For COVID-19 classification, DL methods, notably CNN, have gained considerable favor among AI approaches. On the basis of CXR imaging and CT images, Aggarwal et al. reviewed a number of key research publications on DL-based COVID-19 classification [61]. The contrast limited histogram equalization (CLAHE) method was used to improve the quality of CT images. Md. Robiul et al. devised a novel CNN model to extract the features and then applied it to several ML algorithms, which included Gaussian naive Bayes, SVM, decision tree, logistic regression, and random forest [62].

5.3 CHALLENGES AND FUTURE OUTLOOK

This section discusses current issues and potential directions for DL-based research that can be applied to the diagnosis of various diseases. Although DL models have been successful, there are still a few major challenges and drawbacks that need to be addressed in order to effectively identify and classify a number of diseases. The key challenges identified and future directions for the diagnosis and classification of several diseases with DL are discussed as follows.

5.3.1 Brain Tumor Detection

The challenges associated with brain tumor segmentation include location ambiguity, morphological uncertainty, low contrast, annotation bias, and imbalance problems. While DL-based methods for segmenting brain tumors have demonstrated satisfactory performance, there are still problems that need to be resolved. A large portion of the research methods now employed are fully supervised methods that depend on comprehensive datasets and very valuable annotated segmentation masks [63]. Nevertheless, a substantial amount of work is required to generate a segmentation mask that is devoid of annotation bias. Weak, semi-supervised training with fewer labels is expected to constitute the foundation of future brain tumor segmentation techniques [64]. Neural architecture search algorithms can find efficient brain tumor segmentation networks by combining domain knowledge with search methods. There is also the possibility of converting other CNN networks to hybrid techniques, which could lead to greater outcomes with less time complexity [65].

5.3.2 Breast Cancer Detection

Early disease detection and accurate diagnosis can increase the likelihood of successful treatment and reduce the mortality rate. In fact, an early diagnosis can effectively prevent the disease from spreading and help deter premature victims from getting it. Differentiating benign from malignant tumors and drawing conclusions about early-stage versus advanced breast cancer are difficult tasks for research scientists [66]. The most difficult challenge for breast cancer classification is unsupervised learning. Most studies use supervised learning to categorize breast cancer images. Even though models based on supervised learning produce better results, skilled doctors have difficulty obtaining annotated breast images. The majority of breast images are unlabeled in reality. Indeed, unsupervised learning-based models are essential for identifying and classifying breast cancer images. The imbalanced class problem presents a significant challenge in DL models. The majority class may benefit from a bias in the results. The scarcity of balanced datasets is thus another problem that needs to be addressed. Only a few DL models that are currently in use combine imaging data with non-imaging characteristics. It is necessary to create numerous models that combine radiomic properties with image data.

An additional significant issue for DL models is label noise. Throughout the course of the development of the cancer, breast cancer spreads from one area of the breast to another. Due to the possibility of different breast cancer stages in various areas of the same breast tissue, the same image may have several subcategory annotations. These images can make DL more difficult in a multi-classification problem [67]. Developing a strong DL-based CAD tool is impeded by the expensive nature of medical image acquisition. When training DL algorithms using medical images, it is important to include high-quality, patient-specific annotations. Since abnormal cases outnumber normal cases by a large margin, gathering enough abnormal data would be prohibitively expensive. Data collection in clinical settings is determined by the methods and technology available, as well as the patient volume for a certain examination [68]. The advancement of medical research and the transformation of healthcare could greatly be accelerated by AI. The moral, medical-legal, and regulatory challenges presented by this novel technology are its most challenging features [69]. These are particularly significant for stand-alone AI tools that use breast cancer image analysis to make decisions without the need for human intervention. When data accessibility is complicated, providing a medical report demands additional time. Hence, radiologists and oncologists will be able to easily access DL models through an interactive web application in the future [70].

5.3.3 Skin Disease Diagnosis

A number of studies on the diagnosis of skin diseases using DL methods have been proposed and shown encouraging results as DL has advanced in recent years. However, before DL is widely used to diagnose skin diseases in real-world clinical settings, a number of issues need to be addressed. Previous studies on using DL to diagnose skin diseases frequently trained and tested their models on datasets with a small number of images. Even though huge amounts of data on skin diseases can be obtained from websites or medical institutions without any specific diagnostic information, labeling enormous amounts of data on skin diseases requires extensive knowledge and it can be very difficult due to time and financial constraints. It is well understood that training a DNN necessitates a great amount of labeled data. With a limited dataset, the possibility of overfitting is significant. Therefore, to effectively train a DNN for diagnosing skin diseases, it is essential to use larger datasets that have been labeled. DL algorithms have been discovered to be highly responsive to images obtained from many modalities. Consequently, the identification of skin diseases using DL is hindered by the presence of noisy data from several sources [71]. A substantial amount of research in this area is likely to be carried out in the near future considering the increasing trend of using DL methods to diagnose skin diseases. However, as was already mentioned, there are a number of issues that need to be resolved. There are a few possible future directions that can be investigated in order to deal with the challenges. We have provided potential guidelines and directions for future research in the field of computer vision and pattern recognition, as well as the diagnosis of skin diseases, based on information from the literature.

There is recurrently a lack of labeled data when it pertains to skin disease detection. To address this issue, there are various perspectives from which we can look for solutions. A skilled clinician could be employed to manually label data on skin diseases, but this would be very costly and inefficient. There is a great need for a more capable and accurate system for diagnosing skin diseases that can be modified to examine all types of skin lesions. The effectiveness of diagnosis may also be improved by incorporating human knowledge into current DL algorithms. The geometrical features and elevational characteristics of skin lesions offer crucial reference points for skin disease detection. By incorporating these features with deep features, current DL techniques can be made even more effective. It would be especially promising if the handcrafted feature extraction process could be combined with the deep network learning process. DL can be used to help dermatologists deal with the growing number of patients suffering from skin disorders. A DL-based skin disease recognition system should be available for smart devices to assist a larger population in the future, given the increasing popularity of smartphones, laptops, and wearables [72]. Another challenge in using a mobile application is the image quality captured with a smartphone. This is critical for a precise diagnosis due to the similarities and small size of the lesions. Additionally, a stabilizer and a macro lens in front of the smartphone camera in this direction are highly recommended. In terms of software, we could improve the image and remove noise using AI super resolution techniques. Furthermore, after capturing the image, we recommend flipping it to make it parallel to multiple images taken in the vicinity of the lesion [73].

5.3.4 Cardiovascular Medicine

In cardiology, a number of technical issues must be resolved before AI models can be integrated into clinical care pathways, despite the potential of AI. To optimize value and overcome the complexity, variety, and potential disturbance associated with applying algorithms to external patient cohorts, AI algorithms necessitate substantial quantities of precisely labeled training data sets. The curation of such datasets is a challenging task, and data-sharing agreements frequently impede multicentered collaborations [74]. To handle difficult medical imaging challenges, a CNN and autoencoder have been widely used. This is because the nature of these DL approaches allows them to learn important aspects from data and employ them to generate additional layers of abstraction to reach the desired result. Novel deep feature extractors and deep autoencoders can also be developed in DL models to achieve the best outcomes.

5.3.5 Liver Disease Studies

The current success of DL algorithms for image segmentation, localization, classification, and identification tasks coincides with a significant growth in the amount of medical imaging data available. As image data is easier to analyze for physicians, and is relatively structured and labeled, it has become a high priority. ResUNet demonstrated excellent results in the rapid and accurate diagnosis of liver tumors in recent studies. Future studies can explore a novel DL model at an advanced level to enhance the accuracy of tumor localization, reduce the false negative (FN) rate, and improve the intersection over union (IoU) metric [75]. Numerous algorithms were created exclusively for binary classification and do not support the differentiation of cirrhosis aetiologies. The results of this proof-of-concept study must therefore be supported by larger samples of the relevant subgroups in subsequent research in order to expand its applicability. The clinical benefit of expanding the study to include other aetiologies would be greatly increased [76].

5.3.6 Lung Disease Classification

More information about patients is highly imperative, especially in situations such as clinical prediction provided by medical record data and pathology. When working with numerous sorts of data, the complexity of obtaining data on a big scale increases, particularly when dealing with multiple detection modalities. This is substantially more complex because each patient requires linked data from several data types and patient data must be fragmented. Images are stored in one system, while the clinical data are stored in another system. In working on all the hyperparameters associated with the learning process, any changes in values can result in a massive change in the performance of the model. Therefore, DL models perform substantially worse if they cannot optimize hyperparameters. The process of choosing hyperparameters in a DL model is crucial for achieving optimal performance in the classification of lung diseases [77]. These hyperparameters are optimized to produce empirical results. The Bayesian optimization technique will be utilized in subsequent research for automatic hyperparameter optimization [78]. Various pre-processing strategies can be employed to enhance accuracy in lung disease diagnosis. Experimenting with different networks may yield more precise results [79],[80].

5.4 CONCLUSION

DL and ML have achieved great success in the area of healthcare because they handle large and complex datasets with minimal human intervention. It is possible that DL models will not achieve their intended benefits or may even harm patient care if their accuracy, robustness, and reliability are not systematically assessed. Developing useful AI algorithms will be made easier if we address the challenges described above through research and the adoption of processes that measure clinical impact. Hence, DL has always been proved to represent a promising tool in medicine. This review examined several DL frameworks and models. DL was applied to disease detection and classification, and its performance was compared. Diseases such as brain tumors, breast cancer, cardiovascular complications, ocular problems, dermatological conditions, spinal disorders, liver abnormalities, lung cancer, and infectious diseases were diagnosed and classified using computational approaches of DL. According to the statistical findings of this study, the use of CNN in medical image processing will increase in future applications and trends using DL. The use of physiological signals for diagnosis with DL techniques will become more prominent. In conclusion, DL-based hybrid and ensemble methods produce higher accuracy results than single techniques. By integrating two or more approaches at the same time, these methods improve the process, regardless of the dataset type. Therefore, DL and neural networks are becoming increasingly important in medical applications.

REFERENCES

[1] S. A. Ajagbe and M. O. Adigun. Deep learning techniques for detection and prediction of pandemic diseases: A systematic literature review. *Multimedia Tools Applications*, 83, 5893-5927, 2024. https://doi.org/10.1007/s11042-023-15805-z

[2] S. Kayalvizhi, J. K. Kasthuribha and F. K. Jiavana. Deep learning based micro organism recognition and disease prediction on plants and animals. *Neuro Quantology*, 20(5), 741-746, 2022. http://dx.doi.org/10.14704/nq.2022.20.5.NQ22231

[3] A. S. Ansari. Numerical simulation and development of brain tumor segmentation and classification of brain tumor using improved support vector machine. *International Journal of Intelligent Systems and Applications in Engineering*, 11, 35-44, 2023. https://www.ijisae.org/index.php/IJISAE/article/view/2505

[4] S. Saeedi, S. Rezayi, H. Keshavarz, et al. MRI-based brain tumor detection using convolutional deep learning methods and chosen machine learning techniques. *BMC Medical Informatics Decision Making*, 23, 16, 2023. https://doi.org/10.1186/s12911-023-02114-6

[5] T. C. Hollon, B. Pandian, A. R. Adapa, et al. Near real-time intraoperative brain tumor diagnosis using stimulated Raman histology and deep neural networks. *Nature Medicine*, 26, 52-58, 2020. https://doi.org/10.1038/s41591-019-0715-9

[6] S. Deepak and, P. M. Ameer. Brain tumor classification using deep CNN features via transfer learning. *Computers in Biology and Medicine*, 111, 103345, 2019. https://doi.org/10.1016/j.compbiomed.2019.103345

[7] A. Rehman, S. Naz, M. I. Razzak, F. Akram and M. Imran. A deep learning-based framework for automatic brain tumors classification using transfer learning. *Circuits, Systems and Signal Processing*, 39, 757-775, 2019. https://doi.org/10.1007/s00034-019-01246-3

[8] J. D. Bodapati, N. S. Shaik, V. Naralasetti and N. B. Mundukur. Joint training of two-channel deep neural network for brain tumor classification. *Signal, Image and Video Processing*, 15, 753-760, 2020. https://doi.org/10.1007/s11760-020-01793-2

[9] M. S. Majib, M. M. Rahman, T. M. S. Sazzad, N. I. Khan and S. K. Dey. VGG-SCNet: A VGG net-based deep learning framework for brain tumor detection on MRI omages. *IEEE Access*, 9, 116942-116952, 2021. http://dx.doi.org/10.1109/ACCESS.2021.3105874

[10] A. Zeynettin, A. Galimzianova, A. Hoogi, D. L. Rubin and B. J. Erickson. Deep learning for brain MRI segmentation: State of the art and future directions. *Journal of Digital Imaging*, 30, 449-459, 2017. https://doi.org/10.1007/s10278-017-9983-4

[11] G. Karayegen and M. F. Aksahin. Brain tumor prediction on MR images with semantic segmentation by using deep learning network and 3D imaging of tumor region. *Biomedical Signal Processing and Control*, 66, 102458, 2021. https://doi.org/10.1016/j.bspc.2021.102458

[12] L. Li, M. Wei, B. Liu, K. Atchaneeyasakul, F. Zhou, Z. Pan, S. A. Kumar, J. Y. Zhang, Y. Pu, D. S. Liebeskind and F. Scalzo. Deep learning for hemorrhagic lesion detection and segmentation on brain CT images. *IEEE Journal of Biomedical and Health Informatics*, 25, 1646-1659, 2021. https://doi.org/10.1109/jbhi.2020.3028243

[13] J. Bai, R. Posner, T. Wang, C. Yang and S. Nabavi. Applying deep learning in digital breast tomosynthesis for automatic breast cancer detection: A review. *Medical Image Analysis*, 71, 102049, 2021. https://doi.org/10.1016/j.media.2021.102049

[14] R. Roslidar, et al. A review on recent progress in thermal imaging and deep learning approaches for breast cancer detection. *IEEE Access*, 8, 116176-116194, 2020. https://doi.org/10.1109/ACCESS.2020.3004056

[15] J. V. Tembhurne, A. Hazarika and T.Diwan. BrC-MCDLM: breast Cancer detection using Multi Channel deep learning model. *Multimedia Tools and Applications*, 80, 31647–31670, 2021. https://doi.org/10.1007/s11042-021-11199-y

[16] U. Budak, Z. Comert, Z. N. Rashid, A. Şengur and M. Çibuk. Computer-aided diagnosis system combining FCN and Bi-LSTM model for efficient breast cancer detection from histopathological images. *Applied Soft Computing,* 85, 105765, 2019. https://doi.org/10.1016/j.asoc.2019.105765

[17] L. Shen, L. R. Margolies, J. H. Rothstein, et al. Deep learning to improve breast cancer detection on screening mammography. *Sci*ence *Rep*ort, 9, 12495, 2019. https://doi.org/10.1038/s41598-019-48995-4

[18] E. Deniz, A. Şengur, Z. Kadiroglu, Y. Guo, V. Bajaj and U. Budak. Transfer learning based histopathologic image classification for breast cancer detection. *Health Information Science and Systems*, 6, 18, 2018. https://doi.org/10.1007/s13755-018-0057-x

[19] S. U. Khan, I. Naveed, J. Zahoor, I. Ud Din and J. J. P. C Rodrigues. A novel deep learning-based framework for the detection and classification of breast cancer using

transfer learning. *Pattern Recognition Letters*, 125, 1-6, 2019. https://doi.org/10.1016/J.PATREC.2019.03.022

[20] Y. Yari, T. V. Nguyen and H. T. Nguyen. Deep learning applied for histological diagnosis of breast cancer. *IEEE Access*, 8, 162432-162448, 2020. https://doi.org/10.1109/ACCESS.2020.3021557

[21] L. William, R. D., Abdul, H. Bryan, et al. Robust breast cancer detection in mammography and digital breast tomosynthesis using an annotation-efficient deep learning approach. *Nature Medicine*, 27, 244-249, 2021. https://doi.org/10.1038/s41591-020-01174-9

[22] A. Das, M. Narayan Mohanty, P. K. Mallick, P. Tiwari, K. Muhammad and H. Zhu. Breast cancer detection using an ensemble deep learning method. *Biomedical Signal Processing and Control*, 70, 103009, 2021. http://dx.doi.org/10.1016/j.bspc.2021.103009

[23] R. Krithiga and P. Geetha. Breast cancer detection, segmentation and classification on histopathology images analysis: A systematic review. *Archives of Computational Methods in Engineering*, 28, 2607–2619, 2020. https://doi.org/10.1007/s11831-020-09470-w

[24] M. Desai and M. Shah. An anatomization on breast cancer detection and diagnosis employing multi-layer perceptron neural network (MLP) and Convolutional neural network (CNN). *Clinical eHealth*, 4, 1-11, 2021. https://doi.org/10.1016/j.ceh.2020.11.002

[25] S. Maqsood, R. Damasevicius, F. M. Shah and R. Maskeliunas. Detection of macula and recognition of aged-related macular degeneration in retinal fundus images. *Computing and Informatics*, 40, 957-987, 2021. https://doi.org/10.31577/cai_2021_5_957

[26] G. Kumar, S. Chatterjee and C. Chattopadhyay. DRISTI: A hybrid deep neural network for diabetic retinopathy diagnosis. *Signal, Image and Video Processing*, 15, 1679-1686, 2021. https://doi.org/10.1007/s11760-021-01904-7

[27] A. Das, U. R. Acharya, S. S. Panda and S. Sabut. Deep learning-based liver cancer detection using watershed transform and Gaussian mixture model techniques. *Cognitive Systems Research*, 54, 165-175, 2019. https://doi.org/10.1016/j.cogsys.2018.12.009

[28] M. Chen, B. Zhang and W. Topatana. Classification and mutation prediction based on histopathology H&E images in liver cancer using deep learning. *npj Precision Oncology*, 4, 14, 2020. https://doi.org/10.1038/s41698-020-0120-3

[29] R. A. Priyadharshini, S. Arivazhagan and M. Arun. A deep learning approach for person identification using ear biometrics. *Applied Intelligence*, 51, 2161-2172, 2020. https://doi.org/10.1007/s10489-020-01995-8

[30] S. Yang, J. Kweon, J. H. Roh, J. H. Lee, et al. Deep learning segmentation of major vessels in X-ray coronary angiography. *Scientific Reports*, 9, 16897, 2019. https://doi.org/10.1038/s41598-019-53254-7

[31] Z. Nabulsi, A. Sellergren, S. Jamshy, et al. Deep learning for distinguishing normal versus abnormal chest radiographs and generalization to two unseen diseases tuberculosis and COVID-19. *Science Reports*, 11, 15523, 2021. https://doi.org/10.1038/s41598-021-93967-2

[32] M. Z. C. Azemin, R. Hassan, M. I. M. Tamrin and M. A. M. Ali. COVID-19 deep learning prediction model using publicly available radiologist-adjudicated chest X-ray images as training data: Preliminary findings. *International Journal of Biomedical Imaging*, 2020, 8828855, 2020. https://doi.org/10.1155/2020/8828855

[33] F. Isensee, P. F. Jaeger, S. A. A. Kohl, J. Petersen and K. H. Maier-Hein. nnU-Net: A self-configuring method for deep learning-based biomedical image segmentation. *Nature Methods*, 18, 203-211, 2020. https://doi.org/10.1038/s41592-020-01008-z

[34] A. Comelli, N. Dahiya, A. Stefano, V. Benfante, G. Gentile, V. Agnese, G. M. Raffa, M. Pilato, A. Yezzi, G. Petrucci and S. Pasta. Deep learning approach for the segmentation of aneurysmal ascending aorta. *Biomedical Engineering Letters*, 11, 15-24, 2020. https://doi.org/10.1007/s13534-020-00179-0

[35] X. Du, S. Yin, R. Tang, Y. Liu, Y. Song, Y. Zhang, H. Liu and S. Li. Segmentation and visualization of left atrium through a unified deep learning framework. *International Journal of Computer Assisted Radiology and Surgery*, 15, 589-600, 2020. https://doi.org/10.1007/s11548-020-02128-9

[36] F. Tian, Y. Gao, Z. Fang and J. Gu. Automatic coronary artery segmentation algorithm based on deep learning and digital image processing. *Applied Intelligence*, 51, 8881-8895, 2021. https://doi.org/10.1007/s10489-021-02197-6

[37] F. Grassmann, J. Mengelkamp and C. Brandl, et al. A deep learning Algorithm for prediction of age-related eye disease study severity scale for age-related macular degeneration from color fundus photography. *Ophthalmology*, 125, 1410-1420, 2018. https://doi.org/10.1016/j.ophtha.2018.02.037

[38] R. Sarki, K. Ahmed, H. Wang and Y. Zhang. Automated detection of mild and multi-class diabetic eye diseases using deep learning. *Health Information Science and Systems*, 8, 32, 2020. https://doi.org/10.1007/s13755-020-00125-5

[39] M. H. Strzeleck, M. Strakowska, M. Kozlowski, et al. Skin lesion detection algorithms in whole body images. *Sensors (Basel)*, 21, 6639, 2021. https://doi.org/10.3390/s21196639

[40] F. W. Alsaade, T. H. H. Aldhyani and M. H. Al-Adhaileh. Developing a recognition system for diagnosing melanoma skin lesions using artificial intelligence algorithms. *Computer Mathematical Methods Medicine*, 2021, 9998379, 2021. https://doi.org/10.1155/2021/9998379

[41] M. Nawaz, Z. Mehmood, T. Nazir, R. A. Naqvi, A. Rehman, M. Iqbal and T. Saba. Skin cancer detection from dermoscopic images using deep learning and fuzzy k-means clustering. *Microscope Research Technology*, 85, 339-351, 2022. https://doi.org/10.1002/jemt.23908

[42] A. Ameri. A deep learning approach to skin cancer detection in dermoscopy image. *Journal of Biomedical Physics Engineering*, 10, 801-806, 2020. https://doi.org/10.31661/jbpe.v0i0.2004-1107

[43] M. Y. Sikkandar, B. A. Alrasheadi, N. B. Prakash, G. R. Hemalakshmi, A. Mohanarathinam and K. Shankar. Deep learning based an automated skin lesion segmentation and intelligent classification model. *Journal of Ambient Intelligence and Humanized Computing*, 12, 3245-3255, 2020. https://doi.org/10.1007/s12652-020-02537-3

[44] Z. Merali, J. Z. Wang, J. H. Badhiwala, C. D. Witiw, J. R. Wilson and M. G. Fehlings. A deep learning model for detection of cervical spinal cord compression in MRI scans. *Scientific Reports*, 11, 10473, 2021. https://doi.org/10.1038/s41598-021-89848-3

[45] W. Mbarki, M. Bouchouicha, S. Frizzi, F. Tshibasu, L. Ben Farhat and M. Sayadi. Lumbar spine discs classification based on deep convolutional neural networks using axial view MRI. *Interdisciplinary Neurosurgery*, 22, 100837, 2020. https://doi.org/10.1016/j.inat.2020.100837

[46] K. A. Weber II, R. Abbott, V. Bojilov, A. C. Smith, M. Wasielewski, T. J. Hastie, T. B. Parrish, S. Mackey and J. M. Elliott. Multi-muscle deep learning segmentation to automate the quantification of muscle fat infiltration in cervical spine conditions. *Scientific Reports*, 11, 16567, 2021. https://doi.org/10.1038/s41598-021-95972-x

[47] K. Yasaka, H. Akai, A. Kunimatsu, O. Abe and S. Kiryu. Deep learning for staging liver fibrosis on CT: A pilot study. *European Radiology*, 28, 4578-4585, 2018. https://doi.org/10.1007/s00330-018-5499-7

[48] B. Schmauch, P. Herent, P. Jehanno, O. Dehaene, C. Saillard, C. Aube, A. Luciani, N. Lassau and S. Jegou. Diagnosis of focal liver lesions from ultrasound using deep learning. *Diagnostic and Interventional Imaging*, 100, 227-233, 2019. https://doi.org/10.1016/j.diii.2019.02.009

[49] C. A. Hamm, C. J. Wang, L. J. Savic, et al. Deep learning for liver tumor diagnosis part I: Development of a convolutional neural network classifier for multiphasic MRI. *European Radiology*, 29, 3338-3347, 2019. https://doi.org/10.1007/s00330-019-06205-9

[50] F. Xi, S. Xu, B. J. Wood and P. Yan. Deep learning-based liver segmentation for fusion-guided intervention. *International Journal of Computer Assisted Radiology and Surgery*, 15, 963-972, 2020. https://doi.org/10.1007/s11548-020-02147-6

[51] S. K. Lakshmanaprabu, S. Nandan Mohanty, K. Shankar, N. Arunkumar and G. Ramirez. Optimal deep learning model for classification of lung cancer on CT images. *Future Generation Computer Systems*, 92, 374-382, 2019. https://doi.org/10.1016/j.future.2018.10.009

[52] M. A. Heuvelmans, P. M. A. van Ooijen and S. Ather. Lung cancer prediction by deep learning to identify benign lung nodules. *Lung Cancer*, 154, 1-4, 2021. https://doi.org/10.1016/j.lungcan.2021.01.027

[53] S. Doppalapudi, R. G. Qiu and Y. Badr. Lung cancer survival period prediction and understanding: Deep learning approaches. *International Journal of Medical Informatics*, 148, 104371, 2021. https://doi.org/10.1016/j.ijmedinf.2020.104371

[54] H. Lee, S. Yune, M. Mohammad, et al. An explainable deep-learning algorithm for the detection of acute intracranial haemorrhage from small datasets. *Nature Biomedical Engineering*, 3, 173-182, 2019. https://doi.org/10.1038/s41551-018-0324-9

[55] S. Phan, S. Satoh, Y. Yoshioki, et al. Evaluation of deep convolutional neural networks for glaucoma detection. *Japanese Journal of Ophthalmology*, 63, 276-283, 2019. https://doi.org/10.1007/s10384-019-00659-6

[56] M. Gupta, T.-L. T. Phan, H. Timothy Bunnell and R. Beheshti. Obesity prediction with EHR data: A deep learning approach with interpretable elements. *ACM Transactions on Computing for Healthcare*, 3, 32, 2022. https://doi.org/10.1145/3506719

[57] R. Rashmi, U. Snekhalatha, P. T. Krishnan, et al. Fat-based studies for computer-assisted screening of child obesity using thermal imaging based on deep learning techniques: A comparison with quantum machine learning approach. *Soft Computing*, 27, 583, 2022. http://dx.doi.org/10.1007/s00500-021-06668-3

[58] M. Varma, M. Lu, G. Rachel, et al. Automated abnormality detection in lower extremity radiographs using deep learning. *Nature Machine Intelligence*, 1, 1-6, 2019. https://www.nature.com/articles/s42256-019-0126-0

[59] K. Dev, S. Ali Khowaja, A. Singh Bist, V. Saini and S. Bhatia. Triage of potential COVID-19 patients from chest X-ray images using hierarchical convolutional networks. *Neural Computing and Applications*, 2021, 1-16, 2021. https://doi.org/10.1007/s00521-020-05641-9

[60] Q. Wang. Research on the improved CNN deep learning method for motion intention recognition of dynamic lower limb prosthesis. *Journal of Healthcare Engineering*, 2021, 7331692, 2021. https://doi.org/10.1155/2021/7331692

[61] P. Aggarwal, N. K. Mishra, B. Fatimah, P. Singh, A. Gupta and S. D. Joshi. COVID-19 image classification using deep learning: Advances, challenges and opportunities. *Computers in Biology and Medicine*, 144, 105350, 2022. https://doi.org/10.1016/j.compbiomed.2022.105350

[62] K. D. Padma, P. Harshitha, R. Nafiza, J. F. Lilian and A. Malini. Exploring the potential of machine learning for early diagnosis of Parkinson's disease: A comparative

study. *4th International Conference on Intelligent Engineering and Management, ICIEM 2023*, 2023, 1-6, 2023. http://dx.doi.org/10.1109/ICIEM59379.2023.10167238

[63] Md. R. Islam and Md. Nahiduzzaman. Complex features extraction with deep learning model for the detection of COVID19 from CT scan images using ensemble-based machine learning approach. *Expert Systems with Applications*, 195, 116554, 2022. https://doi.org/10.1016/j.eswa.2022.116554

[64] Z. Liu, L. Tong, L. Chen, et al. Deep learning-based brain tumor segmentation: A survey. *Complex Intelligent System*, 9, 1001-1026, 2022. https://doi.org/10.1007/s40747-022-00815-5

[65] A. Raza, H. Ayub, J. A. Khan, I. Ahmad, S. A. Salama, Y. I. Daradkeh, D. Javeed, A. Ur Rehman and H. Hamam. A hybrid deep learning-based approach for brain tumor classification. *Electronics*, 11, 1146, 2022. https://doi.org/10.3390/electronics11071146

[66] V. Reddy Allugunti. Breast cancer detection based on thermographic images using machine learning and deep learning algorithms. *International Journal of Engineering in Computer Science*, 4, 49-56, 2022. https://doi.org/10.33545/26633582.2022.v4.i1a.68

[67] N. Mohi ud din, R. Ahmad Dar, M. Rasool and A. Assad. Breast cancer detection using deep learning: Datasets, methods, and challenges ahead. *Computers in Biology and Medicine*, 149, 106073, 2022. https://doi.org/10.1016/j.compbiomed.2022.106073

[68] M. Madani, M. M. Behzadi and S. Nabavi. The role of deep learning in advancing breast cancer detection using different imaging modalities: A systematic review. *Cancers*, 14, 5334, 2022. https://doi.org/10.3390/cancers14215334

[69] A. Bhowmik and S. Eskreis-Winkler. Deep learning in breast imaging. *BJR*, 4, 20210060, 2022. https://doi.org/10.1259/bjro.20210060

[70] P. Khanna, M. Sahu, B. Kumar Singh and V. Bhateja. Early prediction of pathological complete response to neoadjuvant chemotherapy in breast cancer MRI images using combined pre-trained convolutional neural network and machine learning. *Measurement*, 22, 1250, 2023. https://doi.org/10.1186/s12885-022-10315-x

[71] H. Li, Y. Pan, J. Zhao and L. Zhang. Skin disease diagnosis with deep learning: A review. *Neurocomputing*, 464, 364-393, 2021. https://doi.org/10.1016/j.neucom.2021.08.096

[72] B. Zhang, X. Zhou, Y. Luo, et al. Opportunities and challenges: Classification of skin disease based on deep learning. *Chinese Journal of Mechancial Engineering*, 34, 112, 2021. https://doi.org/10.1186/s10033-021-00629-5

[73] I. Kousis, I. Perikos, I. Hatzilygeroudis and M. Virvou. Deep learning methods for accurate skin cancer recognition and mobile application. *Electronics*, 11, 1294, 2022. https://doi.org/10.3390/electronics11091294

[74] I. U. Haq, K. Chhatwal, K. Sanaka and B. Xu. Artificial intelligence in cardiovascular medicine: Current insights and future prospects. *Vascular Health Risk Management*, 18, 517-528, 2022. https://doi.org/10.2147/vhrm.s279337

[75] G. K. Sriram, A. Karunasagar, R. Sudharsan and A. Malini. Deep learning approaches for Pneumonia classification in healthcare, *3rd International Conference on Innovative Practices in Technology and Management, ICIPTM 2023*, 2023, 1-6, 2023. https://doi.org/10.1109/ICIPTM57143.2023.10117615

[76] H. Rahman, T. F. N. Bukht, A. Imran, J. Tariq, S. Tu and A. Alzahrani. A deep learning approach for liver and tumor segmentation in CT images using ResUNet. *Bioengineering (Basel)*, 9, 368, 2022. https://doi.org/10.3390/bioengineering9080368

[77] J. A. Luetkens, S. Nowak, N. Mesropyan, et al. Deep learning supports the differentiation of alcoholic and other-than-alcoholic cirrhosis based on MRI. *Science Report*, 12, 8297, 2022. https://doi.org/10.1038/s41598-022-12410-2

[78] Y. Akbulut. Automated pneumonia based lung diseases classification with robust technique based on a customized deep learning approach. *Diagnostics*, 13, 260, 2023. https://doi.org/10.3390/diagnostics13020260

[79] F. Hussein, et al. Hybrid CLAHE CNN deep neural networks for classifying lung diseases from X-ray acquisitions. *Electronics*, 11, 3075, 2022. https://doi.org/10.3390/electronics11193075

[80] K. Ramana, M. R. Kumar, K. Sreenivasulu, T. R. Gadekallu, S. Bhatia, P. Agarwal and S. M. Idrees. Early prediction of lung cancers using deep saliency capsule and pre-trained deep learning frameworks. *Frontiers in Oncology*, 12, 2022. https://doi.org/10.3389/fonc.2022.886739

6 Machine Learning Approach for Different Habitual Activity Versus Sleep Intermittent Stages from Time-Efficient Perspectives based on Facial Features

Krishnakumar K. and S. Latha

6.1 INTRODUCTION

During pandemics, for example, COVID-19, medical experts are required at host places. All life cycles become more intrusively health centric and there is an urge to visit a doctor or have a healthy shadow environment [1]. Our mind and body express our characters through our transmission medium called the skin and its soft tissues. Soft tissues in our face express our illness initially. With reference to the face, it is tested with a basic medical kit considered as a preamble. In hospitals or primary healthcare centers, these measures are taken as an initial assessment and compared with ground truth data [2][3]. In the second stage, a disease-specific test and treatment are performed. Symptoms or metabolic disorders that are not exposed to the naked eye are screened through medical image analysis. In rural, semi-urban, and urban living populations, there are many challenges in getting timely and qualified treatment. The recommendations provided by medical experts in the report have made it easier for doctors to approach symptoms based on patient medical records. The expert's summary relies on medical image retrieval methods, which can be text-based, content-based, or a combination of both [4][5]. In times of pandemics, limitations on travel beyond one's residence are imposed. To evaluate individuals' physical resilience and psychological health based on their routine activities like walking and sports, fitness centers within authorized locations are outfitted to enhance both bodily and mental wellness.. In the past few years, significant attention has been given to investigating innovative methods for assessing human health conditions through the analysis of

 DOI: 10.1201/9781003484233-6

routine activities and comparing this information with established baseline models. This approach enables the non-invasive prediction of an individual's likelihood of falling ill before they reach the stage of requiring ambulatory care [6].

6.1.1 Prior Art: Evolution of AI from Machine Learning Perspectives

In the era of Industry 4.0, also known as the Fourth Industrial Revolution, machine learning (ML) research has garnered significant attention. This period is characterized by the ability to distribute data spaces using Internet of Things (IoT) technologies, coupled with data security measures. The increased availability of data has led to advancements in deep learning, a subset of ML, resulting in the development of intelligent, automated applications across various promising fields. The widespread availability of ML algorithms has led to near-perfect accuracy, steering applications toward cybersecurity, sustainable urban environments, and intelligent farming practices.. Table 6.1 describes services offered by artificial intelligence (AI) with the stated applications. These research applications can explore new avenues in Industry 4.0 [7][8].

ML algorithms categorize data patterns using various labels. They can extract and analyze large-scale data with or without label supervision. Each method is detailed as follows: Within supervised ML, linear regression serves as a technique for forecasting shifts in continuous numerical values with labels. This algorithm offers low computational complexity and finds applications in areas such as predicting real estate prices and stock market trends.

In the unsupervised ML model, the kernel-based clustering algorithm is used and splits n observations into subset (k) cluster attributes of data. It is applied in the medical field for recommending specific treatment to patients. The semi-supervised ML model leverages the good data among labeled and unlabeled data. It is applied in disease subtyping or comorbidities, drug discovery, and medical image analysis. In reinforcement learning (RL), decision-making from data is sequential. RL involves an agent interacting with data to best fit the prediction and is applied in the field of robotics for decision recommendations [9].

In supervised ML, the linear discriminant analysis (LDA) algorithm is primarily used for classification tasks, as well as forecasting the instance's class label based on its features. LDA works by modeling the distribution of features for each class separately and then using Bayes' rule to compute the likelihood that a specific instance

TABLE 6.1
AI services in Industry 4.0

Industry 4.0 applications	Services offered by AI
Cybersecurity systems	Enhancing security through intelligent algorithms
Smart cities	Optimizing urban infrastructure and services
Healthcare	Optimizing diagnostics, treatment, and patient outcomes
E-commerce	Personalizing recommendations and streamlining operations
Agriculture	Enhancing crop yield and resource management

falls into each class. It is predicated on the features having a normal distribution and the classes having a same covariance matrix. [10,11]. LDA is frequently utilized when there are multiple classes to be identified and a linear relationship between the features and the classes is expected. Some common applications of LDA include:

- Face recognition: LDA has been used extensively in facial recognition systems to classify images of faces into different individuals or categories.
- Biometric identification: LDA can be applied to biometric data, such as fingerprints or iris scans, to classify individuals based on their biometric characteristics.
- Medical diagnosis: LDA is used in medical applications to classify patients into different diagnostic categories based on their symptoms or medical test results.
- Speech recognition: LDA can be used in speech recognition systems to classify spoken words or phrases into different categories.

Overall, LDA is a versatile and widely used algorithm in various fields where classification tasks are common and where the relationship between the features and the classes can be assumed to be linear.

The *K*-nearest neighbors (KNN) approach in supervised ML stores training data in terms of instances and predictions based on how similar fresh examples are to existing data points [12]. The KNN algorithm is well-suited for extended periods as it postpones the analysis of training data until a request is made. It retains the complete training dataset instead of learning a discriminative function from the training data. By comparing fresh data points to the labeled data points in the training set, the noise-free KNN classifies data points. Additionally, it selects the majority class among the *k* nearest neighbors of the query point, typically using a distance metric like the Euclidean distance [13] [14]. However, outliers can still affect its performance. One of the challenges of using KNN is selecting the best neighbor (*k*) when making predictions. This can significantly impact the algorithm's performance and often requires empirical testing or cross-validation [11] [15]. The main application of KNN is in classification tasks, but it can also be adapted for regression tasks. It's used in applications where the goal is to classify instances into one of several predefined classes, for example, handwritten digit recognition, email spam detection, and image classification. In regression, the goal is to predict a continuous value based on the features of the data [16] [15], for example, predicting housing prices based on features like location, size, and number of bedrooms, and predicting stock prices based on historical data and market indicators.

The support vector machine (SVM) belongs to the category of supervised ML algorithms and ideates hyperplane(s) to achieve maximum margin separation between different classes [17] [18]. SVM is used in mapping the input features into a higher-dimensional space using a kernel function. This allows SVM to find a hyperplane that separates the classes, even when the decision boundary is nonlinear. SVM is effective in high-dimensional spaces, such as linear, polynomial, radial basis function (RBF), and sigmoid. These kernel functions allow SVM to capture complex relationships between features and improve classification performance. SVM performance may degrade when the dataset contains noise or overlapping classes, as it aims to find the optimal hyperplane that maximizes the margin between classes. Overall, SVMs are powerful and versatile algorithms that can be applied to a wide range of classification, regression, and outlier detection tasks, especially in scenarios where the data are high-dimensional or the decision boundary is complex [19]. Applications of SVM include image classification, text categorization, and bioinformatics, such as protein classification.. SVM can also be used for regression tasks where the goal is to predict a continuous value based on the features of the data. For example, predicting housing prices and predicting stock prices. SVM can be used for outlier detection tasks, where the goal is to identify rare observations that deviate from the majority of the data. For example, fraud detection in financial transactions and anomaly detection in network traffic [20].

One class of supervised ML algorithms is decision tree learning. Its main applications are regression and classification tasks. Since decision trees are non-parametric models, they assume very little about the distribution of the underlying data. Decision trees have a hierarchical structure composed of nodes, where each node represents a decision based on a feature attribute. Decision trees are highly interpretable models, as the rules learned from the data are represented in a tree-like structure that can be easily visualized and understood by humans. Decision trees can provide insights into feature importance, indicating which features are most relevant for making predictions. Decision trees use various criteria for splitting nodes, such as Gini impurity and entropy, to identify the parent node [21] [22]. Decision trees can be applied to a variety of tasks in different domains. They are particularly useful when interpretability and explainability are important, as well as when dealing with both categorical and numerical data. However, decision trees may suffer from overfitting, especially when the trees are deep and complex, which can be addressed through techniques like pruning and ensemble methods like random forests (RF) [23].

The methods discussed are a form of ensemble learning in ML, namely "parallel ensembling" with RF, adaptive boosting (AdaBoost), and extreme gradient boosting (XGBoost). RF makes use of parallel ensembling by training several decision tree classifiers on various dataset subsamples. It combines the predictions of individual trees using majority voting or averaging to make the final prediction. RF minimizes overfitting and increases prediction accuracy by controlling variation through bagging and random feature selection [24]. It's well-suited for handling large datasets, and both categorical and continuous features. It's used in applications such as classification and regression tasks, and both categorical and continuous value predictions. It also combines the predictions of weak classifiers using a weighted sum to produce the final prediction. It improves the efficiency of the classifier by significantly boosting its performance, but can lead to overfitting in some cases. It's used in applications such as binary classification problems to boost the performance of weak classifiers, particularly decision trees. XGBoost utilizes gradient boosting, similar to AdaBoost, to iteratively train decision trees and minimize the loss function [25]. It computes the second-order gradients of the loss function for more detailed approximations and advanced regularization (L1 and L2) to reduce overfitting. It's quick to understand and capable of effectively managing big datasets. It improves model generalization and performance by minimizing loss and considering advanced regularization techniques. Overall, ensemble learning techniques like RF, AdaBoost, and XGBoost are widely used in various ML applications, particularly in classification and regression tasks, to improve prediction accuracy and handle complex datasets [26].

Stochastic gradient descent (SGD) belongs to the category of optimization and introduces randomness by selecting a random training example at each iteration, especially in high-dimensional optimization problems. SGD modifies weights to regulate the magnitude of model parameters. This parameter predetermines the magnitude of the step taken in the direction opposite to the gradient.. Text classification and natural language processing tasks present large-scale, sparse challenges that call for the use of hyperparameters and input in SGD. Despite its sensitivity to hyperparameters and feature scaling, SGD's stochastic nature and computational efficiency make it a popular choice for training ML models on large datasets. It's used in applications such as text classification, language modeling, machine translation, and named entity recognition. SGD is often employed to optimize the parameters of ML models such as linear classifiers (e.g., logistic regression and linear SVM) or neural networks. The model improves its performance on the training dataset by iteratively updating the parameters based on the gradients of the loss function with respect to these parameters. Overall, while SGD itself is an optimization algorithm, it is typically used within the context of supervised ML models to train them effectively on large-scale datasets [27,28].

The classification or regression approach described, which utilizes IF-THEN rules for class prediction, is well-suited for decision trees. Decision trees inherently operate by recursively partitioning the feature space into regions, each associated with a particular class label. At each node of the tree, a decision is made based on the values of one of the input features, leading to a split in the data. This procedure continues until a predetermined end point is reached, like the maximum depth or the minimum amount of instances per node. Here's how the described classification approach aligns with decision trees:

IF-THEN rules: An array of IF-THEN rules can be used to understand decision trees. Descriptive modeling and the explanation of the decision-making process can benefit from the ease of understanding and interpretation of the rules generated by decision trees, which are represented by each path from the parent node to a leaf node [27]. Accuracy: Decision trees can achieve good accuracy on classification tasks while still producing interpretable rules. They are capable of capturing complex relationships between features and class labels, making them suitable for a wide range of classification problems. Overall, decision trees are a natural fit for the described rule-based classification, as well as the regression approach. They excel in generating interpretable rules while maintaining good accuracy and handling high-dimensional data. Their simplicity, interpretability, and ability to produce understandable rules make them a popular choice for rule-based classification tasks [29].

The naive Bayes method is a probabilistic classifier used in supervised ML. It applies Bayes' theorem under the "naive" assumption of feature independence. Predicting a particular instance's class label based on its data properties is mostly utilized for classification jobs [30]. During the training phase, naive Bayes estimates the probability distributions of the features for each class, assuming they are independent of each other given the class attributes. Then, during the prediction phase, it uses these probability distributions to calculate the likelihood of a new instance belonging to each class attribute and selects attributes with the highest probability. Overall, naive Bayes handles small datasets, limited computational resources, or real-time predictions with good accuracy [31].

6.1.2 Face Recognition System

Face feature extraction to detect morphological changes after performing a targeted action involves a dimensionality reduction technique [32,33]. It outputs the most important features from data, which requires a careful evaluation of selected data or a suitable data compression technique, and its types are

- factor evaluation
- analysis of principal components
- analysis of independent components
- a variant of principal component analysis (PCA)

PCA is a technique to implement necessary attributes in the data science domain. Its implementation steps are as follows:

- Ensure data consistency.
- Using a matrix factorization technique, such as the covariance matrix, correlation matrix, or singular value decomposition, get the eigenvectors and eigenvalues used to identify the most important features [34].
- Create a matrix from the chosen k vectors by sorting the eigenvalues in descending order that correspond to the k biggest eigenvalues, where k is the number of dimensions of the new feature subspace ($k \le d$).
- Consider the original dataset X from the k-dimensional feature to introduce the scaled Y.

The drawbacks of PCA include:

Standard PCA struggles to identify critical features in large-scale datasets due to its high demand for computational resources.

While effective for linear patterns, PCA fails to address nonlinear relationships, requiring alternative methods for such data structures.

When datasets have a high number of features (e.g., 50,000) with only a small percentage being significant, PCA may inaccurately detect or disregard important features. Traditional PCA is not a reliable method for achieving perfect or complete extraction of significant features, particularly in complex datasets.

6.1.3 Types of PCA

For real-time systems, a continuous stream of time series data flows in to detect anomalies through facial characteristics. It is crucial that data drift and concept drift do not occur, as this would undermine the entire purpose [35]. Data drift occurs when nonlinear feature identification is overlooked, and insufficient storage or RAM causes data collection to be truncated beyond available space, leading to concept drift. To address this issue, lossless compression is necessary [36]. A new approach should adhere to the principles of incremental learning by performing numerous support vector decompositions (SVD) on numerous batches (let's say *m* batches made from the dataset) consisting of '*n*' samples in order to arrive at the final principal components [32,37]. The data pipeline or data batch, rather than loading all the data into memory, is keyed to avoid lossy compression in kernel PCA (KPCA); however, it can be employed when there is a nonlinear relationship between the various features in the dataset. KPCA for face features is evaluated with root mean square error (RMSE) metrics and five ML models have been analyzed with prediction frequency and training time. The Gaussian process regression (GPR) variant includes rational quadratic GPR (RQ), which is a non-parametric approach to predict data that are linearly/nonlinearly independent of each other. It is involved in applications such as healthcare, security defense, financial markets, and remote explosive detection. This non-parametric technique is more useful in distinguishing samples into different classes when applied to multivariate statistical data applications and performance measures like RMSE [33,38]. The host can be compared with a non-parametric model, such as kernel density estimation, which predicts noisy data from continuous random variables using the probability density function. KNN predicts classification [39,40] among data using the majority class and predicts regression using the mean of the nearest neighbor values. Decision tree identifies less impure data as the parent node and predicts unknowns. RF validates data by providing a subset among data similarities resultant in the prediction of each tree. SVM identifies a hyperplane that suits the classification of data and employs a kernel function to handle the nonlinear relationship among data [41]. Locally weighted regression assigns different weights to the nearest data points. The local pattern is identified on subsequent query points to predict data. Gaussian mixture models employ clustering techniques in two-dimensional (2D) or three-dimensional spaces to analyze data patterns. These models then utilize density estimation methods and subsequently predict various attributes of the data. Isotonic regression or monotonic regression are used to maintain the order of data points and utilize a piecewise constant function to predict data [38,42]. The local outlier factor is a concern that should be considered in biomedical image analysis and statistics. It has to be dealt with using bias and a variance technique. The resultant factor is robust to noise and a greater data density achieves higher prediction accuracy. Kernel method variants, such as kernel SVM (k-SVM) and KPCA, use higher-dimensional space to predict the nonlinear relationship among variables [43,44].

6.2 METHODOLOGY

A person with habitual walking and gym activity is considered and observed for ±30 minutes or within the individual's threshold level. The person's facial features are analyzed and compared with pulse oximeter readings. In the analogy tried here, symptoms for illness are inspected using a basic medical kit, which has been utilized in hospitals (first-stage screening). Then disease-specific treatment is initiated, either

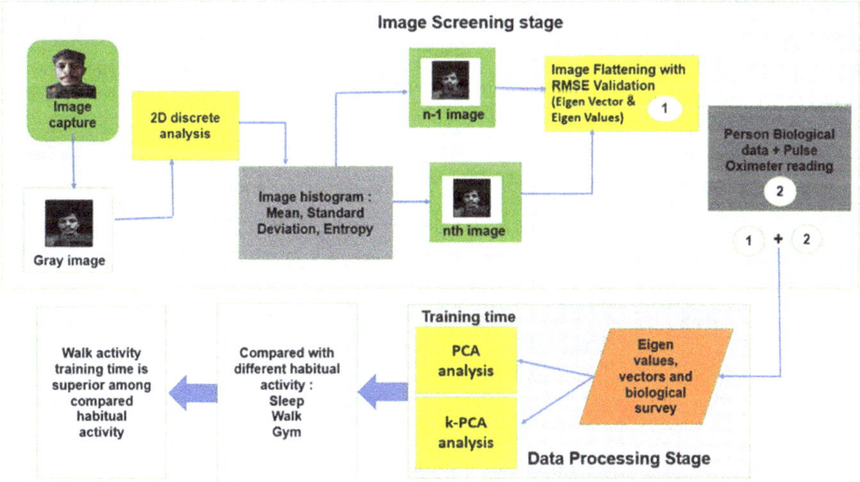

FIGURE 6.1 Block diagram representing different habitual activities optimized for training time using different ML algorithms.

in hospitals or healthcare centers. The development idea behind our proposed system follows the above initiative, which is described systematically in Figure 6.1. It infers a basic health report regarding the individual's health status by comparing facial features after each habitual activity and SpO_2 with reference to the ground truth as sleep activity with six intermittent stages. PCA and KPCA are used to describe essential linear face features and nonlinear face features, and are tabulated in the results.

6.2.1 Face Feature Extraction using Dimensional Reduction Analysis

In a dimensional reduction pattern, a gray image extracted from the RGB of a face image, say n, is taken and a prior gray image (n - 1) face feature acts as a reference for the present gray image to calculate the covariance matrix. Its outcome gives the eigenvector and eigenvalue to explain the amount of variance with respect to the mean. The process known as image flattening is timed, with the duration measured as the log-in time (t) in seconds. The accuracy of the proposed method is evaluated by conducting a statistical analysis, which involves comparing the current gray image to the reference image using a metric like the RMSE value. An RMSE value < 1 acts as metric to determine accuracy and to evaluate the training time for linear PCA, as shown in Table 6.2

6.2.2 Face Feature Extraction using a Kernel Dimensional Reduction Pattern

KPCA allows for nonlinear feature extraction using the following stages. The first stage, stated as dataset preparation, involves each person walking as habitual activity

TABLE 6.2
Supervised ML model using PCA for walking activity – optimizable tree approach

Constraints	Model type	RMSE	MSE	R2	MAE	Prediction speed (observation/sec)	Training time (sec)
PCA – auto	Before	0.608	0.370	-1.55E-15	0.533	999.624	62.427
PCA – manual	walking	**0.599**	0.359	4.22E-15	0.521	**2930.281**	**50.457**
Without PCA		0.608	0.370	-1.55E-15	0.533	2042.767	63.834
PCA – auto	After	0.623	0.388	1.11E-14	0.550	2079.594	103.710
PCA – manual	walking	**0.623**	0.388	1.11E-14	0.550	**1097.996**	**59.706**
Without PCA		0.623	0.388	1.11E-14	0.550	4532.978	84.231

captured at two stages (rest and after walking). In the second stage, stated as image pre-processing, 2D discrete wavelet analysis is used to extract face features for each habitual activity. In the data matrix in the experiment, 310 face image histogram features with their biological data were examined for the training time (70% of n) and results were compared among different habitual activity.

6.2.3 Experimental Setup

6.2.3.1 Supervised Machine Learning for Habitual Activity

For the proposed methodology, persons in the age category between 35 and 55 ±10 performed habitual walking voluntarily. These activities were recorded during the evening with a duration of about ± 30 minutes. Recording activities were performed for different walking stages and observed for only two stages, stated as the start and end of the walking activity.

Face features' statistical data, such as the mean, standard deviation (SD), and entropy, were combined with the person's biological survey data, such as age, sex, and weight. These data were compared with the person's pulse oximeter data, such as beats per minute (BPM) and $SpO_{2,}$ as shown in Table 6.3. The proposed methodology for predicting the morphological changes through face features after/before habitual activity was examined for both ML models. PCA, one of the dimensionality reduction techniques, was applied to predict the essential features during habitual activity through two modes: auto mode (95% variance) and manual mode (selecting components or features). These predictions are necessary in order to calculate the prediction or training time, prediction frequencies, and statistical data obtained through face features, which is traded off by comparing with and without PCA while modeling the equipment. The prediction speed and training time were compared for habitual activity at two-time instances, such as before walking and after walking, and were tabulated as shown in Table 6.2. A supervised ML model, such as decision tree and its variants, was used for both classification and regression, in which a less impure node (feature) was considered as the parent node and compared with new data (feature), and the training time was predicted.

TABLE 6.3
Person's biological survey and face statistical data

Day wise	Biological survey				Face statistical data		
Day 01	Age	Wt	SpO_2	BPM	Mean	SD*	Entropy
P1	46	79	98	95	220.7	75.2376	2.322
P2	65	57	99	88	196.2	69.0771	3.225
P3	54	63	97	76	215.7	81.7338	2.588
P4	48	60	98	87	210	68.2197	3.236

TABLE 6.4
Supervised ML model using PCA for gym activity – optimizable tree approach

Constraints	Model type	RMSE	MSE	R^2	MAE	Prediction speed (observations/sec)	Training time (sec)
PCA – auto	Before	0.803	0.645	0.009	0.679	1835.718	74.486
PCA – manual	gym	0.803	0.645	0.009	0.679	1490.757	56.868
Without PCA	activity	0.804	0.646	0.007	0.679	**2402.083**	**42.016**
PCA – auto	After	0.815	0.664	1.28E-14	0.670	1337.369	84.170
PCA – manual	gym	3.835	14.708	0.082	3.206	**4460.525**	**43.739**
Without PCA	activity	0.815	0.664	1.28E-14	0.670	3102.597	57.556

From Table 6.2, the manual PCA feature selection training time for habitual activity before walking (50.457 secs) and after walking (59.706 secs) was optimized, and for the prediction speed, no trade-off was obtained. Validation accuracy was verified with reference to the RMSE metric, which is more suitable for gray-scale images. The decision tree approach has two drawbacks such as high variance and low bias, hence, an ensemble learning approach, such as ensemble boosted tree and bagged tree, may be used to overcome drawbacks. This method was investigated for habitual activity, such as gym activity, as shown below in Table 6.4, and obtained the optimum training time before gym activity without PCA (42.016 secs) and optimum training time after gym activity with PCA – manual (43.739 secs). Inferences obtained from Table 6.2 in terms of RMSE values before walking activity, 0.599, and after walking activity, 0.623, indicates that the gray-level face image had greater correlation in predicting the computation time with reference to walking as a habitual activity when validated against linear PCA analysis. The inference obtained from Table 6.4 with respect to the RMSE value before gym activity, 0.803, indicates that the gray-level face image had greater correlation in predicting the computation time when validated against PCA analysis.

The after gym activity RMSE value, 3.835, had no such correlation, but indicated a contradiction in the estimation of the training time. The above analysis demonstrates that linear PCA did not achieve a greater result unless the person's habitual activity

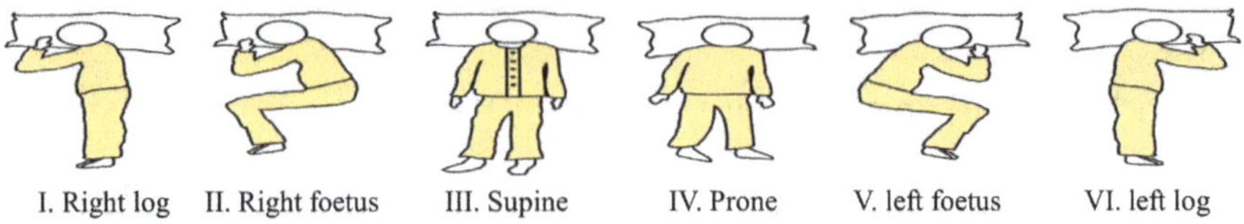

FIGURE 6.2 Free flow and occlusion sleep activity for six intermittent stages [43].

involved more dynamics. The above methodology was described in KPCA and compared with (ground truth model) sleep intermittent stages of both the free flow and occlusion type, as illustrated in Figure 6.2. KPCA applied to walking activity and compared with free flow and occlusion type sleep stages is shown in Figures 6.3 and 6.4.

In Figure 6.3, the bar graph highlighted in orange represents the training time optimized for walking as a habitual activity and is compared with the bar graph highlighted in green using KPCA variants. RQ, squared exponential GPR (SE GPR), Matérn 5/2 GPR (M5/2 GPR), exponential GPR (Ex GPR), and k-SVM are variants of KPCA selected for analysis against free flow sleep intermittent stages. In the bar graph, face features after habitual walking and a free flow sleep model are represented on the *x*-axis and the training time (secs) is represented on the *y*-axis. A total of 310 persons' faces after habitual walking were computed with KPCA variants for both occlusion and the free flow sleep model, as shown in Figures 6.3 and 6.4.

In Figure 6.3, with walking as habitual activity in comparison with the supine stage free flow sleep model, the training time was less for walking activity, and in Figure 6.4, for walking activity with the right fetus occlusion sleep model, the training time was less for walking activity. Additionally, from Figures 6.3 and 6.4, for the left fetus, left log, right fetus, right log, and supine intermittent sleep stages, the training time for addressing nonlinear facial features was greater than that for face features after walking as habitual activity. This infers that walking activity when compared with the occlusion right fetus stage had less training time, which provides no clue for conclusions with reference to static action. The same condition was practiced and described while comparing habitual gym activity with the ground truth, as shown in Figures 6.5 and 6.6. Gym activity compared with left log, right foetus, right log, and supine free flow sleep stages had less training time, as shown in Figure 6.5, and gym activity compared with six occlusion sleep stages had less training time. In summary, a person's habitual activity, such as walking and gym activity, with 309 persons' face features, was compared with six free flow sleep intermittent stages and six occlusion sleep intermittent stages. KPCA computations were performed to address nonlinear face features. The training time was shown as a bar graph that indicated results effectively across KPCA variants. The analysis made concludes that the training time for walking and gym activity was less against sleep postures.

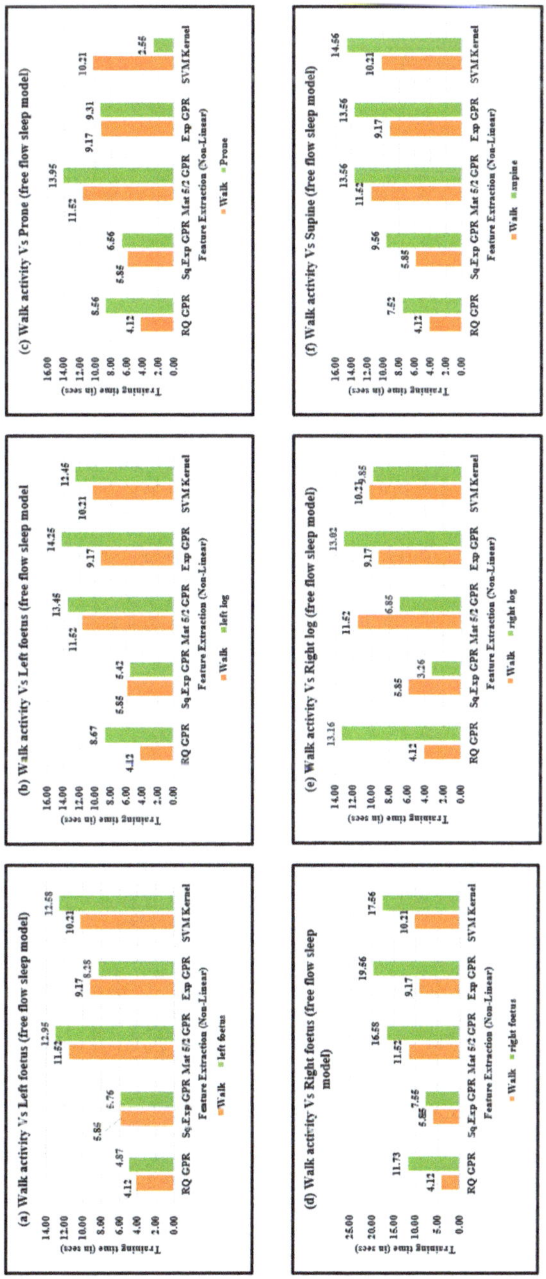

FIGURE 6.3 Walking activity vs. free flow intermittent sleep stages activity.

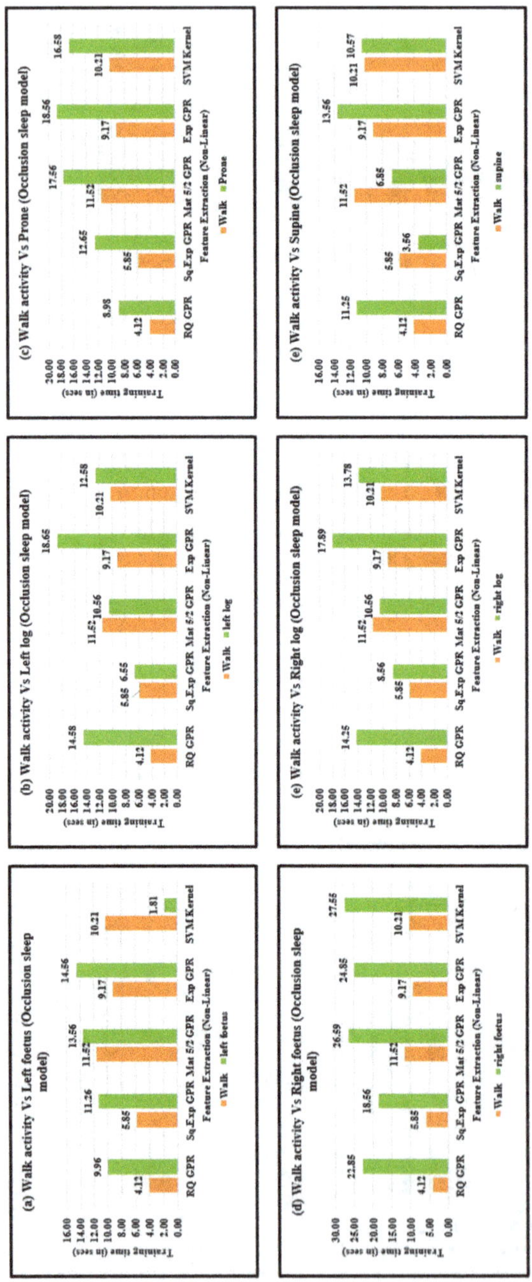

FIGURE 6.4 Walking activity vs. occlusion intermittent sleep stages activity.

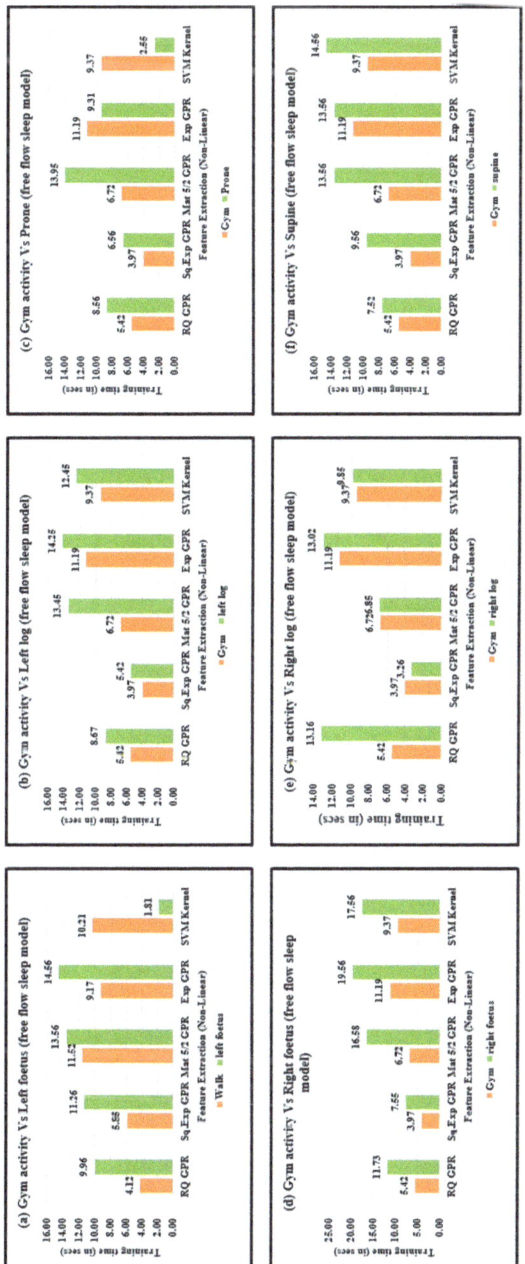

FIGURE 6.5 Gym activity vs. free flow intermittent sleep stages activity.

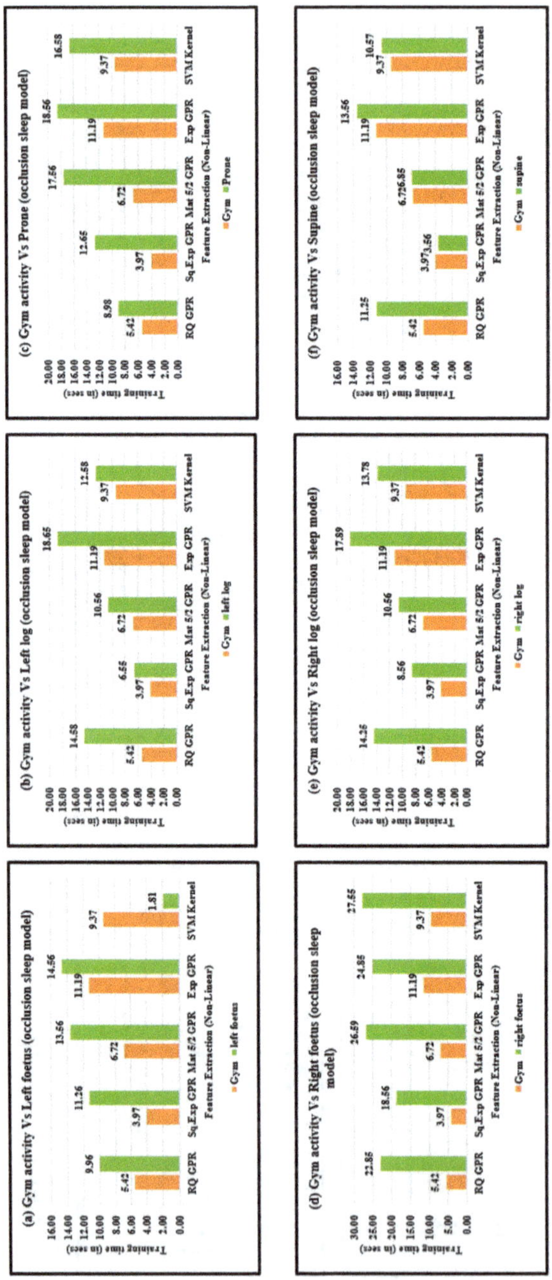

FIGURE 6.6 Gym activity vs. occlusion intermittent sleep stages activity.

6.2.3.2 Unsupervised Machine Learning for Habitual Activity

Habitual activity for the same group of people was analyzed for an unsupervised ML model to address nonlinear features and to find the optimized training time among habitual activities. For this learning type, the clustering of features was validated against benchmark performance metrics.

Face features, along with each person's biological profile, such as age, sex, weight, BPM, and SpO2, were clustered for each habitual activity and processed further to obtain evaluation metrics. Activities were clustered to best suit regression and classification, and justified with metrics such as Pearson's, Spearman's, and Kendall's correlation coefficients, the silhouette score, Calinski–Harabasz index, and Davies–Bouldin index to estimate accuracy based on prediction with new data.

Regression learning, an unsupervised ML technique, trained habitual activity data for 309 individuals. The highest accuracy was scaled to 1, while ridge regression achieved a low positive value of 0.032 for training and a negative value of -0.034 for testing, indicating overfitting. RF obtained a high 0.841 positive value, which indicated a strong linear relationship in the training data, and the value -0.109 for test data inferred an inability to predict new data; hence, overfitting occurred for two different types of regression. In RF regression, raw data for habitual activity should be grouped into a term or subset. It was framed based on similarities among features and obtained the values 0.841 and -0.109, which indicated good correlation during training and poor correlation during testing, which indicated potential overfitting.

Unsupervised learning correlates possible independent features using coefficients such as Pearson's, Spearman's, and Kendall's correlation coefficients to extend support in order to predict a suitable model that fits the new unseen data. Cluster profiling from a person's biological survey data, such as age and SpO_2, was considered. SpO_2 was evaluated against the age category with performance metrics, as shown in Table 6.5, which indicates that age vs. SpO_2 had no potential interference. Dimensionality reduction or PCA identified potential features and clusters using *k*-means with variance as performance metrics, as illustrated in Table 6.6.

The same analysis was visualized in 2D space with reference to data clusters and SpO_2 statistics for walking as habitual activity, as shown in Figure 6.7. Overall, the

TABLE 6.5
SpO_2 prediction vs. SpO_2 in the clustering approach

S. No	Cluster variant	Age ±2.5	SpO_2
1.	Cluster 0	53	98%
2.	Cluster 1	46	
3.	Cluster 2	40	

TABLE 6.6
SpO_2 prediction vs. SpO_2 in the PCA approach

S. No	PCA variant	Variance%	Inferences for SpO_2
1.	PCA1	23.36	No threshold achieved
2.	PCA2	21.63	
3.	PCA3	19.71	
4.	PCA4	18.62	
5.	PCA5	16.69	

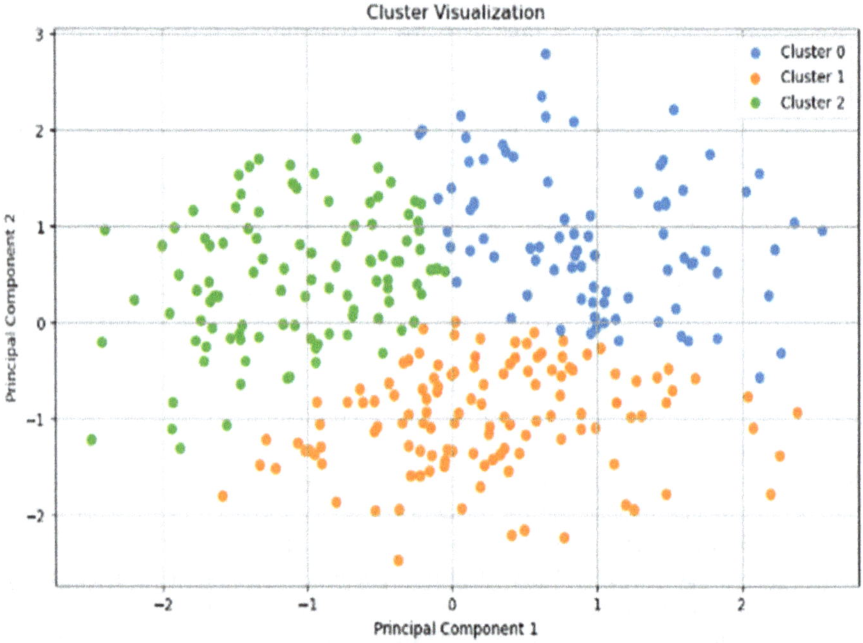

FIGURE 6.7 Cluster approach for SpO_2 prediction using PCA.

unsupervised learning approach for this model indicated the exploration of different clustering algorithms for different habitual activities. Potential conflict in this approach was indicated by the overlap between data clustering in PCA, as shown in Figure 6.8. Ways to improve this depend on various parameters, such as finding object similarity between neighboring clusters, cluster density, and separation. The mean between each cluster and its most similar host was evaluated for different scores using the silhouette score, Calinski–Harabasz index, and Davies–Bouldin index, as shown in Table 6.7. During data training, performance scores indicated a moderate value for clustering performance using the t-distributed stochastic neighbor embedding (t-SNE) component against data features for walking as habitual activity, as

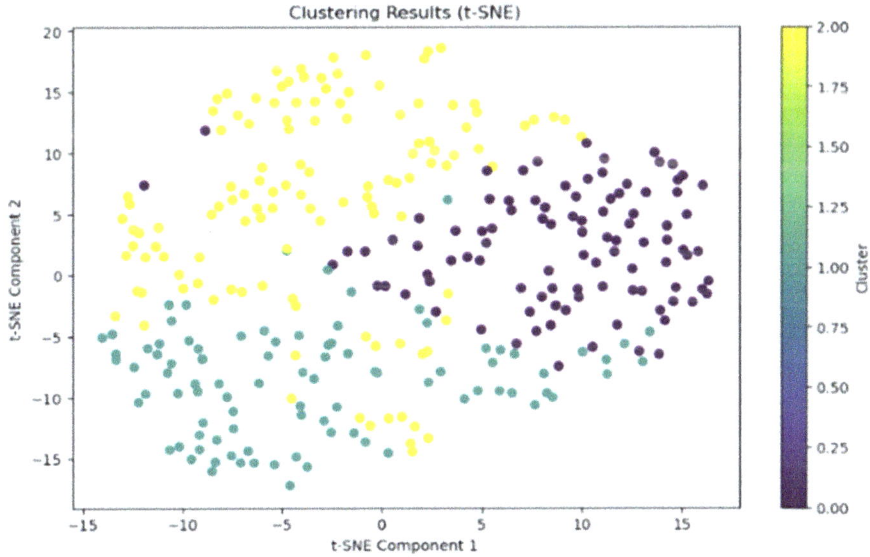

FIGURE 6.8 Cluster approach for SpO_2 prediction using t-SNE (walking activity).

TABLE 6.7
Cluster performances against performance metrics for walking as habitual activity

Performance measures against face for walking activity	Performance metrics	Score	Scale range	Inference
Object similarity between neighbouring cluster	Silhouette score	0.156	±1	Cluster not dense
Cluster density and separation	Calinski–Harabasz index	57.566	0 to 100	Moderate
Mean between each cluster	Davies–Bouldin index	1.869	1 to 2	Moderate

shown in Figure 6.8, and gym activity as habitual activity, as shown in Figure 6.9. The subsequent quartile values, such as 25th, 50th, and 75th, found in the distribution of SpO_2 predicted values based on the face features such as mean and SD are shown in Table 6.8.

The results considering walking as habitual activity for 309 persons and face statistical features, such as mean, SD, as illustrated in Table 6.8 shows 98, 98 and 113 persons' face statistical features after habitual activity confined to SpO_2 as 97% to 99% while clustering and observed in quartiles with threshold level from minimum to maximum. The observed values in Table 6.9 for predicting SpO_2

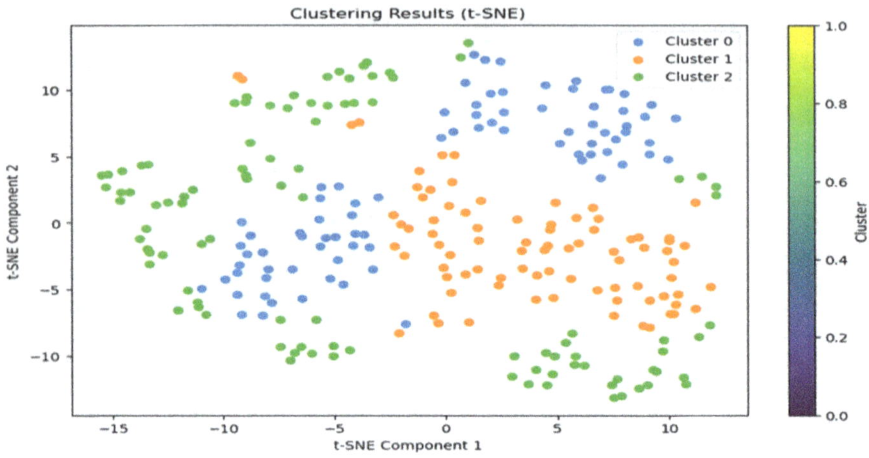

FIGURE 6.9 Cluster approach for SpO_2 prediction using t-SNE (gym activity).

TABLE 6.8
Face statistical features vs. SpO_2 quartiles for walking activity

Cluster	Count*	Mean	SD	Minimum	25%	50%	75%	Maximum
0	98	98.10	0.79	97	97	98	99	99
1	98	97.89	0.76	97	97	98	99	99
2	113	97.97	0.84	97	97	98	99	99

* -309 persons' face features split up count

TABLE 6.9
Cluster performances against performance metrics for gym as habitual activity

Performance measures against face for walking activity	Performance metrics	Score	Scale range	Inference
Object similarity between neighbouring clusters	Silhouette score	0.195	±1	Cluster moderate
Cluster density and separation	Calinski–Harabasz index	62.78	0 to 100	Fair
Mean between each cluster	Davies–Bouldin index	1.614	1 to 2	Good

TABLE 6.10
Cluster performances against performance metrics for left foetus as habitual activity

Performance measures against face for walking activity	Performance metrics	Score	Scale range	Inference
Object similarity between neighbouring clusters	Silhouette score	0.198	±1	Cluster moderate
Cluster density and separation	Calinski–Harabasz index	74.89	0 to 100	Fair
Mean between each cluster	Davies–Bouldin index	1.62	1 to 2	Good

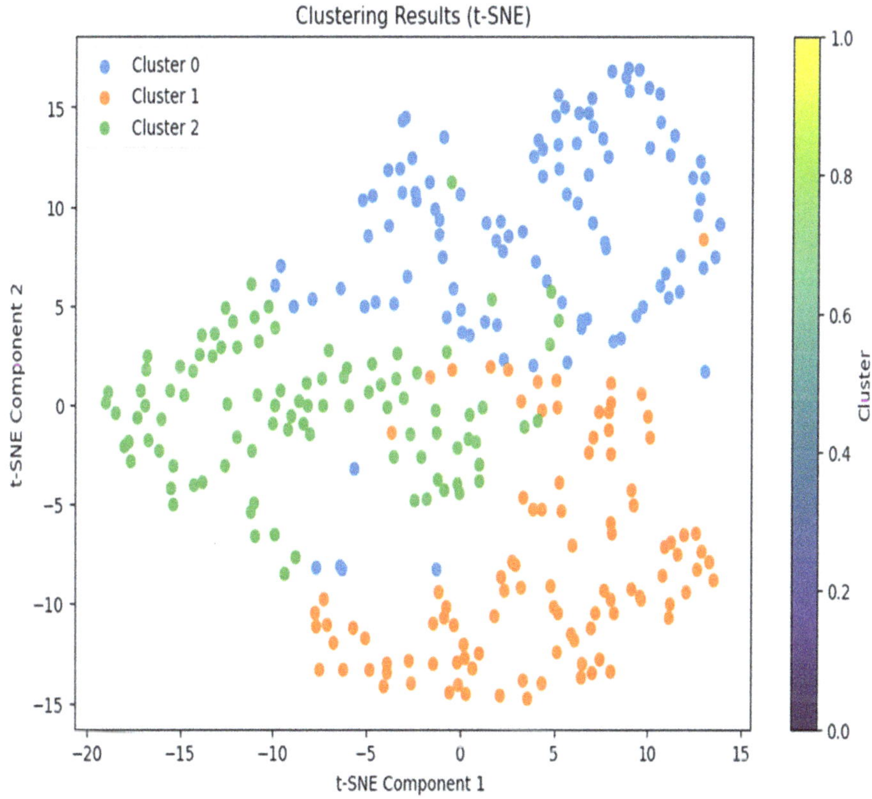

FIGURE 6.10 Cluster approach for SpO_2 prediction using t-SNE (left fetus activity).

TABLE 6.11
Cluster performances against performance metrics for left log as habitual activity

Performance measures against face for walking activity	Performance metrics	Score	Scale range	Inference
Object similarity between neighboring clusters	Silhouette score	0.184	±1	Cluster moderate
Cluster density and separation	Calinski–Harabasz index	70.96	0 to 100	Fair
Mean between each cluster	Davies–Bouldin index	1.65	1 to 2	Good

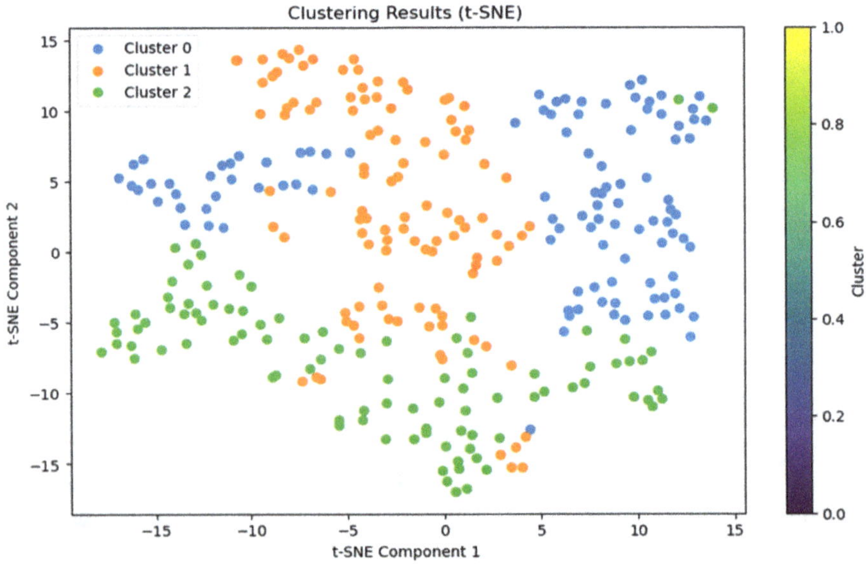

FIGURE 6.11 Cluster approach for SpO_2 prediction using t-SNE (left log activity).

from face features showed improvement and were evaluated for different habitual activities.

Figure 6.10 represents the t-SNE clustering approach for walking as habitual activity. In the 2D scale, clustering results among 309 persons' face features were distributed per quartile, as shown in Table 6.9 with reference to corresponding scores as illustrated in Table 6.8.

In Figure 6.10, clustering analysis using t-SNE for the left fetus sleep stage describes the *k*-means algorithm and its scatter plot for three different clusters. It visualizes the face statistical features, such as mean and SD, using 2D plot and predicts SpO_2. Table 6.10 describes *k*-means clustering against metrics that potentially isolate

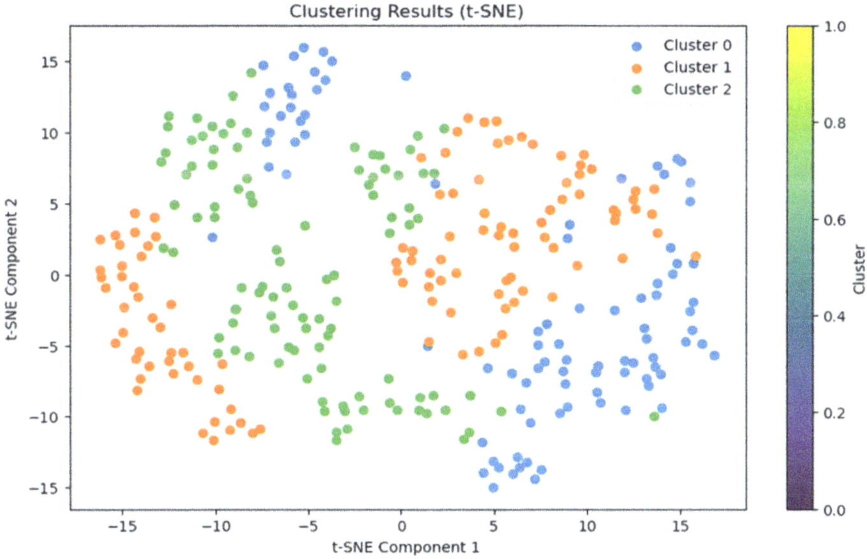

FIGURE 6.12 Cluster approach for SpO_2 prediction using t-SNE (prone activity).

TABLE 6.12
Cluster performances against performance metrics for prone as habitual activity

Performance measures against face for walking activity	Performance metrics	Score	Scale range	Inference
Object similarity between neighbouring clusters	Silhouette score	0.188	±1	Cluster moderate
Cluster density and separation	Calinski–Harabasz index	71.58	0 to 100	Fair
Mean between each cluster	Davies–Bouldin index	1.63	1 to 2	Good

the face features to predict SpO_2. The silhouette score 0.198 describes object similarity between neighboring clusters in a moderate way. The Calinski–Harabasz index of 74.89 infers a fair result regarding cluster density and separation. The Davies–Bouldin index of 1.62 was good enough for mean observation between each cluster.

The t-SNE clustering analysis of left log sleep activity, as depicted in Figure 6.11, employs *k*-means clustering against various metrics to potentially identify facial features for predicting SpO_2. The effectiveness of *k*-means clustering for the left log is confirmed in Table 6.11, which shows a silhouette score of 0.184, indicating the clustering's ability to categorize object similarities among adjacent clusters., the Calinski–Harabasz index of 70.96 describes cluster density and separation, and the Davies–Bouldin index of 1.65 is good enough for mean observation between each

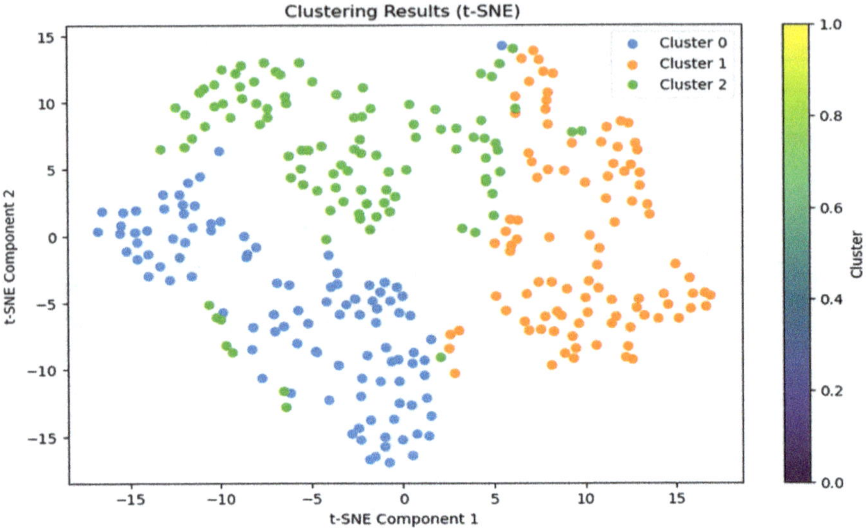

FIGURE 6.13 Cluster approach for SpO_2 prediction using t-SNE (right log activity).

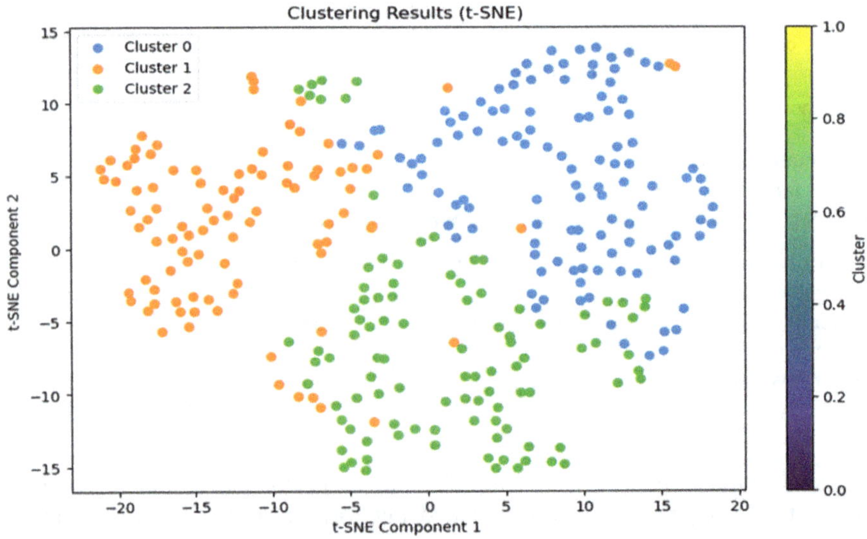

FIGURE 6.14 Cluster approach for SpO_2 prediction using t-SNE (right fetus activity).

cluster. In Figure 6.11, left log sleep activity against *k*-means clustering with the scores in Table 6.10 indicates well-defined clusters among face statistical features. Table 6.12 shows different performance metrics against *k*-means clustering for prone sleep activity as illustrated in Figure 6.12. This infers a compact relationship among features extracted from the face and indicates that moderate clustering took place. The other three stages of sleep activity, as shown in Figures 6.13–6.15, show moderate

TABLE 6.13
Shows sleep stages with *k*-means clustering with performance metrics and inference

Performance criteria evaluated	Performance metrics	Sleep stages with inference					
		Right foetus		Right log		Supine	
Object similarity between neighbouring clusters	Silhouette score	0.202	Fair	0.207	Fair	0.195	Moderate
Cluster density and separation	Calinski–Harabasz index	75.29	Moderate	80.10	Fair	76.65	Moderate
Mean between each cluster	Davies–Bouldin index	1.61	Good	1.54	Moderate	1.58	Moderate

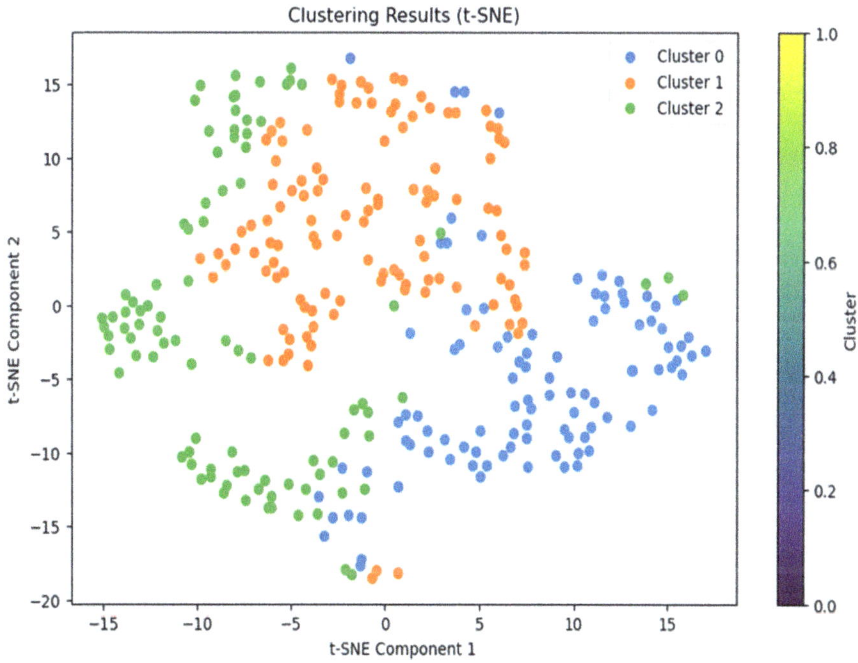

FIGURE 6.15 Cluster approach for SpO_2 prediction using t-SNE (supine activity).

clustering using *k*-means algorithm when validated with performance metrics such as the silhouette score, Calinski–Harabasz index, and Davies–Bouldin index, as shown in Table 6.13.

6.3 CONCLUSION

The suggested method aimed to minimize ambulatory requirement and enhance ongoing health and wellness within individuals' home settings in a comprehensible manner. In this approach, face contours after each activity were discussed with reference to gray-scale image and a suitable probabilistic approach, such as RMSE, R^2, mean absolute error (MAE), and mean square error (MSE) for various activities. By considering PCA, linear face features, as well as nonlinear face features through KPCA, were considered with reference to the training time for different supervised ML algorithms. Habitual walking and gym activity provided less training time compared with the free flow sleep model. For the unsupervised learning algorithm, clustering sleep stages with face features achieved a good score in the Calinski–Harabasz index compared with habitual walking and gym activity.

6.4 FUTURE SCOPE

In a conventional approach, to recover the average value of each image, the inverse of the eigenvalue decomposition matrix is applied. The accuracy of this process is evaluated by comparing the results with a reference grayscale image. The suggested method can be employed to predict the time required before actual system implementation occurs, functioning as a non-destructive testing technique in the field of computing. The unsupervised ML approach for identifying intermittent sleep stages must be validated prior to its recommendation for additional computational processes.

REFERENCES

[1] Hebbar, Pragati B., Angel Sudha, Vivek Dsouza, Lathadevi Chilgod, and Adhip Amin. "Healthcare delivery in India amid the Covid-19 pandemic: Challenges and opportunities." *Indian Journal of Medical Ethics* (2020).

[2] Núñez, Alicia, S. D. Sreeganga, and Arkalgud Ramaprasa. "Access to Healthcare during COVID-19." *International Journal of Environmental Research and Public Health* 18, no. 6 (2021): 2980.

[3] Kapoor, Megha, Karuna Nidhi Kaur, Shazina Saeed, Mohd Shannawaz, and Amrish Chandr. "Impact of COVID-19 on healthcare system in India: A systematic review." *Journal of Public Health* Research 12, no. 3 (2023): 22799036231186349.

[4] Rane, Nitin. "Transformers for medical image analysis: Applications, challenges, and future scope." (2023). http://dx.doi.org/10.2139/ssrn.4622241

[5] Omar Adil Deheyab, A., Mohammed Hasan Alwan, Islam khalid Abdul Rezzaqe, Omar Abdulkareem Mahmood, Yousif I. Hammadi, Ali Noori Kareem and Maha Ibrahim. "An overview of challenges in medical image processing." In *The 6th International Conference on Future Networks & Distributed Systems (ICFNDS '22), December 15, 2022, Tashkent, TAS, Uzbekistan*. New York, NY, USA: ACM, 2022, p. 8.

[6] Haldane, Victoria, Chuan De Foo, Salma M. Abdalla, Anne-Sophie Jung, Melisa Tan, Shishi Wu, Alvin Chua et al. "Health systems resilience in managing the COVID-19 pandemic: Lessons from 28 countries." *Nature Medicine* 27 (2021): 964–980. https://doi.org/10.1038/s41591-021-01381-y

[7] Sarker, I.H. "Machine learning: Algorithms, real-world applications and research directions." *SN Computing Science* 2 (2021): 160. https://doi.org /10.1007/s42979-021-00592

[8] Mazzei, Daniele, and Reshawn Ramjattan. "Machine learning for Industry 4.0: A systematic review using deep learning-based topic modelling." *Sensors (Basel, Switzerland)* 22, no. 22 (2022): 8641.

[9] Hamed Dabiri, Khashayar Rahimzadeh, and Ali Kheyroddin. "A comparison of machine learning- and regression-based models for predicting ductility ratio of RC beam-column joints." *Structures* 37 (2022): 69–81, ISSN 2352-0124.

[10] Yaqub, Muhammad, and Wontae Lee. "Modeling nutrient removal by membrane bioreactor at a sewage treatment plant using machine learning models." *Journal of Water Process Engineering* 46 (2022): 102521.

[11] Srivathsan, K., S. Bharath, A. Malini, R. Kumaravel, and Vandana Sharma. "Extended virtual reality based memory enhancement model for autistic children using linear regression". *International Journal of System Assurance Engineering and Management*. Springer, 2024, pp. 1–11.

[12] Warih Maharani, and Veronikha Effendy, "Big five personality prediction based in Indonesian tweets using machine learning methods." *International Journal of Electrical and Computer Engineering (IJECE)* 12, no. 2 (2022): 1973–1981, ISSN: 2088-8708. DOI: 10.11591/ijece.v12i2.pp1973-1981

[13] Sarker, Suchismita, Robert Tang-Kong, Rachel Schoeppner, Logan Ward, Naila Al Hasan, Douglas G. Van Campen, Ichiro Takeuchi et al. "Discovering exceptionally hard and wear-resistant metallic glasses by combining machine-learning with high throughput experimentation." *Applied Physics Reviews* 9, no. 1 (2022).

[14] Arjaria, Siddhartha Kumar, Abhishek Singh Rathore, and Gyanendra Chaubey. "Developing an explainable machine learning-based thyroid disease prediction model." *International Journal of Business Analytics (IJBAN)* 9, no. 3 (2022): 1–18

[15] Zafra, Amelia, and Eva Gibaja. "Nearest neighbor-based approaches for multi-instance multi-label classification." *Expert Systems with Applications* 232 (2023): 120876.

[16] Agarwal, Govind, Chirag Goel, Chunduru Sri Abhijit, and Alok Chauhan. "Development and comparative analysis of an instance-based machine learning classifier." *SPAST Reports* 1, no. 2 (2024).

[17] Ayats, H. Ambre, Peggy Cellier, and Sébastien Ferré. "Concepts of neighbors and their application to instance-based learning on relational data." *International Journal of Approximate Reasoning* 164 (2024): 109059.

[18] Alhussan, Amel Ali, Fatma M. Talaat, El-Sayed M. El-kenawy, Abdelaziz A. Abdelhamid, Abdelhameed Ibrahim, Doaa Sami Khafaga, and Mona Alnaggar. "Facial expression recognition model depending on optimized support vector machine." *Computers, Materials & Continua* 76, no. 1 (2023).

[19] Subudhiray, Swapna, Hemanta Kumar Palo, and Niva Das. "Effective recognition of facial emotions using dual transfer learned feature vectors and support vector machine." *International Journal of Information Technology* 15, no. 1 (2023): 301–313.

[20] Zhang, Xian, J. Adam Noah, Rahul Singh, James C. McPartland, and Joy Hirsch. "Support vector machine prediction of individual Autism Diagnostic Observation Schedule (ADOS) scores based on neural responses during live eye-to-eye contact." *Scientific Reports* 14, no. 1 (2024): 3232.

[21] Rajasekaran, Umamaheswari, G. K. Sriram, P. Ramyavarshini, and A. Malini. "XAI-based light-weight CNN-HAR model using random sampling." In *Lecture Notes in Networks and Systems*, 2023, 730 LNNS, pp. 377–388.

[22] Rumahorbo, Brilyan Nathanael, Kenjovan Nanggala, Gregorius Natanael Elwirehardja, and Bens Pardamean. "Analyzing important statistical features from facial behavior in human depression using XGBoost." *Communication Mathematical Biology Neuroscience* 2023 (2023): Article-ID.

[23] Saeed, Vaman Ashqi. "A framework for recognition of facial expression using HOG features." *International Journal of Mathematics, Statistics, and Computer Science* 2 (2024): 1–8

[24] Khan, Talha Ahmed, Rehan Sadiq, Zeeshan Shahid, Muhammad Mansoor Alam, and Mazliham Bin Mohd Su'ud. "Sentiment analysis using support vector machine and random forest." *Journal of Informatics and Web Engineering* 3, no. 1 (2024): 67–75.

[25] Wu, Lei-jie, Xu Li, Ji-dong Yuan, and Shuang-jing Wang. "Real-time prediction of tunnel face conditions using XGBoost Random Forest algorithm." *Frontiers of Structural and Civil Engineering* (2024): 1–19.

[26] Kshatri, Sapna Singh, Deepak Singh, Bhavana Narain, Surbhi Bhatia, Mohammad Tabrez Quasim, and Ganesh Ram Sinha. An empirical analysis of machine learning algorithms for crime prediction using stacked generalization: An ensemble approach. *IEEE Access* 9 (2021): 67488–67500.

[27] Mukta, Md Saddam Hossain, Jubaer Ahmad, Akib Zaman, and Salekul Islam. "Attention and meta-heuristic based general self-efficacy prediction model from multimodal social media dataset." *IEEE Access* (2024).

[28] Jiao, Liuyang, and Jianan Yao. "Design of an Olympic performance prediction system based on optical sensing technology and facial expression recognition." (2024).

[29] Lee, Dong Yun, Narae Kim, ChulHyoung Park, Sujin Gan, Sang Joon Son, Rae Woong Park, and Bumhee Park. "Explainable multimodal prediction of treatment-resistance in patients with depression leveraging brain morphometry and natural language processing." *Psychiatry Research* (2024): 115817.

[30] Yong Sun, Yanfang Zhao, Jifa Wu, Nan Liu, Xuming Kang, Shanshan Wang, and Deqing Zhou. "An explainable machine learning model for identifying geographical origins of sea cucumber Apostichopus japonicus based on multi-element profile." *Food Control*, 134 (2022): 108753, ISSN 0956-7135.

[31] Sungil Hong, Junghyun Kim, and Eunhwa Yang. "Automated text classification of maintenance data of higher education buildings using text mining and machine learning techniques. *Journal of Architectural Engineering* V, no. 28 (2022). DOI: 10.1061/(ASCE)AE.1943-5568.0000522

[32] Veerashetty, Sachinkumar, Virupakshappa, and Ambika. "Face recognition with illumination, scale and rotation invariance using multiblock LTP-GLCM descriptor and adaptive ANN." *International Journal of System Assurance Engineering and Management* 15, no. 1 (2024): 174–187.

[33] Safdar, Sadia, Muhammad Rizwan, Thippa Reddy Gadekallu, Abdul Rehman Javed, Mohammad Khalid Imam Rahmani, Khurram Jawad, and Surbhi Bhatia. Bio-imaging-based machine learning algorithm for breast cancer detection. *Diagnostics* 12, no. 5 (2022): 1134.

[34] Latha, S., P. Muthu, Samiappan Dhanalakshmi, R. Kumar, Khin Wee Lai, and Xiang Wu. "Emerging feature extraction techniques for machine learning-based classification of carotid artery ultrasound images." *Computational Intelligence and Neuroscience* 2022 (2022).

[35] Lu, Min, Ruijie Yin, and X. Steven Chen. "Ensemble methods of rank-based trees for single sample classification with gene expression profiles." *Journal of Translational Medicine* 22, no. 1 (2024): 140.

[36] Dujaili, Mohammed Jawad Al. "Survey on facial expressions recognition: Databases, features and classification schemes." *Multimedia Tools and Applications* 83, no. 3 (2024): 7457–7478.

[37] Hidayat, Fadhil, Ulva Elviani, George B. Situmorang, Muhammad Zaky Ramadhan, Figo Agil Alunjati, and Reza Fauzi Sucipto. "Face recognition for automatic border control: A systematic literature review." *IEEE Access* (2024).

[38] Grimmer, Marcel, Christian Rathgeb, and Christoph Busch. "Pose impact estimation on face recognition using 3d-aware synthetic data with application to quality assessment." *IEEE Transactions on Biometrics, Behavior, and Identity Science* (2024).

[39] Marukatat, Sanparith. "Tutorial on PCA and approximate PCA and approximate kernel PCA." *Artificial Intelligence Review* 56, no. 6 (2023): 5445–5477.

[40] Abdullah, Azween, S. Nithya, M. Mary Shanthi Rani, S. Vijayalakshmi, and Balamurugan Balusamy. "Stacked LSTM and Kernel-PCA-based ensemble learning for cardiac arrhythmia classification." *International Journal of Advanced Computer Science and Applications* 14, no. 9 (2023).

[41] Latha, S., Dhanalakshmi Samiappan, P. Muthu, and R. Kumar. "Fully automated integrated segmentation of carotid artery ultrasound images using DBSCAN and affinity propagation." *Journal of Medical Biology Engineering* 41 (2021): 260–271. https://doi.org/10.1007/s40846-020-00586-9

[42] Hsiao, Rong-Shue, Tian-Xiang Chen, Mekuanint Agegnehu Bitew, Chun-Hao Kao, and Tzu-Yu Li. "Sleeping posture recognition using fuzzy c-means algorithm." *Biomedical Engineering Online* 17 (2018): 1–19.

[43] Islam, Samiul, Saman Hassanzadeh Amin, and Leslie J. Wardley. "A supplier selection & order allocation planning framework by integrating deep learning, principal component analysis, and optimization techniques." *Expert Systems with Applications* 235 (2024): 121121.

[44] Yazdani, Hamid Reza, and Ali Reza Shojaeifard. "Facial recognition system using eigenfaces and PCA." *Mathematics and Computational Sciences* 4, no. 1 (2023): 29–35.

7 A Survey of Interoperability and Security Challenges in the IoT Healthcare Environment

Parthiban S. and Saranya J.

7.1 INTRODUCTION

Interoperability, that is, integration between many systems and devices, is an essential feature of apps. Terms like standards, middleware, integration, and interoperability are often used interchangeably. Interoperability simplifies the integration of diverse devices, enabling the creation of innovative and flexible services and facilitating efficient application development. Non-interoperability leads to inefficiency, particularly in handling crises or unique requirements. This survey offers a comprehensive overview of methods and tactics addressing interoperability issues, including a taxonomy of potential solutions for compatibility challenges [1, 2]. Blockchain technology has recently come to light as a potential solution to these kinds of problems and breaches. In view of the Internet of Things' (IoT's) wider practical application in the medical industry, we investigate the security implications of its layered design in this chapter [3, 4]. We categorize the various layers of security concerns that IoT faces, along with the special dangers and security problems that IoT-based healthcare systems must deal with in terms of computation, authentication, and communication [5, 6]. We then discuss the use of blockchain technology to assist healthcare businesses in overcoming various IoT security challenges [7, 8].

7.2 INTEROPERABILITY: A GLIMPSE INTO THE FUTURE OF HEALTHCARE INTEROPERABILITY

IoT has opened the door to a new world of intelligence and user adaptability. It has mechanized and electronically changed many routine tasks and given rise to sentient items that can perceive and interact with their environment. Additionally, these gadgets are accessible at any time and from any location [9], [10].

 DOI: 10.1201/9781003484233-7

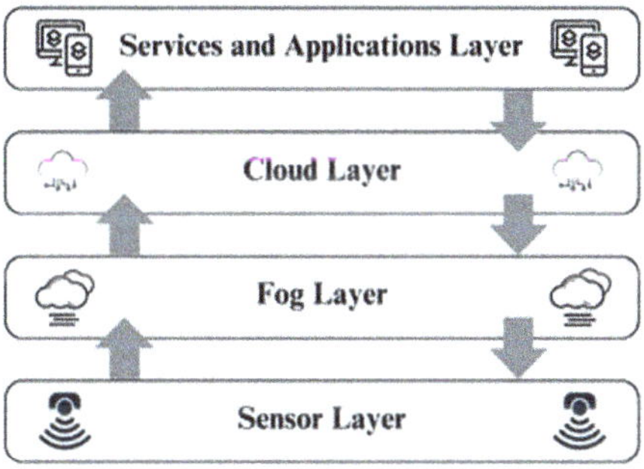

FIGURE 7.1 General IoT architecture.

As ideas for smart buildings, smart cities, and other IoT-enabled concepts emerge, academics, developers, and consumers are all very interested in IoT. However, proprietary goods that are incompatible are causing the rise of these IoT devices to lag behind in the market [11].

IoT currently lacks a precise standard structure, although Figure 7.1 [12] illustrates a generic hierarchical IOT architecture.

7.2.1 Definitions of Interoperability

There are several definitions of interoperability that usually associate qualities related to its significance and potential advantages, but there isn't a single, accepted definition of interoperability.

To develop a definition, we may utilize the following:

- Without requiring any work from the end user, interoperability offers methods of connectivity, collaboration, and partnership for the interchange and transfer of data [13]-[14].
- The process of integrating disparate platforms and building an extensive database through interoperability lowers costs, facilitates the creation of new services, and creates open marketplaces for data processing [15].
- Interoperability refers to the capacity to communicate data in a particular setting, and receive and comprehend it in another [16], [17].
- Interoperability is the process of standardizing the structure of information collected from different sensors so that it may be exchanged, analyzed in real-time, and queried consistently [18].
- The process of fostering interoperability among developers allows them to work together to construct broadly accepted solutions [19], [20].
- One of the most significant design criteria for a smart city is interoperability, which is essential for cutting expenses related to systems, data, and applications [21], [22].

- When service providers don't want to work together on a single platform, interoperability acts as a mediator [23], [24].
- Policies, standardized practices, and shared ideas that support resource cooperation and data uniformity are known as interoperability [25], [26].

7.2.1.1 IoT Development Stages [27], [28], [29], [30], [31]

This is an overview of IoT devices.

- Radio frequency signals or physical connections enable human users to directly manage equipment [32].
- In order to establish a gateway between them, humans have control of their gadgets while they are online [33, 34].
- When devices need to be directly linked to the Internet, this is when the concept of smart devices should be presented.
- These gadgets are getting more features to improve their memory and computational power.

The most recent IoT hierarchy (Dev, Fog, Core Fog, Cloud, and Apps) is created using Core Fog Nodes [35, 36]. Using various protocols, data formats, languages, ideas, and other tools, many firms are experimenting with IoT in many domains [37, 38].

7.2.2 Interoperability Properties

Interoperability is associated with a number of attributes, such as the source of data formats, stages, actions, situations, appropriate levels, and context.

7.2.2.1 Interoperability Types [15], [39], [40]

- Horizontal communication with many databases, devices, platforms, and providers (e.g., Azure, AWS, Google, and IBM).
- Vertical communication between the system, data source, and user. One way to lower machine-to-machine (M2M) costs related to open platform integration protocols could be to produce cars with interoperability compatibility.

7.2.2.2 Levels of Interoperability

- Foundation level: Disinfecting various infrastructures [15].
- Functional collaboration refers to the technical (hardware and software) aspects of data exchange via portals without the need for general functionality, that is, the capacity to understand the data [16].
- Structural level: The description of grammar, syntax, and data structure at the scale of sensible data transmission in standard formats [41].
- Semantic level: Using standard data models, the systems comprehend the precise meaning of the data that are transferred [42].

7.2.2.3 Types of Data Sources [15], [43]

- Make data accessible to everybody.
- Information that needs permission to be accessed by a third party.
- The exchange of data between cities and other entities.
- Static information, like a place or structure's position.
- Real-time information gathered via wireless network sensors, for example.

7.2.2.4 Conditions for Achieving Interoperability [41], [44]

- Generality, which allows for use in a variety of sectors.
- Effectiveness, which guarantees that the use cases have a suitable solution.
- Consistency, when using the same application again yields the same outcome.
- Transparency that conceals intricate technical details.
- Scalability that makes big data analytics accessible to all users.
- The ability to operate with several layers thanks to its verticality.
- Horizontality, which facilitates working with many application domains.
- Security, privacy, and trust that guarantee a secure, reliable, and intrusion-free environment [45].

7.2.2.5 IoT Interoperability Activities [46], [20]

- Learn about the various locations in cities.
- It is possible to access shared resources by utilizing the same formats for data storage.
- Platform independence, enabling usage across many geographies and cooperation tools [47].
- The service can connect to multiple platforms by standardizing the service's interface; these platforms each offer distinct data and work together to create new services.

7.2.3 Driven Thought and Importance

True integration provides essential data for achieving various goals, ideas, thoughts, and approaches [13]. Smart cities, characterized by open data platforms, collaborative e-government data centers, and individuals acting as sensors, face challenges due to numerous outdated, incompatible, and non-standard systems operated by public or private entities [48]. The lack of interoperability in these technologies limits the potential for interesting and practical applications in smart cities [14]. Currently, smart cities rely on closed systems with restricted capabilities, hindering expansion and integration due to accessibility and data exchange limitations [15]. The diverse data generated by different components of smart cities presents challenges, requiring standardization and real-time processing using standardized query methods [16, 18]. While smart city development focuses on intelligent, secure, and environmentally friendly services, the absence of a unified ontology results in disjointed services that resemble private property, complicating their integration with other smart city services [19, 21]. A powerful video compressive sensing encryption technique based on bit-level, pixel-level, and nucleotide sequence functions, as well as the fractional order hyperchaotic Chen system, has been proposed and implemented. The suggested method ensures enhanced security and efficient video compression [49].

Collaboration and compatibility across smart city applications and systems are crucial, as highlighted by various instances [23]. Interoperability is vital in disaster response, fostering collaboration among teams and agencies to expedite actions and mitigate consequences. It enables the quick transfer of resources, even to inaccessible locations [25].

The belief is that smart cities will advance civilization by extensively employing sensors and robotics, especially in healthcare and humanitarian assistance. For this vision to materialize, these robots must effectively communicate and collaborate with leadership or decision-support centers and with each other to fulfill their responsibilities [50]. Enhanced healthcare, relying on constant monitoring through various sensors to measure vital signs accurately, demands data exchange and the resolution of format disparities. For instance, during a home ambulance visit, the immediate unification of all electronic health data is critical for patient safety [51].

The complexity of smart healthcare arises from information heterogeneity and the requirement for cross-departmental, cross-technological, cross-location collaboration [26]. Smart sensor and cloud service operations need to be connected with the standard applications that these apps offer [52].

The complexity of smart healthcare stems from diverse data and the requirement for cooperation between many departments, devices, and locations [26]. This also holds true for the transportation industry. For smart cities to facilitate the creation of novel services and apps that might solve traffic congestion and air pollution, open data and open architecture are essential [53]. In addition to providing typical applications (e.g., parking management, garbage segregation, healthcare applications, security, and power metering), these applications must function with smart sensors and cloud services operations [52].

It is necessary for them to be in the same place for a solution to facilitate cross-platform interaction [54]. Since most service providers utilize sensors that are maintained across several platforms, interoperability is required since certain sensors are unable to function on a single, shared platform. Consequently, the data may be stored as big data, and time series forms on a cloud [24]. Due to the scattered nature of IoT and its applications, real-time big data processing is challenging because of the significant gap in the standard type of data [28, 40, 41].

The public should achieve sustainability in various areas within smart cities, covering monitoring, safety, collaboration, health services, marketing, facility management, transportation, traffic congestion, environmental preservation, green services, and more. Smart city innovations must be rooted in open data usage. To enhance service quality, performance, flexibility, and intelligence, tight integration with context is essential [55, 56].

7.2.4 Interoperability: Historical Solutions and Approaches

The necessity to tackle interoperability gaps in application processing has intensified, notably with the surge in millions of services and apps for IoT-related smartphones, devices, and systems. Several attempts have been made to address this issue. Research suggests various approaches to support interoperability, including incorporating it into device designs from the beginning [57].

However, challenges like ownership issues, middleware complexities, collaboration-facilitating application programming interfaces (APIs), and the establishment of common concept dictionaries make this task challenging. Finally, we present and go over a list of primary or branching techniques [58].

The following examples serve as a broad summary of interoperability assistance strategies:

7.2.4.1 Mapping

The process of translating data between formats and establishing an abstraction at the data level allows the systems to work together. This is known as data mapping [13]. In [51], researchers explored the concept of a mapper code that translates JavaScript Object Notation (JSON) from Extensible Markup Language (XML).

7.2.4.2 Middleware

In order to accommodate various sources, the mediator may operate at the database level or at the level of communications between applications. Similar to a broker, this is a publish-subscribe system. These mechanisms are effective in resource-constrained environments and typically rely on the Message Queuing Telemetry Transport (MQTT) protocol, which offers data protection, but lacks i006E site discovery capabilities in Symantec Web technologies [13], [15], and [25]. One suggested method for acting as a middleman between apps and services is the cloud [20].

7.2.4.3 Translator

At the application level (between the sender and the recipient), a translator – which can be one-way or two-way is commonly used to convert data between different formats so that the recipient can understand it [13].

7.2.4.4 Wrapper

By acting as a bridge between external systems and legacy systems, the wrapper helps to encase these systems in a layer that facilitates communication with them [13].

7.2.4.5 Data Adapter

A data adapter is a middleman that provides a single private query interface in standard formats for connecting a large number of databases. This enables the creation of a web service to enable users across several frameworks and databases to access data without worrying about the heterogeneity of those databases or the range of applications that utilize them [24]. In [50], researchers created the Robot Operating System (ROS) platform to enable communication between robotic devices and drones and the unified command center. The platform uses an adapter to act as a means of communication among the web service and the drone.

7.2.4.6 Message Exchange

On the platform of a particular data exchange, services or apps collaborate on message exchange by using mutually understood standard data representations, such as XML and JSON [13], [25]. The notion of an event-messaging system within smart cities was introduced by the authors of [57].

7.2.4.7 APIs

APIs enable programs providing open methods that may be accessed from other applications and systems to deliver particular services or information in the format that the caller requests [13]. A single, unified standard must be used, and an API is typically only appropriate for reaching consensus on particular, shared focus areas [15]. Emphasis is placed on the need and importance of making it easier to collect and share data using open APIs in [30].

7.2.4.8 Bridge

Applications themselves serve as the foundation for bridges or external gates, which are preferable to application modification. Since applications are developed for a variety of purposes, the bridge maps data between multiple common formats and translates protocols [25]. The authors of [21] proposed using three interoperable business models (Proxy, Standard APIs, and Semantic Web) to find a consensus platform or bridge. The agent must adapt the information among them if the criteria differ.

7.2.4.9 Service-Oriented Architecture (SOA)

In order to enable automation with REST, SOA emulates the API gateway principle and makes it easier for IoT services to be reused. A software framework for apps and services, an intermediary layer, interaction coding, a layer of abstraction, and a visualizer are the layers that make up the platform [31]. A basic web service called "InterSensor," introduced by researchers in [40], offers a way to link to many platforms and their models of data in order to integrate data from various sensors. According to [59], standard web apps may make the process of integrating data easier.

7.2.4.10 Dictionary

Ontology or dictionary adoption by system developers can use a common vocabulary to handle the issue for new systems. To support the above, whenever feasible, it is best to depend on expanding and utilizing an existing ontology. A common dictionary was proposed in [41] as a means of integrating diverse data. Research in [26] highlights the necessity of creating guidelines, norms, and shared ideas to support source collaboration and data uniformity.

7.2.4.11 Ontology

Ontology supports catalog workers by creating a dictionary of concepts, facilitating the establishment of shared concepts for effective communication, collaboration, and data comprehension among services and applications. It is often recommended to enhance existing ontologies rather than creating new ones from scratch, aiming to increase compatibility and support for earlier systems [60, 61]. Several well-known libraries demonstrate the ontological concept of creating an intelligent city that ensures interoperability on various stages (OpenSensingCity, VoC, Ready4SmartCity, Lov4IoT, etc.) in [22]. Domain-specific data, including the climate, wellness, water, intelligent homes, transport, parking areas, and environmental issues, is the main focus of these catalogs [62].

7.2.4.12 Semantics

Semantics is a technique that helps services and apps work together more effectively when exchanging data by using gestures or tokens to interpret messages. It relies on ontology and indirectly utilizes methods from natural language processing, data processing, and retrieval [13]. One platform that provides terminology and ideas shared by billions of web pages and search engines is Schema.org, which may be customized for particular areas or circumstances [20]. Joint modeling, suggested in [41], uses heuristics to build new triads, linking concepts and enriching content via semantic web technologies. The concept of a Resource Description Framework-based repository, where users can access and use vocabulary, was introduced in [63]. In [46], semantics is investigated to improve configuration and service quality. According to [64], data annotation utilizing the RDF trinity is advised for improved comprehension while transferring information between systems. In order to establish shared standards and concepts inside the same metropolis or between different metropolises, the investigation in [19] uses the framework and ontology.

7.2.4.13 Standardizing

Processing that is required is sped up by data standardization and profiling. This kind of real-time processing of big data is possible. Data manipulation, analysis of context, the ontology, web-based semantic approaches, and semantic annotations are some of the procedures and techniques in data profiling that we must perform in order to determine semantics for objects [18]. It is important to remember that the cloud can offer several support tiers, including the virtual, application, application interface, central services, and application layers [42].

The concept of normalizing data for completeness and similarity, making it easier to handle, is discussed in [28]. This involves actions like adding or removing duplication, treatment, resizing, managing time, and queuing up data. TabDoc, a novel technique that shows how to extract additional information from documents, is presented in [17]. These documents need to be represented in one of the commonly used formats (Document Type Definition (DTD), XML, or XML Schema Definition (XSD). In order to enhance mobile app interoperability in the smart metropolises, particularly in the field of smart transports [65], two standards, O-M1CO-DF and O-M1CO-DF, are investigated in [66].

7.2.4.14 Distributed Intelligent Digital Archive

In [67], researchers recommended the use of an intelligent digital archive that is distributed, and enables many users and organizations to share information that is modeled according to a consistent or stipulated manner. To provide particular kinds of data, in [24], researchers looked into Twitter, in addition to other platforms (OpenSensors, ThinkSpeak, Fireware, and Weather Underground). By the way highlighted in [63], complete data accessibility improves system sustainability and opens up new uses for public information in smart metropolises [56]. The concept of using an open government to achieve sustainable development in smart towns is covered in [68].

7.2.4.15 Open Data

Access to public or centralized information and data is facilitated by a platform that provides publicly available data for many applications and services. This platform can operate as an e-participation hub, crucial for e-governments [48]. Ideally, an open standard on a specific data format should be the basis for the efficient management of data access, storage, and coordination [25]. Using URLs to define, grant access to, and query different objects and connections, the LoV project from the European Union is highlighted in [63].

In addition to connecting common interfaces, defining the contexts necessary for interoperability, and allowing syntactical threading throughout prevalent information and messaging protocols like Symantec and XML, with semantics threaded execution determined by the meaning of the content, a citation is provided in [42] to emphasize the significance of agreement on syntax, semantics, and concepts. One such technique, put out in [51], makes use of cloud computing to create a single data center with the goal of offering a centralized data repository.

Central platforms for the IoT ecosystem have been proposed by other academics [16]. It is important to have a shared language and communication protocols. Creating a single data platform that facilitates data management and interchange across several applications is advised in [26]. It carries out several tasks, such as (i) central connection, which serves as a coordinator amongst the various systems; (ii) self-care, where each system applies the information at the centralized platform and manages itself; and (iii) knowledge: certain apps and systems were given tasks by the centralized system to handle particular data segments on the centralized platform [69].

7.2.4.16 Three-Level Hybrid

Three degrees of resolution are provided in [15], as opposed to just one, and they handle the following:

- Foundational Level: A method that eliminates the need for data interpretation in order to communicate or obtain information via gateways or APIs.
- Structural Level: Using common languages or protocols, similar-format data sharing defines the syntax, data structure, and format, as seen in the JSON, MQTT and XML formats.
- Semantic Level: Contributing systems need to use standard data formats and the Internet in order for them to comprehend the precise meaning of the data being delivered.

7.2.4.17 Web of Things (WoT)

Using a smart pilot framework for city temperature control as an example, WoT mission investigated the benefits and disadvantages regarding open systems [44], [70]. By using open standard technologies, WoT enables consumers to engage with IoT over the web; interoperability platforms such as Ready4SmartCity, OpenSensingCity, Lov, and Lov4IoT are a few examples [44], [70]. The Federation, as stated in [25], aims to accomplish integration through the use of uniform interfaces, agreement on data model standards, restrictions on design engineering, and standardized communication messages across collaborating systems including components. Standardized protocols (SOAP and REST) and standard data description formats (XML and JSON) are used [25].

The creation of smart cities requires the use of well-defined rules and standards [51]. According to a suggestion in [41], a federal structure should be established to combine current systems and provide developers with a framework for constructing cohesive projects. This approach addresses syntactic, semantic, and technical interoperability challenges. The notion of an union layer is introduced at the database platform level [71], which is very helpful when working with several data representation types. It is also advised to use "Open Information" and "Smart Metropolitan Profile" [71].

7.2.4.18 Platform for Development

In order to locate more suitable apps and services, developers can modify and establish unified APIs by using common pattern models of information, which are created by the development platform [20]. It offers a platform that satisfies a number of crucial requirements, which are listed below:

- Establish a standard web interface for semantic descriptions of services and resources at the cloud or fog level, like BigIoT [27, 72].
- Resources employing standardized formats for data representation are accessible through a common framework.

7.2.4.19 Abstraction

A comprehensive framework called abstraction is employed to categorize smart city infrastructure into different fields. Using a full-service operator and a central smart control, this combines the advantages of smart metropolitan priorities (health, safety, cooperation, monitoring, daily services, and parking utilities) [71].

Examples of standard applications that leverage shared protocols and solutions across several domains are provided in [52], such as the GreenIoT framework. A set of separate files called the SOS approach is presented in [14]. These files enable heterogeneous systems to work together toward a shared goal.

7.2.4.20 Publishing and Marketplace System

Econo-API has implemented a revised protocol for developing apps and distributing services and products via a publisher platform. A platform for facilitating the exchange of services and data has been built [44].

The structure is composed of the subsequent levels:

- Network Things: All devices or systems that are linked with the internet.
- Access Layer: Examples of unified protocols that let devices and apps compete with one another are Hypertext Transfer Protocol (HTTP), Constrained Application Protocol (CoaP), MQTT, Presence Protocol (XMPP), and Extensible Messaging.
- Find Layer: This layer uses adaptable semantic models and content-aware messaging to present data in a manner that simplifies the process of indexing and searching.
- Share Layer: The type of data, its safe publication through a publisher or customer, incentives for service provider stakeholders to engage, and processing transparency.
- Compose Layer: Offers an integrated development environment (IDE) so that anybody without programming experience may create suitable services and apps.
- Using interfaces, rules, permissions, and access control to integrate security management.

7.3 BLOCKCHAIN

7.3.1 Introduction

Over the past decade, the healthcare industry has experienced a significant advancement as a result of the widespread use of IoT, especially with wearables and mobile devices, which have improved health data interchange for accurate diagnosis. However, the existence of sensitive patient data raises security and privacy issues. As a potential remedy for these issues, blockchain technology has surfaced and provides a strong foundation for protecting health data in healthcare systems based on IoT.

7.3.2 IoT Integrated with Healthcare Systems

IoT-enabled remote health monitoring offers advantages over traditional methods. Radio-frequency identifications (RFIDs) and portable sensors streamline health checks and device identification. These devices bridge the virtual and physical realms, continuously transmitting real-time health data of virtual patients. The proactive nature of IoT-driven remote health monitoring revolutionizes the healthcare industry by facilitating effective data collection for disease risk maps, surveillance, and health statistics [73].

Patients' bodies have sensors that transmit data to health monitoring devices, which save it in the cloud for effective administration. Security is still a major worry, though, particularly when it comes to encrypting data from low-resource devices to guarantee integrity and secrecy throughout transmission [74].

7.3.3 Security Issues in IoT-Based Healthcare Applications

Despite advancements in scalability, challenges remain in data security and transmission reliability, with concerns about data sharing and leakage in the IoT ecosystem [75, 76].

This section discusses security difficulties with IoT-based healthcare systems, including issues with authentication, storage, communication, time synchronization, and sensing layer problems. The sensing layer is mainly used for security defense, employing time source nodes to prevent inaccuracies [77]. Detailed discussions on specific issues can be found in subsequent subsections.

7.3.3.1 Security Threats on Sensing Nodes

IoT sensors and actuators comprise the sensing layer, which is responsible for detecting physical activity in its surroundings [78, 79]. The sensors pick up data in a range of circumstances.

The node capture and bogus data injection codes, which an attacker used to carry out these nefarious actions, are described in Figures 7.2 and 7.3, respectively. Such risks affect temperature sensors, ultrasonic sensors, and other kinds of sensors.
The sensing layer is linked to the following issues:

Node Capture: In the sensing layer, a major challenge is node capture. These nodes, often low-power actuators and sensors, can be easily breached and taken control of by attackers. The malicious node becomes part of the IoT system, and the attacker only needs to engage in malicious activity to gain control [80].

Malicious Code Injection Attack: An attacker can simply modify and alter data by introducing malicious code into the sensing layer node. An attacker may utilize this technique to get access to the IoT system [81].

Attack Involving the Injection of False Data: The assailant gains control of the endpoints and falsifies data from an IoT system. The IoT system's-controlled nodes all produce false and inaccurate data, which can cause the system to fail [82].

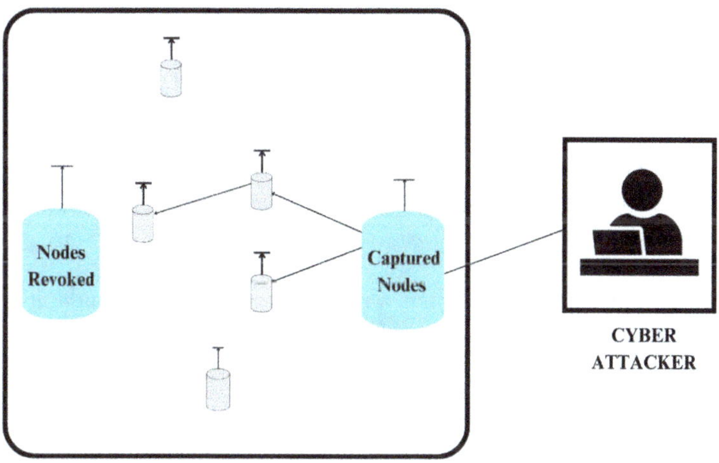

FIGURE 7.2 Acquiring nodes and injecting false data.

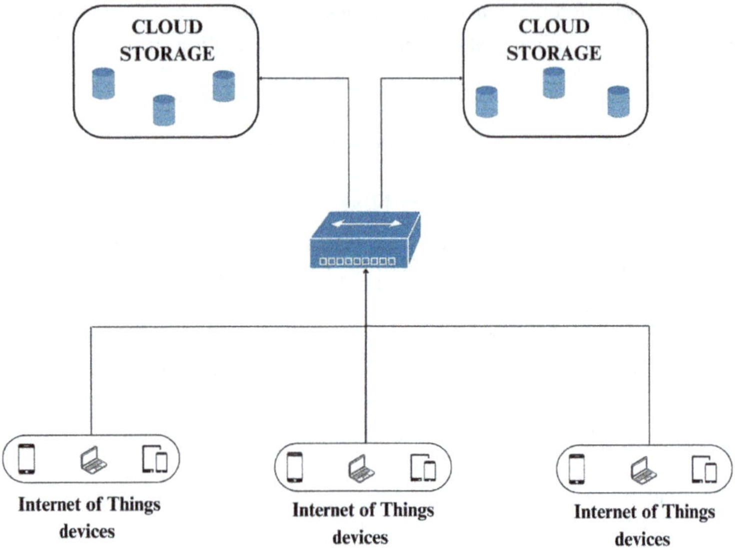

FIGURE 7.3 Network based on IoT.

Side-Channel Attacks: Side-channel attacks happen when adversaries attack nodes directly with the intention of taking private data from them and giving it to a third party. Third parties are also given access to power usage data. An illustration of a side-channel attack is in [83].

Eavesdropping and Interference: The terms "eavesdropping" and "interference" describe how attackers obtain information from multiple sources and disrupt different stages of the process, like data transfer and authentication processes [84].

Sleep Deprivation Attacks: Attackers that target a node and insert malware that throws IoT into an endless loop are known as sleep deprivation attackers. This affects the sensing layer's sensors, causing rapid depletion of battery power due to infinite loops [83].

Phishing Site Attack: Attackers using phishing sites may target several IoT devices with a minimum of effort. A person may encounter a phishing attempt when they visit a different webpage [81].

Access Attack: When someone enters a network without authorization, it's known as an access attack. In this kind of assault, the unauthorized person steals important network data [85].

DDoS Attack: A distributed denial of service (DDoS) attack occurs when an individual deliberately makes a large number of unauthorized requests to a network, resulting in a slowdown and disruption of its normal functioning [86].

Attack on Data Transition: Attacks using data transition occur if the information is moved between locations. The attacker only targets the network and steals vital information from it. It's also known as a cyber-attack at times [85].

Attacks by Routing: In the context of routing attacks, a malevolent node inside the larger network may try to manipulate the route that each piece of information follows when moving between two specific locations [86].

Theft of Data: Data transfer through multiple phases in an adversary's acquisition of user data is referred to as data theft. When using a seemingly trustworthy IoT application, users will be reluctant to provide their personal information. These applications make it simple to steal data [86].

Sniffing Out Attacks: Through the use of several applications, attackers monitor everything that occurs within the network. Furthermore, they use the software to steal personal data [82].

Reprogram Attack: Attackers could easily reprogram IoT devices because the programming process is not secure [83].

7.3.3.2 Issues with a Centralized System

In numerous IoT applications, including the medical field, constant information flow is essential to maintaining the patient's medical record. But if IoT devices proliferate, the server may become slower, which would affect how well patient data are updated and perhaps result in data loss. The use of a centralized storage system poses a risk of sensitive patient data loss due to cyberattacks [87]. An IoT-based network's design is shown in Figure 7.3.

Cloud storage systems are commonly used for outsourcing patient health records in the personal health data exchange system. However, relying on a single large company as a third party creates a potential single point of failure when data volume and connected devices increase [73]. The constant data requests from numerous IoT devices can strain centralized storage, and even with backups, cloud service providers may face unforeseen events, preventing clients from accessing their data [88].

7.3.3.3 Issues with Time Synchronization and Incentive

For medical IoT applications to provide accurate monitoring and prompt patient care, time synchronization is essential. On the other hand, if data are not sent promptly, a rogue node inside the network might cause significant problems by upsetting synchronization. For instance, if a patient's heart rate data are not synchronized, it might have potentially lethal consequences [77].

Service providers continuously exchange data, but privacy concerns often hinder data providers from releasing information. The lack of a compensation mechanism for these valuable services and support for future developments can be addressed more effectively with blockchain technology [88].

7.3.4 IoT with Blockchain

Blockchain is a decentralized record-keeping system that uses a hash function to connect each transaction to the first one in a sequential way, along with timestamps. The process of aggregating transactions is done through the use of a Merkle tree, while blockchain technology maintains the resulting root hash. Simply, the root hash is required to be verified in order to preserve security since changes made to one transaction impact all hashes. Due to the inclusion of cryptographic keys in each block, it becomes arduous and tedious for attackers to manipulate the data [89]. Further, testing and validation are crucial in addressing security issues with respect to blockchain technology [90].

Blockchain technology is advocated as a reliable and tamper-proof data format for IoT data, meeting specific needs [91, 92]. The process of circulating transactions on the blockchain is called mining. Organizations are developing platforms like Ethereum, Hyperledger, Fabric, and Ripple to simplify the development and maintenance of blockchain systems [93].

In 2015, the Linux Foundation introduced Hyperledger Fabric, a permissioned blockchain platform with identity management and access control features, customizable for diverse business requirements. Consensus algorithms guarantee a uniform methodology for the storage and implementation of consensus-requiring transactions, such as smart contracts. Transactions deemed invalid [94, 95] are those that do not satisfy consensus requirements. Every new block that gets added to the blockchain using consensus techniques guarantees that it reflects the consensus reached by all nodes [92]. Achieving consensus is a key protocol goal, and each node must participate, with consensus algorithms seeking solutions beneficial to the entire network [96].

1. **Proof of Work (PoW):** The miner for the subsequent batch of blocks is chosen by the consensus mechanism depending on how well they solve a difficult mathematical puzzle. The node that exerts the highest computational capacity in solving this challenge is granted the privilege of mining the subsequent block. Bitcoin is an example of a blockchain that employs the PoW consensus mechanism [97].
2. **Proof of Stake (PoS):** The majority favors PoS over PoW. The Ethereum network utilizes PoW as its consensus method. Instead of investing resources in deriving a solution to a difficult problem, validators take part in this version by staking a portion of their currencies. An incentive structure is used by PoS to encourage validators to come to an agreement [97].
3. **Delegated Proof of Stake:** Delegated PoS (DPoS) is a variation of PoS where users stake tokens to endorse certain delegates who are responsible for validating the following block. Without transferring tokens between wallets, staking services enable users to pool their tokens and earn interest [97].
4. **Proof of Importance (PoI):** In the context of bitcoin, PoI means an attempt to demonstrate nodes' values inside the system so they may produce blocks [96].
5. **Proof of Elapsed Time (PoET):** PoET is a fair consensus technique that is frequently employed in blockchain networks that need user identification. With an equal chance of creating a block for every network validator, it guarantees fairness in the selection of the next block to create. In blockchain

technology, the proof phase is won by the validator whose timer value is the lowest; its user's block is then added [96].

6. **Practical Byzantine Fault Tolerance (PBFT):** The goal of PBFT is to solve problems with existing Byzantine Fault Tolerance techniques for low-overhead asynchronous systems [97]. The establishment of consensus, communication, and authentication node insertion are the points of security concern in IoT for intelligent navigation. Composition and authenticity are not in harmony when using the Byzantine consensus method, which is based on gossip policy and chronology. Nonetheless, the Byzantine consensus method protocol poses difficulties due to its extensive message size set and unstable connectivity [98]. Hu et al.'s approach [99] accomplishes decentralization, disability, and Byzantine error tolerance. However, if a node needs to transmit more data than the message capacity, it can lead to a deterioration in delivery quality. In order to ensure effective distribution, venues must refrain from gossiping about certain information elements beyond a predetermined number of times [91]. The gossip protocol used in the method can also slow down the program due to sluggish processing, raising concerns about speed.

Smart contracts, or self-triggered programs, run on blockchains like Ethereum, eliminating the need for central intermediaries in contracts. Ethereum is a secure

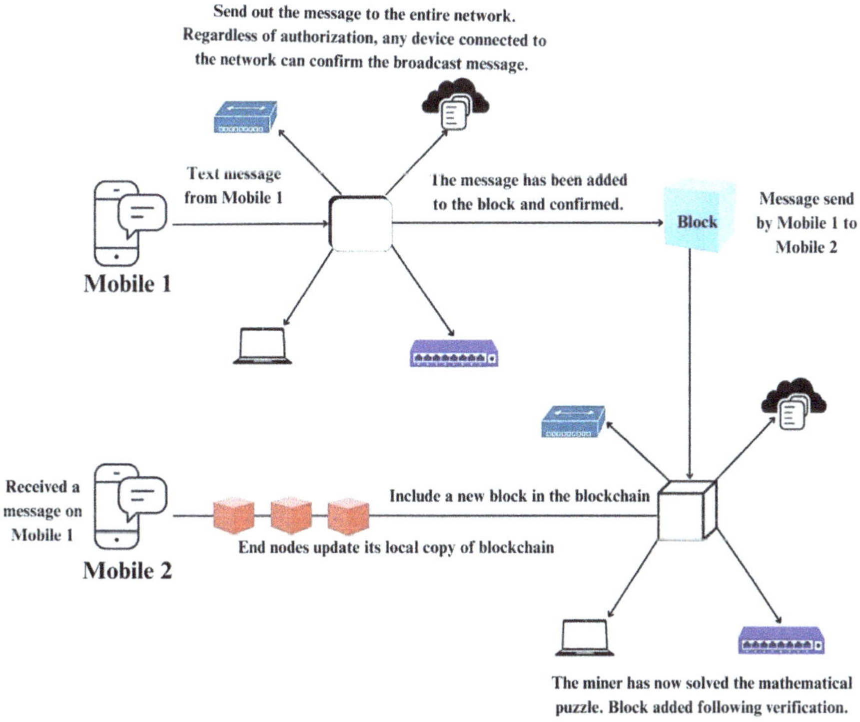

FIGURE 7.4 Blockchain working process.

platform for executing these contracts and gas represents the transaction cost. Miners determine gas prices based on network demand. A normal Ether (ETH) transaction has a minimum gas limit of 21,000 units. The "gas limit" refers to the upper limit of ETH that a user is willing to allocate for a transaction [85, 100].

Merkle trees add security to the blockchain ledger, safeguarding private data on IoT devices and potentially reducing the number of blocks. Resembling a binary tree, Merkle trees store hash values in roots and transfer data through leaf nodes [101], as in Figure 7.4. The number of blocks might be lowered by treating each root hash as a separate block. Multiple hashing layers at each tree node enhance data security [94]. Combining blockchain with Merkle tree manipulation could be a strategy given IoT device interconnectedness.

The blockchain's operation and the path a message takes from device M1 to device M2, passing via several middlemen, are depicted in Figure 7.4.

7.3.5 Securing Blockchain-Based Healthcare Systems

7.3.5.1 Keeping Sensing Equipment Safe

IoT devices, due to their constant data movement and connection to various networks, face security challenges. The vulnerability arises from their interaction with a cloud server accessible from anywhere. Implementing blockchain technology addresses this issue by ensuring data security and integrity through unchangeable hashes in each communication block. Moreover, the reliance on a single central cloud server creates a sole point of failure. By dispersing and safely keeping data, blockchain provides a remedy and reduces the hazards connected with centralized storage.

IoT devices face security risks from potential interference and misinformation. Blockchain technology, with its use of public and private keys, offers a solution by ensuring registered participants communicate securely. Even if encrypted data is accessed, malicious actors cannot exploit it. To address resource limitations, a proxy-based blockchain architecture allows efficient storage of encrypted resources, enabling quick retrieval for IoT devices.

7.3.5.2 Blockchain as a Security Solution for Centralized System Problems

A reliable and secure decentralized framework is created by blockchain technology. The revolutionary solution to privacy, security, and centralized storage problems has been recognized as blockchain [81]. Because of the volume of data that IoT devices transit, it is less secure and more likely to be misused. This is because their connectivity to a cloud server and a collection of other gadgets allows them to communicate from any location. But since every communication has a block in the blockchain that has a unique hash that is immutable, the utilization of blockchain technology may guarantee the integrity and privacy of data. Additionally, there is a potential vulnerability due to the fact that the vast amounts of data exchanged by IoT devices are kept on a centralized server that might fail. In order to address this problem, the data could be disseminated and kept safely by utilizing the blockchain system.

7.3.5.3 Blockchain-Based Time Synchronization and Incentive Problem Security

When IoT devices were initially constructed, time synchronization presented a security vulnerability. IoT devices addressed this flaw by implementing a blockchain-based solution, which established security. The recommended method is an approximation of documenting, recording, and broadcasting time via a publicly certified ledger. Developing a better PBFT consensus technique can be an effective way to use time synchronization [77]. Service providers are incentivized to continue offering valuable services and connecting with gadgets in the decades to come because IoT devices reward them for their efforts after they obtain services from them [102].

7.3.5.4 An Answer Amid the Fog and Edge Layers

The fog level uses a number of techniques to safeguard data and computations throughout the network. An intrusion detection system has been put in place to keep an eye out for any unusual behavior occurring on the network. Data may be safely sent between locations with the fog layer [81, 103]. Edge computing refers to the utilization of computing and cognitive resources at the periphery of a network. The fog and the user are separated by a small edge server. Edge layer experiences similar dispensation [103]. Low-cost connection is made possible by edge computing, which also stops data from being sent to the cloud or fog [103].

7.4 SECURITY ASPECTS ON INTEROPERABLE HEALTHCARE SECTOR: A HYBRID APPROACH

Due to a number of laws and rules, including the Healthcare Portability and Accountability Act (HIPAA), developing a strong, transparent, and interoperable e-healthcare infrastructure has proven to be impossible. Healthcare service providers prefer to keep patient data locked up in silos behind firewalls and security measures that are frequently insufficient.

Such a method restricts the capacity to obtain a comprehensive picture of a patient's medical history and leads to data breaches. This article described a national blockchain architecture for managing patient money, control of access, and Electronic Health Records (EHRs) within the context of India's national healthcare program [104]. High unpredictability and a wealth of dynamic phenomena in the fractional order hyperchaotic Chen system improve encryption, while DNA operations further boost algorithm efficiency [105]. Recent advances in the field of machine learning have produced advanced findings that show how quantum computers may be used to tackle artificial intelligence problems more quickly than traditional approaches [106].

This study involves evaluating the maturity of blockchain interoperability in multi-party and multi-chain ecosystems, deciding whether to implement new blockchain solutions based on their interoperability in order to develop new multi-chain use cases, or comparing the interoperability of various ecosystems in order to determine which ones to collaborate on across multiple chains.

7.5 CONCLUSION

An extensive summary of the strategies and techniques employed to address interoperability-related problems is given by this review of the literature. Along with this, the chapter offers a taxonomy of possible workarounds for the lack of compatibility. The advantages and disadvantages of the existing interoperability-promoting strategies have been identified in this study. A thorough literature analysis was done to look at the architectural processes supporting blockchain-based health management systems' interoperability and security. Several scenarios that highlight the possible uses of these mechanisms in connection to their history, issues, and other architectural concerns (e.g., security and interoperability) were developed in light of the findings.

REFERENCES

[1] R. S. Romaniuk, "IoT – Review of critical issues," *International Journal of Electronics and Telecommunications*, vol. 64, no. 1, pp. 95–102, 2018.

[2] I. Lee and K. Lee, "The Internet of Things (IoT): Applications, investments, and challenges for enterprises," *Business Horizons*, vol. 58, no. 4, pp. 431–440, Jul. 2015.

[3] C. C. Sobin, "A survey on architecture, protocols and challenges in IoT," *Wireless Personal Communications*, vol. 112, no. 3, pp. 1383–1429, Jun. 2020.

[4] M. Noura, M. Atiquzzaman, and M. Gaedke, "Interoperability in Internet of Things: Taxonomies and open challenges," *Mobile Networks and Applications*, vol. 24, no. 3, pp. 796–809, 2019.

[5] R. Liu and J. Wang, "Internet of Things: Application and prospect," in Proc*eedings of the* MATEC Web Conf*erences*, vol. 100, Les Ulis, France: EDP Sciences, 2017, p. 02034.

[6] F. Wortmann and K. Fluchter, "Internet of Things," *Business & Information Systems Engineering*, vol. 57, no. 3, pp. 221–224, 2015.

[7] B. Farahani, F. Firouzi, and K. Chakrabarty, "Healthcare IoT," in *Intelligent Internet of Things*, Cham, Switzerland: Springer, 2020, pp. 515–545.

[8] D. A. Gandhi and M. Ghosal, "Intelligent healthcare using IoT: An extensive survey," in *Proceedings of the 2nd International Conference Inventive Communications and Computational Technology (ICICCT)*, IEEE, Coimbatore, India, Apr. 2018, pp. 800–802.

[9] S. H. Shah and I. Yaqoob, "A survey: Internet of Things (IOT) technologies, applications and challenges," Proceedings of the *2016 IEEE Smart Energy Grid Engineering (SEGE)*, IEEE, Oshawa, ON, Canada, 2016, pp. 381–385.

[10] S. Li, L. D. Xu, and S. Zhao, "The internet of things: A survey," *Information Systems Frontiers*, vol. 17, no. 2, pp. 243–259, 2015.

[11] A. Malini, A. B. Yugakiruthika, S. P. Gunasekar, and R. Preethi, "Testing as a service focused on semantic interoperability: An approach," in *IEEE 4th Biennial International Conference on Nascent Technologies in Engineering*, IEEE, New York, NY, USA, 2021.

[12] P. P. Ray, "A survey on Internet of Things architectures," *Journal of King Saud University – Computer and Information Sciences*, vol. 30, pp. 291–319, 2016.

[13] A. Costin and C. Eastman, "Need for interoperability to enable seamless information exchanges in smart and sustainable urban systems," *Journal of Computing in Civil Engineering*, vol. 33, no. 3, May 2019, Art. no. 04019008, pp. 1-2.

[14] F. Lopes, S. Loss, A. Mendes, T. Batista, and R. Lea, "SoS-centric middleware services for interoperability in smart cities systems," in *Proceedings of the* 2nd International Workshop Smart, Association for Computing Machinery, New York, USA, Dec. 2016, pp. 1–6.
[15] M. Buchinger, P. Kuhn, A. Kalogeropoulos, and D. Balta, "Towards interoperability of smart city data platforms," in *Proceedings of the* Annual Hawaii International Conference on System Sciences (HICSS), 2021, IEEE, New York, USA, pp. 2454.
[16] A. Brutti, P. De Sabbata, A. Frascella, N. Gessa, R. Ianniello, C. Novelli, S. Pizzuti, and G. Ponti, edited by S. S. Shajahan and D. P. Acharjya, "Smart city platform specification: A modular approach to achieve interoperability in smart cities," in *The Internet of Things for Smart Urban Ecosystems.* Cham, Switzerland: Springer, 2019, pp. 25–50.
[17] S. Yang and R. Wei, "Semantic interoperability through a novel cross-context tabular document representation approach for smart cities," *IEEE Access*, vol. 8, pp. 70676–70692, 2020.
[18] S. Balakrishna, V. K. Solanki, V. K. Gunjan, and M. Thirumaran, edited by D. K. Sharma and R. Bhatia, "A survey on semantic approaches for IoT data integration in smart cities," in *Proceedings of the* International Conference on Intelligent Computing and Communication Technologies. Singapore: Springer, Jan. 2019, pp. 827–835.
[19] P. Espinoza-Arias, M. Poveda-Villalón, R. García-Castro, and O. Corcho, "Ontological representation of smart city data: From devices to cities," *Applied Sciences*, vol. 9, no. 1, p. 32, Dec. 2018.
[20] A. Bröring, S. Schmid, C.-K. Schindhelm, A. Khelil, S. Käbisch, D. Kramer, D. Le Phuoc, J. Mitic, D. Anicic, and E. Teniente, "Enabling IoT ecosystems through platform interoperability," *IEEE Software*, vol. 34, no. 1, pp. 54–61, Jan./Feb. 2017.
[21] J. Hwang, J. An, A. Aziz, J. Kim, S. Jeong, and J. Song, "Interworking models of smart city with heterogeneous Internet of Things standards," *IEEE Communications Magazine*, vol. 57, no. 6, pp. 74–79, Jun. 2019.
[22] A. Gyrard, A. Zimmermann, and A. Sheth, "Building IoT-based applications for smart cities: How can ontology catalogs help?" *IEEE Internet of Things Journal*, vol. 5, no. 5, pp. 3978–3990, Oct. 2018.
[23] W. M. da Silva, A. Alvaro, G. R. H. P. Tomas, R. A. Afonso, K. L. Dias, and V. C. Garcia, "Smart cities software architectures: A survey," in *Proceedings of the* 28th Annual ACM Symposium on Applied Computing, Association for Computing Machinery (ACM), New York, Mar. 2013, pp. 1722–1727.
[24] K. Chaturvedi and T. H. Kolbe, "InterSensor service: Establishing interoperability over heterogeneous sensor observations and platforms for smart cities," in Proceedings of the IEEE International Smart Cities Conference (ISC2), IEEE, New York, Sep. 2018, pp. 1–8.
[25] M. Pradhan, N. Suri, C. Fuchs, T. H. Bloebaum, and M. Marks, "Toward an architecture and data model to enable interoperability between federated mission networks and IoT-enabled smart city environments," *IEEE Communications Magazine*, vol. 56, no. 10, pp. 163–169, Oct. 2018.
[26] S. Liu, W. Li, and K. Liu, "Pragmatic oriented data interoperability for smart healthcare information systems," in *Proceedings of the* 14th IEEE/ACM International Symposium on Cluster, Cloud and Grid Computing, IEEE, New York, NY, USA, May 2014, pp. 811–818.
[27] A. A. A. Sen and M. Yamin, "Advantages of using fog in IoT applications," *International Journal of Information Technology*, vol. 13, no. 3, pp. 829–837, Jun. 2021.

[28] M. Babar and F. Arif, "Smart urban planning using Big Data analytics to contend with the interoperability in Internet of Things," *Future Generation Computer Systems*, vol. 77, pp. 65–76, Dec. 2017.

[29] A. A. A. Sen, F. A. Eassa, K. Jambi, and M. Yamin, "Preserving privacy in Internet of Things: A survey," *International Journal of Information Technology*, vol. 10, no. 2, pp. 189–200, Jun. 2018.

[30] A. Sharma, S. Acharya, V. Rajaraman, R. Ramesh, A. Babu, and B. Amrutur, "Schemas for IoT interoperability for smart cities," in *Proceedings of the 4th ACM International Conference on Systems for Energy-Efficient Built Environments*, Association for Computing Machinery, New York, Nov. 2017, pp. 1–2.

[31] O. Uviase and G. Kotonya, "IoT architectural framework: Connection and integration framework for IoT systems," March 2018, arXiv:1803.04780.

[32] H. Landaluce et al., "A review of IoT sensing applications and challenges using RFID and wireless sensor networks," *Sensors (Basel, Switzerland)*, vol. 20 , no. 9, art. no. 2495, pp. 1-25, 2020.

[33] L. B. Campos and C. E. Cugnasca, "Applications of RFID and WSNs technologies to Internet of Things," in *Proceedings of the IEEE Brazil RFID Conference*, IEEE, Sao Paulo, Brazil, Sep. 2014, pp. 19–21.

[34] M. Yamin and Y. Ades, "Crowd management with RFID and wireless technologies," in *2009 First International Conference on Networks & Communications*, IEEE, Bangalore, India, 2009, pp. 439–442.

[35] S. Yi, C. Li, and Q. Li, "A survey of fog computing: Concepts, applications and issues," in *Proceedings of the Workshop Mobile Big Data*, IEEE, Hong Kong, China, Jun. 2015, pp. 37–42.

[36] M. Iorga, L. Feldman, R. Barton, M. Martin, N. Goren, and C. Mahmoudi, *Fog Computing Conceptual Model, Special Publication (NIST SP)*. Gaithersburg, MD, USA: National Institute Standards Technology, 2018. DOI: 10.6028/NIST.SP.500–325.

[37] M. M. Sadeeq, N. M. Abdulkareem, S. R. M. Zeebaree, D. M. Ahmed, A. S. Sami, and R. R. Zebari, "IoT and cloud computing issues, challenges and opportunities: A review," *Qubahan Academic Journal*, vol. 1, no. 2, pp. 1–7, Mar. 2021.

[38] A. Hosseinian-Far, M. Ramachandran, and C. L. Slack, "Emerging trends in cloud computing, big data, fog computing, IoT and smart living," in *Technology for Smart Futures*, Cham, Switzerland: Springer, 2018, pp. 29–40.

[39] F. Ayadi, I. Colak, and R. Bayindir, "Interoperability in smart grid," in *Proceedings of the* 7th International Conference on Smart Grid (icSmartGrid), IEEE, New York, NY, USA, Dec. 2019, pp. 165–169.

[40] K. Chaturvedi and T. Kolbe, "Towards establishing cross-platform interoperability for sensors in smart cities," *Sensors*, vol. 19, no. 3, p. 562, Jan. 2019.

[41] A. Gyrard and M. Serrano, "Connected smart cities: Interoperability with SEG 3.0 for the Internet of Things," in Proceedings of the 30th International Conference on Advanced Information Networking and Applications Workshops (WAINA), Mar. 2016, IEEE, New York, NY, USA. pp. 796–802.

[42] A. Zeid, S. Sundaram, M. Moghaddam, S. Kamarthi, and T. Marion, "Interoperability in smart manufacturing: Research challenges," *Machines*, vol. 7, no. 2, p. 21, Apr. 2019.

[43] E. Palomar, X. Chen, Z. Liu, S. Maharjan, and J. Bowen, "Component-based modelling for scalable smart city systems interoperability: A case study on integrating energy demand response systems," *Sensors*, vol. 16, no. 11, p. 1810, Oct. 2016.

[44] J. Robert, S. Kubler, N. Kolbe, A. Cerioni, E. Gastaud, and K. Främling, "Open IoT ecosystem for enhanced interoperability in smart cities – Example of métropole de Lyon," *Sensors*, vol. 17, no. 12, p. 2849, Dec. 2017.
[45] O. Soultatos, M. Papoutsakis, K. Fysarakis, G. Hatzivasilis, M. Michalodimitrakis, G. Spanoudakis, and S. Ioannidis, "Pattern driven security, privacy, dependability and interoperability management of IoT environments," in Proc*eedings of the* IEEE 24th International Workshop on Computer Aided Modeling Design and Communication Links in Networks (CAMAD), IEEE, Athens, Greece, Sep. 2019, pp. 1–6.
[46] D. Tektonidis and A. Koumpis, "Accessible Internet-of-Things and Internet-of-Content services for all in the home or on the move," *International Journal of Interactive Mobile Technologies*, vol. 6, no. 4, pp. 25–33, 2012.
[47] M. Bagheri and S. H. Movahed, "The effect of the Internet of Things (IoT) on education business model," in *Proceedings of the* 12th International Conference on Signal-Image Technology & Internet-Based Systems (SITIS*)*, IEEE, Marrakech, 2016, pp. 435–441.
[48] J. Cano, C. E. Jimenez, and S. Zoughbi, "A smart city model based on citizen-sensors," in Conference Proc*eedings of the* IEEE 1st International Smart Cities Conference (ISC2), IEEE, Washington, D.C., USA Oct. 2015, pp. 173–175.
[49] S. Kayalvizhi, and S. Malarvizhi "Video transmission secrecy improvement based on fractional order hyper chaotic system," *Computer Systems Science and Engineering*, vol. 46, no. 1, pp. 1201–1214, Jan. 2023.
[50] M. Pradhan and S. Devaramani, "Enabling interoperability for ROS-based robotic devices for smart city HADR operations," in *Proceedings of the* IEEE Military Communications Conference (MILCOM*)*, IEEE, New York, Nov. 2019, pp. 1–6.
[51] A. Jaleel, T. Mahmood, M. A. Hassan, G. Bano, and S. K. Khurshid, "Towards medical data interoperability through collaboration of healthcare devices," *IEEE Access*, vol. 8, pp. 132302–132319, 2020.
[52] B. Ahlgren, M. Hidell, and E. C.-H. Ngai, "Internet of Things for smart cities: Interoperability and open data," *IEEE Internet Computing*, vol. 20, no. 6, pp. 52–56, Nov./Dec. 2016.
[53] P. S. Saarika, K. Sandhya, and T. Sudha, "Smart transportation system using IoT," in *Proceedings of the International Conference* Smart Technol*ogy* Smart Nation (SmartTechCon), IEEE, Bengaluru, India, Aug. 2017, pp. 1104–1107.
[54] C. E. Jimenez, A. Solanas, and F. Falcone, "E-government interoperability: Linking open and smart government," *Computer*, vol. 47, no. 10, pp. 22–24, 2014.
[55] J. Satyakrishna and R. K. Sagar, "Analysis of smart city transportation using IoT," in *Proceedings of the* 2nd Int*ernational* Conf*erence* Inventive Syst*em* Control (ICISC), IEEE, Coimbatore, India, Jan. 2018, pp. 268–273.
[56] T. Lodato, E. French, and J. Clark, "Open government data in the smart city: Interoperability, urban knowledge, and linking legacy systems," *Journal of Urban Affairs*, vol. 43, no. 4, pp. 586–600, Apr. 2021.
[57] A. Zabasta, N. Kunicina, K. Kondratjevs, A. Patlins, L. Ribickis, and J. Delsing, "MQTT service broker for enabling the interoperability of smart city systems," in Proceedings of the Energy Sustainability in Small Developing Economies (ES2DE), IEEE, New York, Jul. 2018, pp. 1–6.
[58] S. Anand and S. K. Routray, "Issues and challenges in healthcare narrowband IoT," in *Proceedings of the 2nd International Conference Inventive Communications and Computational Technology* (ICICCT), IEEE, Coimbatore, India, Mar. 2017, pp. 486–489.

[59] D. Buhalis and R. Leung, "Smart hospitality – Interconnectivity and interoperability towards an ecosystem," *International Journal of Hospitality Management*, vol. 71, pp. 41–50, Apr. 2018.
[60] Y. U. Devi and M. S. S. Rukmini, "IoT in connected vehicles: Challenges and issues – A review," in *International Conference* Signal Process*ing* Commun*ications* Power Embedded Syst*ems* (SCOPES), IEEE, Bangalore, India, Oct. 2016, pp. 1864–1867.
[61] N. H. Motlagh, M. Mohammadrezaei, J. Hunt, and B. Zakeri, "Internet of Things (IoT) and the energy sector," *Energies*, vol. 13, no. 2, p. 494, Jan. 2020.
[62] A. Sharma, S. Acharya, V. Rajaraman, R. Ramesh, A. Babu, and B. Amrutur, "Schemas for IoT interoperability for smart cities," in Proceedings of the 4th ACM International Conference on Systems for Energy-Efficient Built Environments, Association for Computing Machinery (ACM), New York, Nov. 2017, pp. 1–2.
[63] N. Kolbe, S. Kubler, J. Robert, Y. Le Traon, and A. Zaslavsky, "Towards semantic interoperability in an open IoT ecosystem for connected vehicle services," in Proceedings of the Global Internet of Things Summit (GIoTS), IEEE, New York, NY, USA, Jun. 2017, pp. 1–5.
[64] S. Jabbar, F. Ullah, S. Khalid, M. Khan, and K. Han, "Semantic interoperability in heterogeneous IoT infrastructure for healthcare," *Wireless Communications and Mobile Computing*, vol. 2017, Mar. 2017, Art. no. 9731806, pp. 1-10.
[65] A. Alnahdi and S.-H. Liu, "Mobile Internet of Things (MIoT) and its applications for smart environments: A positional overview," in Proc*eedings of the* IEEE International Congress on Internet of Things (ICIOT), IEEE, San Francisco, CA, USA, Jun. 2017, pp. 151–154.
[66] A. Karpenko, T. Kinnunen, T. Madhikermi, M. Robert, J. Främling, K. Dave, and A. Nurminen, "Data exchange interoperability in IoT ecosystem for smart parking and EV charging," *Sensors*, vol. 18, no. 12, p. 4404, Dec. 2018.
[67] P. Brizzi, D. Bonino, A. Musetti, A. Krylovskiy, E. Patti, and M. Axling, "Towards an ontology-driven approach for systems interoperability and energy management in the smart city," in *Proceedings of the* International Multidisciplinary Conference on Computer and Energy Science (SpliTech), Jul. 2016, pp. 1–7.
[68] C. E. Jiménez, F. Falcone, A. Solanas, H. Puyosa, S. Zoughbi, and F. González, "Smart government: Opportunities and challenges in smart cities development," in *Civil and Environmental Engineering: Concepts, Methodologies, Tools, and Applications*, Spain: IGI-Global, 2016, pp. 1454–1472. DOI: 10.4018/978-1-4666-9619-8.ch066.
[69] Y. Mehmood, F. Ahmad, I. Yaqoob, A. Adnane, M. Imran, and S. Guizani, "Internet-of-Things-based smart cities: Recent advances and challenges," *IEEE Communications Magazine*, vol. 55, no. 9, pp. 16–24, Sep. 2017.
[70] P. Murdock et al., "Semantic interoperability for the Web of Things," *Ph.D. dissertation*, Dépt. Réseaux et Service Multimédia Mobiles, Institut Mines-Télécom-Télécom SudParis, Tech. Rep. hal-01362033, 2016, p. 18.
[71] J.-Y. Ahn, J. S. Lee, H. J. Kim, and D. J. Hwang, "Smart city interoperability framework based on city infrastructure model and service prioritization," in Proceedings of the 8th International Conference on Ubiquitous Future Networks (ICUFN), IEEE, New York, Jul. 2016, pp. 337–342.
[72] R. Mahmud, R. Kotagiri, and R. Buyya, "Fog computing: A taxonomy, survey and future directions," in *Internet of Everything*. Singapore, Springer, 2018, pp. 103–130.
[73] A. R. Rajput, Q. Li, M. T. Ahvanooey, and I. Masood, "EACMS: Emergency access control management system for personal health record based on blockchain," *IEEE Access*, vol. 7, no. 7, pp. 84304–84317, 2019. DOI: 10.1109/ACCESS.2019.2917976.

[74] M. Hassanalieragh, A. Page, T. Soyata, G. Sharma, M. Aktas, G. Mateos, B. Kantarci, and S. Andreescu, "Health monitoring and management using Internetof- Things (IoT) sensing with cloud-based processing: Opportunities and challenges," in *IEEE International Conference on Services Computing, SCC*, IEEE, pp. 285–292, 2015. DOI: 10.1109/SCC.2015.47.
[75] N. Bui and M. Zorzi, "Healthcare applications: A solution based on the internet of things," in *Proceedings of the 4th International Symposium on Applied Sciences in Biomedical and Communication Technologies*, Wiley in Hoboken, NJ, USA, pp. 131–138, 2018. DOI: 10.5958/0974-360X.2018.00580.2.
[76] B. Lee, "Healthcare framework on the IoT open platform," service model, architecture," *International Journal of Applied Engineering Research*, vol. 9, no. 2, pp. 29783–29792, 2014. DOI: 10.1016/j.future.2016.02.020.
[77] K. Fan, "Blockchain-based secure time protection scheme in IoT," *IEEE Internet of Things Journal*, vol. 6, no. 3, pp. 4671–4679, 2019. DOI: 10.1109/jiot.2018.2874222.
[78] C. Crisan and B. Butunoi, "An IoT based smart home automation system," *International Symposium on Electronics and Telecommunications ISETC*, vol. 12, no. 4, pp. 321–334, 2021. DOI: 10.3390/s21113784.
[79] K. Salih, T. Rashid and N. Bacanin, "A comprehensive survey on the internet of things with the industrial marketplace," *Sensor*, vol. 22, pp. 321–341, 2022. DOI: 10.3390/s22030730.
[80] K. Zhao and L. Ge, "A survey on the internet of things security," in *Computational Intelligence and Security (CIS), 9th International Conference*, pp. 663–667, 2013. DOI: 10.1109/ACCESS.2018.2851611.
[81] Z. Lu, W. Liu, Q. Wang, G. Qu, and Z. Liu., "A privacy-preserving trust model based on blockchain for VANETs," *IEEE Access*, vol. 6, no. 4, pp. 45655–45664, 2018. DOI: 10.1155/2020/8831611.
[82] C. Kolias, G. Kambourakis, A. Stavrou, and J. Voas, "DDoS in the IoT: Mirai and other Botnets," *Computer*, vol. 50, no. 7, pp. 80–84, 2017. DOI: 10.1109/MC.2017.201.
[83] S. N. Swamy, D. Jadhav, and N. Kulkarni, "Security threats in the application layer in IoT applications," in *Proceedings of the International Conferences IoT Social, Mobile, Analytics Cloud (I-SMAC)*, pp. 477–480, 2017. DOI: 10.1109/ACCESS.2022.3205351.
[84] H. M. Hamad and M. Al-Hoby, "Managing intrusion detection as service in cloud networks," *International Journal of Computer Applications*, vol. 41, no. 1, pp. 35–40, 2012. DOI: 10.1372/Access.2021.897765.
[85] APWG. Phishing Activity Trends Report. Available: https://docs.apwg.org/reports/apwg_trends_report_q4_2017.pdf. [Accessed Feb. 12, 2019].
[86] C. Li and C. Chen, "A multi-stage control method application in the ght against phishing attacks," in *Proceedings of the 26th Computerised Security Academy Communication Across Country*, Frontiers Media, Switzerland, pp. 145–157, 2021. DOI: 10.3389/fcomp.2021.5630.
[87] Y. Chen, S. Ding, Z. Xu, H. Zheng, and S. Yang, "Blockchain-based medical records secure storage and medical service framework," *Journal of Medical Systems*, vol. 43, no. 4, pp. 1–9, 2018. DOI: 10.1007/s10916-018-1121-4.
[88] S. Wang, Y. Zhang, and Y. Zhang, "A blockchain-based framework for data sharing with fine-grained access control in decentralized storage systems," *IEEE Access*, vol. 17, no. 6, pp. 38437–38450, 2018. DOI: 10.1109/ACCESS.2018.2851611.
[89] H. Abie and I. Balasingham, "Risk-based adaptive security for smart IoT in eHealth," in *Proceedings of the 7th International Conference on Body Area Networks*, Institute for Computer Sciences, Social-Informatics and Telecommunications Engineering, Brussels, Belgium, pp. 269–275, 2012. DOI:10.4108/icst.bodynets.2012.250235.

[90] A. B. Yugakiruthika, and A. Malini, "A comprehensive tool survey for blockchain to IoT applications," in *Data Engineering for Smart Systems. Lecture Notes in Networks and Systems*, vol. 238. Springer, 2022. ISBN: 978-981-16-2640-1.

[91] E. Oyekanlu, C. Nelatury, A. O. Fatade, O. Alaba, and O. Abass, "Edge computing for industrial IoT and the smart grid: Channel capacity for M2M communication over the power line," in *Proceedings of the IEEE 3rd International Conference Electro-Technology National Development (NIGERCON)*, pp. 1–11, 2017. DOI: 10.1109/ACCESS.2019.2924045.

[92] T. Aste, P. Tasca, and T. D. Matteo, "Blockchain technologies: The foreseeable impact on society and industry," *Computer*, vol. 50, no. 9, pp. 18–28, 2017. DOI: 10.1109/MC.2017.3571064.

[93] R. Henry, A. Herzberg, and A. Kate, "Blockchain access privacy: Challenges and directions," *IEEE Security and Privacy*, vol. 16, no. 4, pp. 38–45, 2018. DOI: 10.1145/3133956.3134093.

[94] J. Wang, M. Li, Y. He, H. Li, K. Xiao, and C.Wang, "A blockchain based privacy-preserving incentive mechanism in crowdsensing applications," *IEEE Access*, vol. 6, pp. 17545–17556, 2018. DOI: 10.1109/ACCESS.2018.2805837.

[95] G. Asma. S. Aafety, *Privacy and security of sensitive data*, Springer, pp. 211–221, 2019. DOI: 10.5623/security.2019.2951.

[96] P. Arul and S. Renuka, "Blockchain technology using consensus mechanism for IoT-based e-healthcare system," *IOP Conferences Series Materials Science Engineering*, vol. 1055, no. 1, p. 012106, 2021. DOI: 10.1088/1757-899x/1055/1/012106.

[97] A. Jain and D. S. Jat, "A review on consensus protocol of blockchain technology," *Lectures Notes Networks Systems*, vol. 334, pp. 813–829, 2022. DOI: 10.1007/978-981-16-6369-7-72.

[98] W. Hu, Y. Hu, W. Yao and H. Li, "A blockchain-based byzantine consensus algorithm for information authentication of the internet of vehicles," *IEEE Access*, vol. 7, pp. 139703–139711, 2019. DOI: 10.1109/ACCESS.2019.2941507.

[99] E. Oyekanlu, C. Nelatury, A. O. Fatade, O. Alaba, and O. Abass, "Edge computing for industrial IoT and the smart grid: Channel capacity for M2M communication over the power line," in *Proceedings of the IEEE 3rd International Conference on Electro-Technology for National Development (NIGERCON)*, IEEE, New York, NY, USA, pp. 1–11, 2017. DOI: 10.1109/ACCESS.2019.2924045.

[100] R. Kandaswamy and D. Furlonger, *Blockchain-based transformation*, WITSC, pp. 312–334, 2021. www.gartner.com/en/doc/3869696-blockchain-based-transformation-a-gartner-trend-insight-report 43

[101] D. Koo, Y. Shin, J. Yun, and J. Hur, "An online data-oriented authentication based on Merkle tree with improved reliability," in *Proceedings of the IEEE International Conferences Web Services (ICWS)*, IEEE, New York, NY, USA, pp. 840–843, 2017. DOI:10.3390/app8122532.

[102] S. Chandrasekhar and M. Singhal, "Efficient and scalable query authentication for cloud-based storage systems with multiple data sources," *IEEE Transaction Services Comput*ing, vol. 10, no. 4, pp. 520–533, 2015. DOI: 10.1109/ACCESS.2022.3209355.

[103] M. Alrowaily and Z. Lu, "Secure edge computing in IoT systems: Review and case studies," in *Proceedings of the IEEE/ACM Symp. Edge Comput. (SEC)*, IEEE, New York, NY, USA,pp. 440–444, 2018. DOI: 10.1109/SEC.2018.00060.

[104] A. I. Taloba et al., "A blockchain-based hybrid platform for multimedia data processing in IoT-Healthcare," *Alexandria Engineering Journal*, vol. 65, pp. 263–274, 2023.

[105] S. Kayalvizhi, and S. Malarvizhi "A novel encrypted compressive sensing of images based on fractional order hyper chaotic Chen system and DNA operations," *Multimedia Tools and Applications*, pp. 1–18, Apr. 2019. DOI: 10.1007/s11042-019-7642-0

[106] A. Kumar, B. Surbhi, K. Keshav, S. Manjula Gandhi, S. Gayathri Devi, D. A. De J. Pacheco, and A. Mashat, "Survey of promising technologies for quantum drones and networks," *IEEE Access*, vol. 9, 2021, pp. 1-5.

[107] G. Bedi, G. K. Venayagamoorthy, R. Singh, R. R. Brooks, and K.-C. Wang, "Review of Internet of Things (IoT) in electric power and energy systems," *IEEE Internet of Things Journal*, vol. 5, no. 2, pp. 847–870, Apr. 2018.

[108] S. S. I. Samuel, "A review of connectivity challenges in IoT-smart home," in Proceedings of the 3rd MEC International Conference on Big Data Smart City (ICBDSC), IEEE, New York, NY, USA, Mar. 2016, pp. 1–4.

[109] E. Avelar, L. Marques, D. D. Passos, R. Macedo, K. Dias, and M. Nogueira, "Interoperability issues on heterogeneous wireless communication for smart cities," *Computer Communications*, vol. 58, pp. 4–15, Mar. 2015.

[110] J. Nilsson and F. Sandin, "Semantic interoperability in industry 4.0: Survey of recent developments and outlook," in Proceedings of the IEEE 16th International Conference on Industrial Informatics (INDIN), IEEE, New York, NY, USA, Jul. 2018, pp. 127–132.

[111] V. Hassija, V. Chamola, V. Saxena, D. Jain, P. Goyal, and B. Sikdar, "A survey on IoT security: Application areas, security threats, and solution architectures," *IEEE Access*, vol. 7, pp. 82721–82743, 2019. DOI: 10.1109/access.2019.2924045.

8 Automated Cardiovascular Disease Prediction Using Ant Colony Optimization with a Deep Learning Improved Neural Network

K. Sathya, R. Shanthi, J. Esther, C. Selvi, and M. Pandiyan

8.1 INTRODUCTION

Cardiovascular disease (CVD) is the major cause of death globally [1] and late diagnosis significantly increases CVD mortality. The early prediction of CVD risk has great potential to improve this devastating condition [2]. CVDs include heart disease, coronary artery disease, stroke, and hypertension. Globally, they are the leading disability and cause of death [3]. Lifestyle choices and genetics are the major risk elements. Health professionals are crucial in prevention and early detection education to prevent the spread of CVD. A healthy lifestyle and regular exploration are encouraged.

CVD symptoms can vary greatly. Chest pain, dyspnea, fatigue, and irregular heartbeat are common symptoms of heart failure and coronary artery disease [4]. On the other hand, the symptoms of muscle pain and nausea can include headaches, slurred speech, blurred vision, and paralysis on one side of the body. Many CVDs have such symptoms, making it hard to distinguish between them using these characteristics alone. For instance, chest pain may indicate heart failure or myocardial infarction. Furthermore, other than specific symptoms of CVDs, fatigue and dyspnea can also be symptoms of heart disease or high blood pressure (hypertension) Diagnosing and treating CVD requires a medical evaluation completed including imaging, laboratory tests, and physical examination. Special tests may sometimes be required [5]. This

 DOI: 10.1201/9781003484233-8

highlights the importance of maintaining cardiovascular health through a functional and customized approach.

CVDs affect the blood vessels of the heart, such as arteries and veins. With CVD on the rise, it has become known as the "second epidemic" in many countries, surpassing contagious diseases worldwide as the growing disability and cause of death among those older than 65 years [6]. Early detection is essential to reduce mortality. Echocardiography is a valuable tool and a useful method for diagnosing heart disease. This non-invasive technique uses sound waves to image the heart, showing information regarding the shape, size, and function of its valves and chambers. It is used to detect cardiac irregularities in infants and young children [7].

An effective approach to diagnose and evaluate CVD signs and symptoms after observation is to use longitudinal deep learning (DL) vectors to characterize the impact of variable risk factors. Study protocols are used to accurately detect cardiovascular symptoms. Study findings can enhance cardiovascular health in the United Arab Emirates (UAE) by enabling early detection and truculent treatment interventions [8,9].

Patient-supplied electronic medical records (EMRs) generate a wealth of medical data that can transform early CVD diagnosis and aggressive treatment, ultimately saving countless lives. This convention on the timely detection and effective management of CVD is expected to usher in a new era marked by significantly improved patient outcomes [10]. With error detection, critical condition identification, patient data analysis, and timely action, this decision support system (DSS) aims to provide indispensable information and support to e-health professionals. The need for more accurate and effective methods, such as DSS, has been emphasized by the laborious and common errors associated with the traditional manual assessment of CVD data [11].

Due to the increasing importance of big data in healthcare, artificial intelligence (AI) approaches, especially those based on machine learning (ML) and DL, are increasingly being applied to solve problems, and in intensive diagnostic and prognostic management [12]. In contrast to manual diagnostic approaches, AI systems are highly accurate in diagnosing the closeness of certain diseases because they analyze large amounts of health information. ML-driven diagnostic methods can predict diseases based on individual complication factors and be easily integrated into clinical DSSs, which is particularly noteworthy [13]. Due to their great potential, ML tools are useful for improving patient outcomes and diagnostic accuracy, especially in cardiology. ML is based on successive model input (text, images, etc.) and is particularly responsive to the desired prognosis (positive, pathological, or non-pathological). These models can provide more accurate and resource-efficient diagnosis of cardiomyopathy because they are trained on raw EMRs collected from inexpensive wearable devices [15].

Recently, DL has become important in the study of CVDs [16]. DL algorithms belonging to the artificial neural network (ANN) subtype are accurate at recognizing learning and patterns from complex and large datasets. DL is widely used in diagnostic research and imaging in medicine in all cases. DL has been shown to be surprisingly effective for cardiovascular health, especially its ability to identify correct patterns in complex data to diagnose heart disease and use imaging modalities, such as magnetic resonance imaging (MRI), angiogram, and echocardiogram.

DL systems are particularly good at identifying certain patterns and symptoms found in the medical images of cardiac problems. Using imaging analysis, abnormalities can be detected in the structure of the vasculature, blood flow, and heart [17]. In addition, DL is used to analyze cardiovascular data, including electrocardiograms (ECGs) and patient health records, in addition to image analysis. These systems use ECG data functions to predict the likelihood of certain cardiac events, including simple heart failure. DL systems also analyze patients' medical data to calculate the risk of heart disease, taking into account variables such as age, sex, lifestyle, and family history. Although DL for the diagnosis of cardiomyopathy is still at its growing level, early findings are so promising. DL is poised to play an important role in continuing the fight against CVD as information becomes more accessible and technological advances continue [18].

DL, mainly in natural language processing and image analysis, has shown tremendous potential in the medical field [19, 20]. DL applies ANNs to mine large datasets for patterns and predictions. DL's ability to independently extract features from unstructured data eliminates the need for time-consuming human factor engineering, which is one of its major advantages. DL models are well-suited to real-world healthcare applications due to their proficiency in big data and capacity to better adapt to new services [21, 22].

Regression analysis is used to extract features from DL-based data models for CVD prediction [23]. A unique study uses ML algorithms to identify prevalent chronic diseases where disease prevalence is high [24]. To predict outcomes, this study uses latent component modeling to identify clinical difference data collected in China from 2013 to 2015. The authors use a convolutional neural network (CNN) algorithm to extract features from statistical data and unstructured text. They identify the most common chronic diseases found in this area. Finally, a multi-disease risk estimation method is proposed for both structured and unstructured data based on the CNN. This study highlights the flexibility and potential of DL across a variety of healthcare contexts.

A statistical modeling technique called regression analysis is used to predict continuous outcomes based on predictor variables. Return, blood pressure, cholesterol, other related symptoms, etc., can be used for heart disease (CVD) diagnosis [25]. Usually, the testing of the dataset, validation, and training set are included to ensure the generalizability of the model. Subsequently, the experimental set-up is applied to analyze the performance of the model. Cross-validation methods are further effective in performance estimation. Regression models are needed to determine who is more likely to develop CVD. These models use variables related to cardiovascular risk to facilitate educated choices about preventive medication options [26].

Finding the best model for the task, and handling multiple factors, are challenges in CVD diagnosis. Research has shown that hyperparameter tuning and feature selection (FS) are two important techniques to significantly improve the performance of CVD detection systems. The main goal of FS is to find a highly suitable element for the CVD identification task. This is important because using too many factors can lead to overfitting, which makes the sample less applicable to a larger number of people. The model is able to make accurate predictions by selecting the most important attributes and focusing on the most informative data [27, 28].

Hyperparameter tuning fine-tunes the parameters of the model to maximize performance and ensure that they are optimized for the specific task of detecting CVDs. Hyperparameter tuning is important for accurate CVD detection, good generalization performance, less overfitting, and increased accuracy, in addition to FS This chapter presents an intelligent CVD diagnosis model (ACVD-ACOIDL). It combines advanced methods for DL and ant colony optimization (ACO). ACO is used for selecting features, min-max scaling is used for pre-processing the data, and a DL-improved neural network (DLINN) classifier is used for CVD classification in the ACVD-ACOIDL system. The hyperparameters of the DLINN classifier are optimized using Bayesian techniques. The efficacy of ACVD-ACOIDL can be evaluated using reference data from medical sources.

A number of notable advances have occurred in CVD assessment. Among these are the new concepts of positive CVD assessment integrated into the ACVD-ACOIDL approach and DLINN classification, the implementation of minimum-maximum normalization, ACO-based FS, and Bayesian optimization. It should be noted that there are currently no records of this combined method for CVD detection in the literature. The ACVD-ACOIDL method using ACO uses a novel technique called "ACO-based FS," which selects the best subset of features. This method attempts to reduce the computational cost when it improves model performance. In addition, the DLINN classifier uses Bayesian optimization, where hyper-criteria are optimized through a cross-validation process. Through optimization, the prediction accuracy of the method is still enhanced for the observed data, which can improve the evaluation of the model for CVD.

The remainder of the chapter is structured as follows: The algorithmic data measurement model, ACO-based FS technique, CVD classification using the optimal DLINN method, and additional steps of the proposed model. Analysis is provided on deep neural network classifiers for CVD and ACO. The final section of this chapter compares and evaluates the overall strengths of the models in the performance validation section.

8.2 RELATED WORK

Nagavelli et al. [29] examined a number of ML approaches for CVD identification. Automatic ischemia detection by analytical methods, weighted systems for naive Bayes estimation, and accurate classification by a combination of a support vector machine (SVM) and extreme gradient boosting were observed. These methods encourage the accurate diagnosis and prognosis of CVD. The improved SVM model developed for the dual-based method is used to detect cardiac arrest by SVM optimized with the dual-optimized method of cardiac arrest. Several methods are used to diagnose heart disease, each with its own advantages and disadvantages. Processing power, accuracy requirements, and data availability are some of the factors that determine the best option for an application.

The review in [30] looked at two approaches to determining adequate cardiovascular fitness. First, it uses sensitive sensors to collect data in real-time for risk assessment, including blood oxygenation and ECG readings. Second, it uses an optimized ANN (OANN) that combines distance-based misclassified instance extraction (DBMIR) and teaching–learning-based optimization (TLBO) to analyze CVD. This method, which includes training available online and offline together, works in phases of the risk assessment, delivering practical solutions for continuous monitoring and risk forecasting [31].

Ali et al.'s study [32] aimed to identify the best ML methods for CVD (heart disease) prediction. The usefulness of the features of each algorithm was evaluated and contrasted between supervised ML methods for heart disease prediction, except *K*-nearest neighbors (KNN) and the multilayer perceptron (MLP). The study [33] uses the UCI Repository database and health sensors to develop a powerful framework for heart disease prediction. The proposed method analyzes patient data and uses classifier algorithms to inform heart disease patients. The classifier is trained on the benchmark dataset during the training phase. In the next phase of testing, patient data are used to confirm the presence of heart disease.

Using a standard database, the study investigates the working principle of different classifiers, like J48, SVM, MLP, and logistic regression (LR), and the ML method of cardiac and neural analysis introduced by Li et al. [34]. Their method uses traditional options, like relief, the lower absolute shrinkage selection operator (LASSO), minimum-redundancy maximum relevance (MRMR), and many local learning and classification techniques, such as SVM, LR, ANN, KNN, naive Bayes, and decision trees. By eliminating irrelevant and redundant symptoms, this combined approach seeks to improve cardiac screening. Based on accessible clinical trials, Atallah and Al-Moussa [35] developed a robust ensemble algorithm for cardiovascular event prediction. Using real patient data, the system combined predictions from multiple ML algorithms in an effort to improve physician confidence and diagnostic accuracy. The findings showed that accuracy increased compared with relying on individual methods alone. It offered a more accurate prediction of cardiac fit.

Noele et al. studied the prevalence of CVDs in adults aged 65 years and older. [36]. Their study focused on risk factors, such as obesity, cholesterol, smoking, diabetes, lack of physical activity, high blood pressure, and a higher complication of acute stroke, connected to the most common problem of death and disability in this age group. Furthermore, in their study [37], they evaluated the use of CVD risk prediction models.

An overview of wearable photoplethysmography (PPG) and its research was provided by Charlton et al. [38]. The growing demand for smart wearable elements equipped with PPG sensors has made it possible to directly monitor cardiac health noninvasively. The study explored the PPG signal of arterial blood pressure measurement and it looked at several proposed combinations for effective assessment.

Chieng and Kistler developed the benefits of regular tea and coffee consumption in preventing CVD [39]. According to their research, people with metabolic syndrome benefit from two to three moderate cups of coffee a day, which can also reduce the complication of heart disease. Furthermore, the problem of a 9% reduction in blood pressure is associated with seven cups of coffee a day. Drinking tea and coffee may also help lower the risk of many CVDs, including atrial fibrillation, cardiac arrest, stroke, and death from CVD.

The triglyceride-glucose (TyG) index was examined by Tao et al. [40] as a potential biomarker for insulin resistance (IR), a known problem for CVD. By fusing fat and sugar elements, the TyG index provides a reliable and beneficial method for monitoring IR and controlling diseases such as hypertension and obesity prediction. Studies show that the TyG index outperforms the widely used HOMA-IR in evaluating IR in diabetic and non-diabetic subjects. The authors found that the optimization of the TyG score may enhance the stratification of risk factors and prediction of CVD outcome.

A study to analyze the efficiency of telemedicine in standardized care for CVD prevention was conducted by Battineni et al. [41]. The telemedicine system incorporates precise medical principles into the routine examination of patients with CVD as the disease progresses. Telemedicine enables secure telephone or video conversations through text, audio, and video exchanges of clinical information between patients and healthcare providers. Telecardiology, especially cardiology, offers many advantages in remote patient care. This study highlights the importance of telemedicine for providing quality care to patients with CVD.

In their paper, Bays et al. [42] provided information on problem factors integrated with CVD. They detected ten major problem factors, that is, hyperglycemia, cholesterol, obesity, renal disease, hereditary/familial cholesterol, hypertension, thrombosis/smoking, older age, race/ethnicity, and sex, and other demographic variables differ because CVD patients have various problem factors. To reduce the risk of CVD, the book emphasized the benefits of regular exercise, a balanced diet, and intermittent fasting.

To enhance prevention strategies, a study highlighting the importance of detecting and addressing problem factors integrated with CVD through comprehensive self-care considerations was conducted by Dixon et al. [43], who examined the effect of work-related factors on older people with CVD and self-care practices. Based on this theory, self-monitoring is a natural decision-making process. Research on the connection between illness markers and depressive symptoms was conducted by Ellis et al. [44]. As part of this study, 46 respondents in 61 eligible groups were interviewed, with a particular focus on older patients with serious illness, who frequently exhibit somatic symptoms of depression [45].

Although the exact nature of the association between dyspepsia and gastroesophageal reflux disease (GERD) is still unknown, Hsu et al. [46] suggested that the two conditions frequently coexist in the general population, although symptoms of these types were absent in 761 individuals in the study. This was reported in combination with epigastric pain or burning. Those with GERD-D exhibited more severe GERD symptoms and were more frequently associated with GERD-alone (IBS) syndrome [47]. It can be difficult for patients and physicians to attribute concomitant cause or activity to cardiovascular symptoms, such as palpitations, dyspnea, and chest tightness, in highly active individuals in stressful situations with generalized anxiety [48]. Even when not fitting the official criteria for a diagnosis of disorder, widespread anxiety about routine activities has been associated with promoting and accelerating CVD [49]. This includes stress and distress.

8.3 PROPOSED MODEL

This study proposes a novel ACVD-ACOIDL approach for better detection of CVD. Data scaling, feature subset selection applying ACO, classification with DLINN, and parameter optimization by Bayesian optimization are all included. The steps of the ACVD-ACOIDL method are illustrated in Figure 8.1, which also shows the natural flow of the research process. More efficient FS is possible with this new approach, which combines DL with DLINN for robust classification, uses ACO for FS, and uses Bayesian optimization to drive the overall accuracy of the CVD analysis, and provides adequate hyperparameter tuning.

8.3.1 Data Scaling Process

The first step in the ACVD-ACOIDL method is to fix the clinical data with a min-max scalar. This scalar transforms the original data linearly applying the min-max normalization technique. The variable is determined by the maximum (*MaxY*) and minimum (*MinX*) values of attribute A. Min-max normalization converts the attribute to a value M' in the specified range by using the limit values *N_MinX1* and *N_MaxX1*, usually zero to one. By standardizing and normalizing the data, this procedure ensures that it is suitable for use in subsequent analyses:

$$M' = \frac{M1 - MinX1}{MaxX1 - MinA1}\left(N\_MaxX1 - N\_MinX1\right) + N\_MinX1 \tag{1}$$

8.3.2 Algorithmic Design of the ACO-Based FS Technique

The ACO algorithm derives from the fact that ants find the most efficient routes to food sources through group foraging. Conventional selection techniques based on ACO are common and rely on prior knowledge of objects. On the other hand, the proposed algorithm presents a different approach by using the length and classifier performance of the important feature vectors as heuristic data for ACO. This modification makes the FS process more flexible, resulting in dynamic and efficient algorithms. To use ACO, the problem must be represented as a graph connected by nodes and edges. Figure 8.2 shows the procedure of the ACO method: 1. heuristic

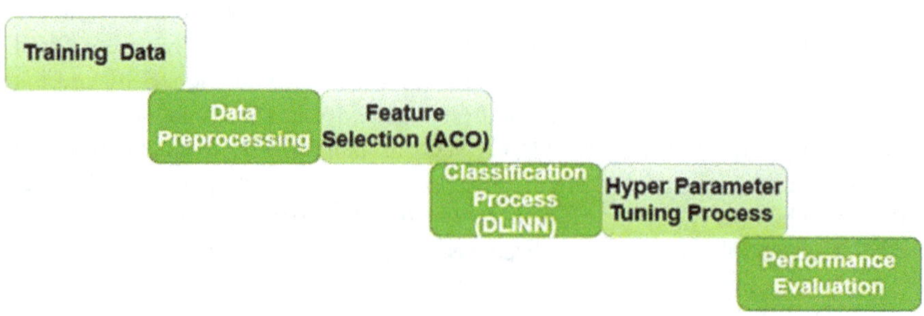

FIGURE 8.1 Workflow of the ACVD-ACOIDL algorithm.

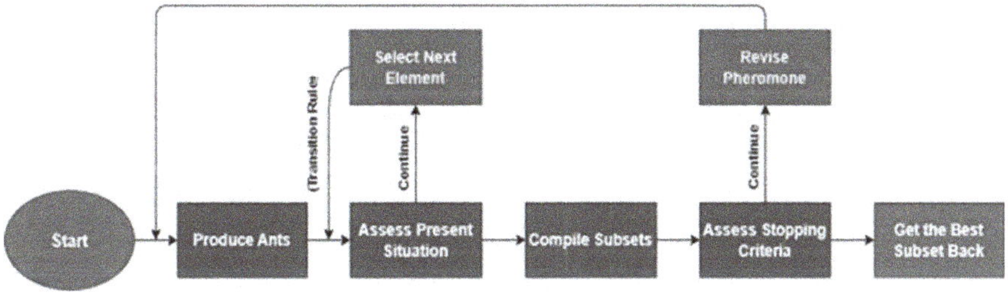

FIGURE 8.2 Flow diagram of the ACO method.

desirability (η), 2. construction of feasible solutions, 3. pheromone updating rule, and 4. probabilistic transition rule.

The problem depends on determining the appropriate method for ACO in terms of FS. The ACO design needs a graph representation in which the elements are indicated as edges and nodes that indicate that the next feature is selected. Figure 8.2 illustrates this process by visiting as many nodes as possible to find the best feature subset that matches the ant searching the graph. At node 'a', the ant can choose to add the next object (indicated by a dotted line) to its traverse.

According to the probabilistic transition rule, initially the ant chooses feature 'b', then 'c', and finally 'd'. The fused heuristic attraction of traversal and edge pheromone levels is the basis for such selection. The traversal ends when the current subset {a, b, c, d} reaches 'd' and satisfies the traversal stop requirement with sufficiently high classification accuracy. Then this feature subset is output as a possible path for data that will be reduced by the ant. The probabilistic transition rule tells us the probability that the ant at feature '*i*' will move to feature '*j*' at time '*t*':

$$\tau C_{ij}^{n}(l) = \begin{cases} t1 \\ 0 \end{cases} \frac{\left[\mu_{ij}(t1)\right]\vartheta 1 . \left[\delta_{ij}\right]\sigma 1}{\sum_{k \in f_i^n}\left[\mu_{ik}(t1)\right]\vartheta . \left[\delta_{ik}\right]\sigma 1} \quad \text{if} \;\; \mathrm{j}1 \in f1_i^n \tag{2}$$

where k is the number of flies and μ_{ij} is the heuristic desirability of selecting feature j when it is among feature i in the ACO FS process. An optional but critical parameter to ensure the efficiency of the algorithm is δ_{ij}. The neighboring node i whose ant n has not yet passed is identified by the set $f1_i^n$. The virtual pheromone concentration at edges (i, j), and so on, is represented by the parameters β, α, θ, and σ, which are all greater than 0 (where $\theta > 0$ and $\sigma > 0$). $\mu_{ij}(t1)$, θ, and σ are chosen experimentally.

The method starts by creating k ants, each of which is randomly placed on the graph starting with a particular random attribute. Another approach is to set the number of flies over the number of objects and start building paths from individual parts. Worms follow a possible path at the edge until the stationary condition is satisfied. The process searches the resulting subsets and stops when the best subset is found or reaches a predetermined number of iterations, and then generates the best feature subset. The process repeats, generating new flies and an additional dose of pheromone if there is no condition. The formula determines how each edge's pheromone is renewed:

$$\mu 1_{ij}(t1+1) = (1-\varnothing 1).\mu 1_{ij}(t1) + \varnothing 1.\Delta\mu 1_{ij}(t1) \tag{3}$$

where:

$$\Delta\mu 1_{ij}(t1) = \sum_{n=1}^{m} (\partial 1'(F1^n)/|F1^n| \tag{4}$$

If the edge has been traversed, the pheromone update on edge (i, j) takes place; if not, (t) $\Delta\mu 1_{ij}(t)$ is 0. The rate of pheromone evaporation is denoted by the decay constant, $\varnothing 1$ ($0 \le \varnothing 1 \le 1$). F^n represents the feature subset that ant n discovered. The "goodness" measure ($\partial 1'$) of the ant's feature subset and the subset's size both influence the pheromone update. By this concept, every ant participates in the pheromone update.

8.3.3 CVD Classification Using the Optimal DLINN Model

The study uses the DLINN classifier to classify CVD, which is shown in Figure 8.3. At the input layer of the classification, the inputs are sent to various nodes, each with a separate characteristic [50]. Each input has a weighted average assigned randomly. The next layer, called the hidden layer, combines the input product values of the hidden nodes with the weighted vectors of the linked input node. DLINN weighted value optimization can be solved by DLINN and kernel harmony search algorithm (KHOA) methods. In order to improve its performance, the new surface propagation (backpropagation (BP)) scheme is introduced by adding random weighted values to the optimizing method. This layer distributes the results to other layers and uses activation functions. The algorithmic steps of the DLINN method

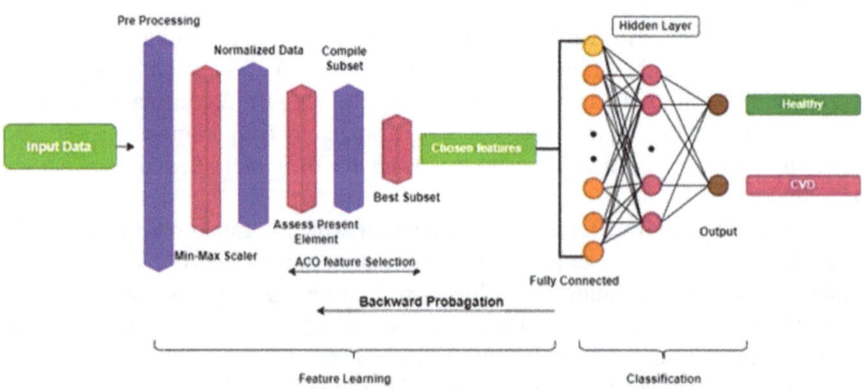

FIGURE 8.3 Model of the DLINN classifier.

are as follows and classification results are largely determined by the effects of the weights.

Step 1: Provide the score values and corresponding weights of the selected elements as follows:

$$U1_i = \{U1_1, U1_2, U1_3 \ldots\ldots U1_n\} \tag{4}$$

$$V1_i = \{V1_1, V1_2, V1_3 \ldots\ldots V1_n\} \tag{5}$$

Step 2: Give a weight vector (which can be taken randomly) to the input and then run the whole equation:

$$\mathbf{Y1} = \sum_{i=1}^{n} U1_i V1_i \tag{6}$$

where:
$V1_i$ – weight values,
Y1 –total value,
$U1_i$ – value of the input entropy.

Step 3: Calculate the activation function by applying

$$F1_j = f1\left(\sum_{i=1}^{n} U1_i V1_i\right) \tag{7}$$

Step 4: Evaluate the hidden layers' result as

$$P1_i = b1_i + \Sigma H1_i V1_i \tag{8}$$

where:
$H1_i$ – values that are modified when AF's are given,
$b1_i$ – bias value,
$V1_i$ – hidden layers and the input are both given equal weight.

Step 5: For each layer in the DLINN, follow steps 2–4. Finally, add the weighted inputs to calculate the resulting unit and calculate the value of the output layer neuron:

$$O1_i = b1_i + \Sigma Q1_i V1_i \tag{8}$$

where:
$V1_i$ – weighted hidden layer,
$O1_i$ – output unit,
$Q1_i$ – final layer .

Step 6: Compare the objective values with the network effects. Abnormal data are represented by the difference between these two values. The mathematical term for this difference is

$$R1_i = T1_i - O1_i \tag{9}$$

where:

$T1_i$ – aimed target output,
$O1_i$ – classifier present output,
$R1_i$ – error signal.

Step 7: The objective value is now measured by the resulting unit. Consequently, the relative error is defined. Based on this error, a value of δ_i can be determined to backward propagate the error to each unit in the network:

$$\varphi 1_i = R1_i \left[f1\left(O1_i\right)\right] \tag{10}$$

Step 8: Weighted corrections are calculated using the BP method. This relationship is expressed as follows:

$$\tau 1 v 1 c 1_i = \omega 1 \varphi 1_i \left(U1_j\right) \tag{11}$$

where:

$\varphi 1_i$ – error that is distributed from the network,
$\tau 1 v 1 c 1_i$ – weighted correction,
$U1_j$ – input vector,
$\omega 1$ – momentum term.

Finally, the best way to select hyperparameters is to use the Bayesian optimization technique. Bayesian optimization is an efficient method for solving problems through global optimization [51]. The goal of global optimization is to find an input that minimizes or maximizes the value of a particular objective function (OF). Because they can be high-dimensional, noisy, non-convex, computationally expensive, and nonlinear, OFs can be difficult to estimate using purchasing function Bayesian optimization. The conditional probability of event X1 given another event Y1, or Q(X1 | Y1), can be estimated using Bayes' theorem as follows:

$$Q1\left(X1 \| \mathrm{Y1}\right) = \mathrm{Q1}\left(\mathrm{Y1} \| \mathrm{X1}\right) * \frac{Q\left(X1\right)}{Q\left(Y1\right)} \tag{12}$$

By removing the marginal likelihood Q1(Y1) from the conditional probability calculation, Bayes' theorem is modified for the sake of this case. This leads to the following:

$$Q1\left(X1 \| \mathrm{Y1}\right) = \mathrm{Q1}\left(\mathrm{Y1} \| \mathrm{X1}\right) * Q1\left(X1\right) \tag{13}$$

The marginal probability Q1(X1) is called the prior probability, the probability is called the inverse conditional probability Q1(X1 | Y1), and the posterior probability is usually associated with the conditional probability Q1(X1 | Y1). Consequently, the following represents Bayes improved form of the theory:

$$posti = p1_b * priori \tag{14}$$

where:

$p1_b$ –probability.

In Bayesian optimization, the next sample in the search space is selected based on the posterior probability, which is used to compute the OF.. Procurement functions are used for evaluation and subsequent policy selection to optimize site exploration. Bayesian optimization is a method of learning that constantly improves its understanding of the OF. First, the OF is calculated using a substitution function. This study uses a Gaussian method with a Matérn 5/2 kernel for this purpose.

The OF is the evaluation of F(also known as x) at random points in the search space (x_1, x_2,..., x_n) and the process of estimating it. This model can be compiled by processing the analyses to form the dataset M = {(x_1, F(x_1)), (x_2, F(x_2)),..., (x_n, F(x_n))} and the number of samples, denoted by n, in this case.

Backward and forward functions can be derived from this dataset. Eq. (15) shows how the background function measures the probability of observing data given the OF. The Bayesian framework for revising our confidence in the OF in light of the observed data is captured in this equation:

$$Q1(\text{I1|J1}) = Q1(\text{J1|I1}) * Q1(J1) \tag{15}$$

The posterior is then updated by estimating probabilities and priorities. Then, as stated in Eq. (16), the purchase function, represented as L1, is subsequently transformed into a Gaussian ordered replacement function for sample selection x_n:

$$x_n = a1x_i L1(x|J_{1:n-1} \tag{16}$$

In this case, the procurement process is completed using the prospective growth method:

$$L1(x) = \varepsilon\left[\max 1\left(f(x) - Q1(x1^a), 0\right)\right] \tag{17}$$

where x^a denotes the location of the optimal model in the search space, $L1(x)$ denotes the value of the OF for the optimal model, and ε represents the expectation function, and then the cycle repeats until the OF reaches the specified minimum or smallest value at the specified runtime. As usual, in this case, the OF is specified as greater than 30. Each probe is run in one customized iteration. After a predetermined threshold is met, the observed value is based on the release criteria.

8.4 PERFORMANCE VALIDATION

This section uses a dataset from Kaggle [20] to analyze the CVD classification performance of the ACVD-ACOIDL algorithm. The dataset contains 629 diseased samples and 561 non-diseased samples. Characteristics include variables such as age, sex, type of chest pain, heart rate, resting ECG results, lipid levels, exercise-induced angina, exercise-induced ST depression, number of large muscles, maximal exercise, effects of thallium stress, and objectives. The ACO algorithm identified heart rate, lipid profile, ECG, type of chest pain, and resting blood pressure as the most suitable classifiers among the 14 available features in the 19th century.

The ACVD-ACOIDL method identified 522 samples as normal and 602 as disease group. Table 8.1 shows the distribution of CVD associated with the ACVD-ACOIDL method at different historical periods (Table 8.2).

The classification performance of the first 400 iterations of the ACVD-ACOIDL method is shown in Figure 8.4a. It claims to be able to distinguish between healthy and diseased samples. The method achieves high recall (94.11%), F1 score (94.79%),

TABLE 8.1
Complete results of CVD categorization using the ACVD-ACOIDL method

Class	@accuracy (a_b)	@precision (p_n)	@recall (r_l)	@f-score (f_s)	@g-measure (g_m)
@400 epochs					
Non-diseased	94.010	97.120	94.110	94.790	94.060
@Diseased	97.040	94.930	97.010	97.030	95.320
@mean	95. 530	96.330	95.560	95.910	94.690
800 epochs					
Non-diseased	95.110	97.990	95.180	95.990	95.560
@Diseased	98.140	95.510	98.120	97.880	96.120
@mean	96.630	96.750	96.650	96.940	95.840
1200 epochs					
Non-diseased	88.110	97.990	88.180	93.190	93.160
@Diseased	98.440	90.510	98.820	94.980	94.120
@mean	93.280	94.250	93.500	94.080	93.640
1600 epochs					
Non-diseased	95.510	96.010	95.380	95.790	95.560
@Diseased	96.140	95.810	98.120	96.880	96.420
@mean	95.830	95.910	96.750	96.340	95.990
2000 epochs					
Non-diseased	94.010	96.190	94.180	95.290	95.160
@Diseased	97.140	95.110	97.210	96.080	96.100
@mean	95.580	95.650	95.700	95. 690	95. 630
2400 epochs					
Non-diseased	99.110	99.890	98.980	99.490	99.560
@Diseased	99.940	99.130	99.940	99.580	99.520
@mean	99. 530	99. 510	99.460	99. 540	99.540

TABLE 8.2
Dataset information

Class	No. of instances
@Healthy	561
@Diseased	629
@Total instances	1190

precision (97.12%), and Matthews correlation coefficient (94.06%) in the normal category for an equally impressive disease group. The results are 97.04% accuracy, 94.93% precision, 97.01% recall, 97.03% F1 score, and 95.32% Matthews correlation coefficient. These results demonstrate the effectiveness of the method for classifying samples with common diseases.

Classification observed during the first 800 epochs of the ACVD-ACOIDL method is shown in Figure 8.4b, which shows the effectiveness of the method in correctly classifying healthy or diseased samples. The method has a high recall (95.18%), accuracy (95.11%), and precision (97.99%) in the conventional class, and obtains an F1 score (95.99%) and Matthews correlation coefficient (95.56%). In the same range, the disease group exhibits strong performance values, such as 98.14% accuracy, 95.51% accuracy, 98.12% residuals, 97.88% F1 score, and 96.12% Matthews correlation coefficient. These results confirm the robustness and accuracy of the classification of diseased and healthy samples during the first 800 epochs.

The classification results from the first 1200 iterations of the ACVD-ACOIDL method are shown in Figure 8.4c, which illustrates the accuracy of the method in classifying healthy and disease-related events. The ACVD-ACOIDL algorithm achieves 88.11% accuracy ($a1_b$), 97.99% precision ($p1_n$), 88.18% recall ($r1_l$), 93.19% F1 score (f_s), and 93.16% Matthews correlation coefficient ($g1_m$), and the ACVD-ACOIDL method achieves 98.44% accuracy ($a1_b$), 90.51% precision ($p1_n$), 98.82% recall ($r1_l$), 94.98% F1 score ($f1_s$), and 94.12% Matthews correlation coefficient ($g1_m$). These findings highlight the ability of the method to correctly classify healthy and diseased samples in the first 1200 samples.

The classification results for the first 1600 iterations of the ACVD-ACOIDL method are shown in Figure 8.4d, indicating that the method can effectively classify healthy or diseased cases. The ACVD-ACOIDL model achieves 95.51% accuracy ($a1_b$), 96.01% precision ($p1_n$), 95.38% recall ($r1_l$), 95.79% F1 score ($f1_s$), and 95.56% Matthews correlation coefficient ($g1_m$), and obtains the following results for the disease class by the ACVD-ACOIDL method in the same order: 96.88% F1 score ($f1_s$), 96.14% accuracy, 96.42% Matthews correlation coefficient ($g1_m$), 95.81% accuracy, and 98.12% for recall. These findings highlight the ability of the method to correctly classify healthy and diseased samples in the first 1600 seasons.

The classification output of the ACVD-ACOIDL approach for the first 2000 epochs are depicted in Figure 8.4e, which shows the ability of the algorithm to correctly classify healthy and diseased samples. The ACVD-ACOIDL system achieves 94.01% accuracy ($a1_b$), 96.19% accuracy ($p1_n$), 94.18% residual ($r1_l$), 95.29% F1 score ($f1_s$),

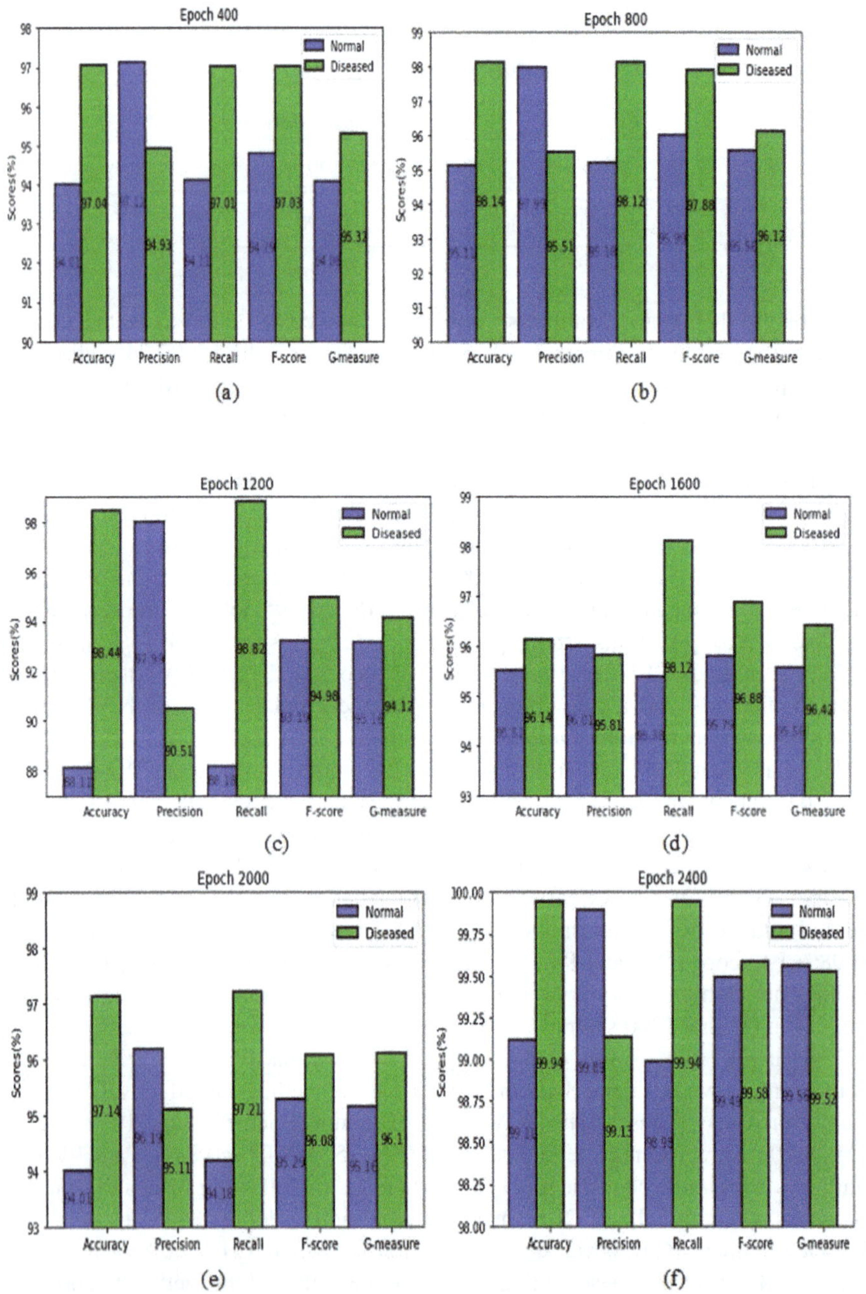

FIGURE 8.4 ACVD-ACOIDL approach's algorithm results for the first 400 epochs (a), the initial 800 epochs (b), the first 1200 epochs (c), the first 1600 epochs (d), the first 2000 epochs (e), and the first 2400 epochs (f).

and 95.16%. Matthews's correlation coefficient ($g1_m$). In the same range, the ACVD-ACOIDL method achieves the following results in the disease group: 96.10% for the Matthews correlation coefficient ($g1_m$), 96.18% precision ($a1_h$), 95.11% accuracy ($p1_n$), 97.21% recall ($r1_l$), and 96.08 F1 score ($f1_s$). These findings highlight the effectiveness of the method in correctly classifying normal and diseased samples in the first 2000 seasons.

The classification performance during the first 2400 epochs of the ACVD-ACOIDL method is shown in Figure 8.4f, which reveals the accuracy of the method in classifying healthy and pathological cases. The ACVD-ACOIDL algorithm achieves 99.11% accuracy ($a1_b$).), 99.89% precision ($p1_n$), 98.98% residual ($r1_l$), 99.49% F1 score ($f1_s$), and 99.56% Matthews correlation coefficient ($g1_m$) for normal samples. For the same approach, the ACVD-ACOIDL method obtains the following results for the disease group: 99.94% accuracy, 99.13% precision, 99.94% recall, 99.58% F1 score, and 99.52% Matthews correlation coefficient. These data suggest that, for the first 2400 seasons, the method was robust in correctly classifying samples from both the relevant time and disease.

Cholesterol levels are an important metric for diagnosing CVD, and Figure 8.5 shows their test. Chest pain can be classified into four categories according to CVD. There are four types of angina: specific angina, caused by minimized blood flow to the heart; atypical angina that is not associated with cardiac problems; non-cardiac chest pain, usually due to cooking dullness; and asymptomatic chest pain, which is chest discomfort not associated with any disease. Figure 8.6 predicts and illustrates the probability of CVD occurrence through such chest pain.

Under the correlation between the independent variables, the confusion matrices generated by the ACVD-ACOIDL method show that 522 samples were classified as normal and 602 as disease-related. This study provides context for the independent variables that are likely to affect the target variables. Detailed correlation statistics for each variable are presented in Figure 8.7. High positive values indicate an increased probability of correlation between the variables, while high negative values indicate the possibility that the relationship will decline. A deeper understanding of the dataset and its underlying parameters is facilitated by this information, which helps explain the correlations and dependencies between objects

The performance of the ACVD-ACOIDL method in classifying CVD is compared with current models based on a_y [52], [53] in Figure 8.8a where the accuracies of the SVM and REPTree models are 85.19% and 93.41%, respectively. Meanwhile, the accuracies of ANN and the bagging model are slightly better at 95.95% and 95.19%, respectively. Moreover, the accuracy values of the SC and J48 models are comparable, that is, 99.16% and 98.11%, respectively. The ACVD-ACOIDL method gives remarkably good results, with a high accuracy of 99.71%. This demonstrates the efficiency of the ACVD-ACOIDL method in CVD classification compared to other models.

The CVD classification results of the ACVD-ACOIDL techniques are compared with existing methods in Figure 8.8b, based on accuracy ($p1_n$). The results show that the SVM and REPTree models have the lowest accuracies of 85.15% and 93.32 %, respectively. Meanwhile, the accuracies of the bagging and ANN methods increased slightly, reaching 95.18% and 95.96%, respectively. Moreover, close

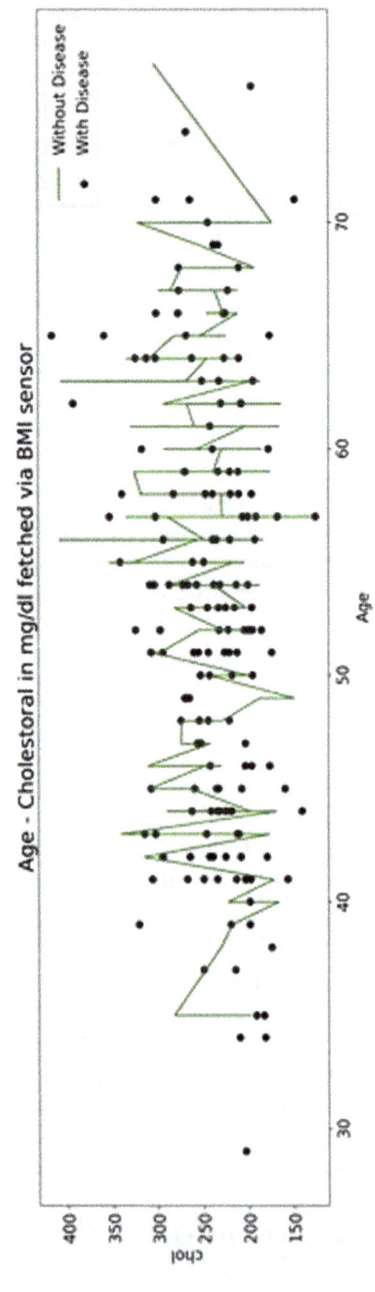

FIGURE 8.5 CVD based on cholesterol level and age.

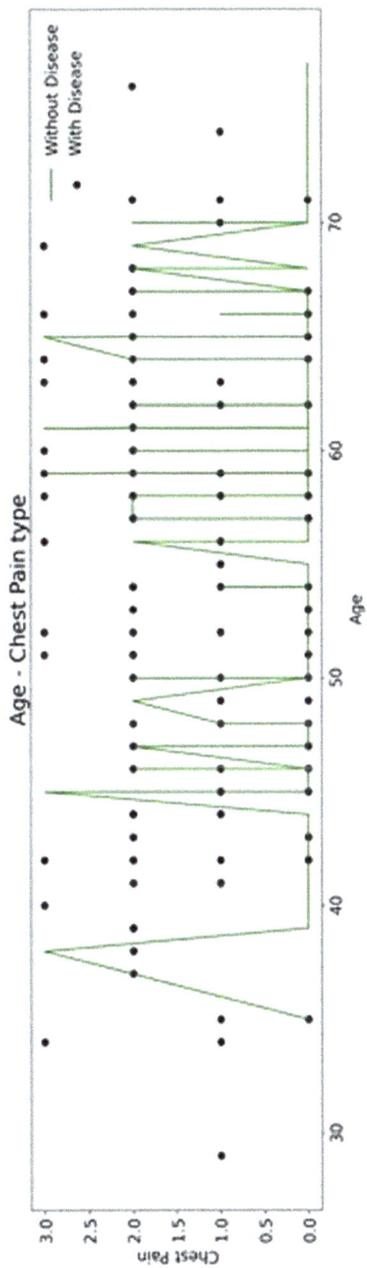

FIGURE 8.6 CVD based on chest pain type and age.

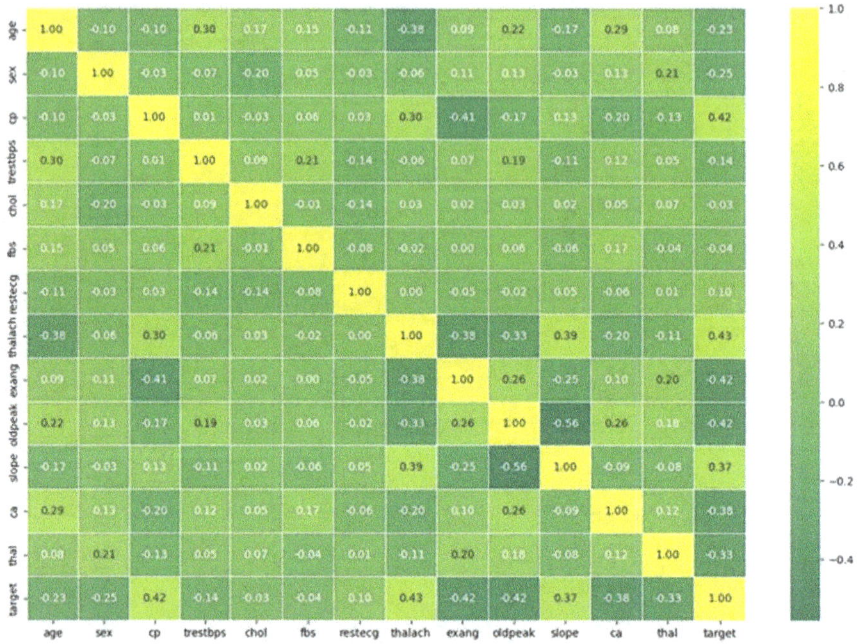

FIGURE 8.7 ACVD-ACOIDL method's confusion matrices based on the correlation between independent variables.

accuracy values of 98.02% and 99.05% are obtained by the J48 and SC methods, respectively. Importantly, the ACVD-ACOIDL algorithm gives good results, with an accuracy increase of 99.44%. This highlights the effectiveness of the ACVD-ACOIDL algorithm in CVD classification, as it outperforms existing methods in terms of accuracy.

A comparative analysis of CVD classification results resulting from the ACVD-ACOIDL approach is shown in Figure 8.8c, focusing on recall ($r1_l$). The observed analysis indicates that the decreased recall values for the SVM and REPTree models obtained were 84.18% and 93.47%, respectively. ANN and the bagging method get slightly better recall values of 95.15% and 94.29%, respectively. Furthermore, the J48 and SC methods achieve close recall values of 99.11% and 97.91%, respectively. Finally, the ACVD-ACOIDL method shows excellent results, with a recall rate of 99.71%. This indicates the memory efficiency of the ACVD-ACOIDL method in CVD classification compared to other methods.

An analysis of the CVD classification results from the ACVD-ACOIDL method is shown in Figure 8.8d. The findings of the F1 score ($f1_s$) show a decrease of the F1 score value of 84.29% and 94.78% by the SVM and REPTree methods, respectively. At the same time, ANN and the bagging methods obtain slightly improved F1 score values of 96.07% and 95.14%, respectively. Moreover, the F1 score values of 98.82% and 98.97%, respectively, are close to those obtained by the SC and J48 methods. Finally, the ACVD-ACOIDL model shows the best results, with an improved F1 score

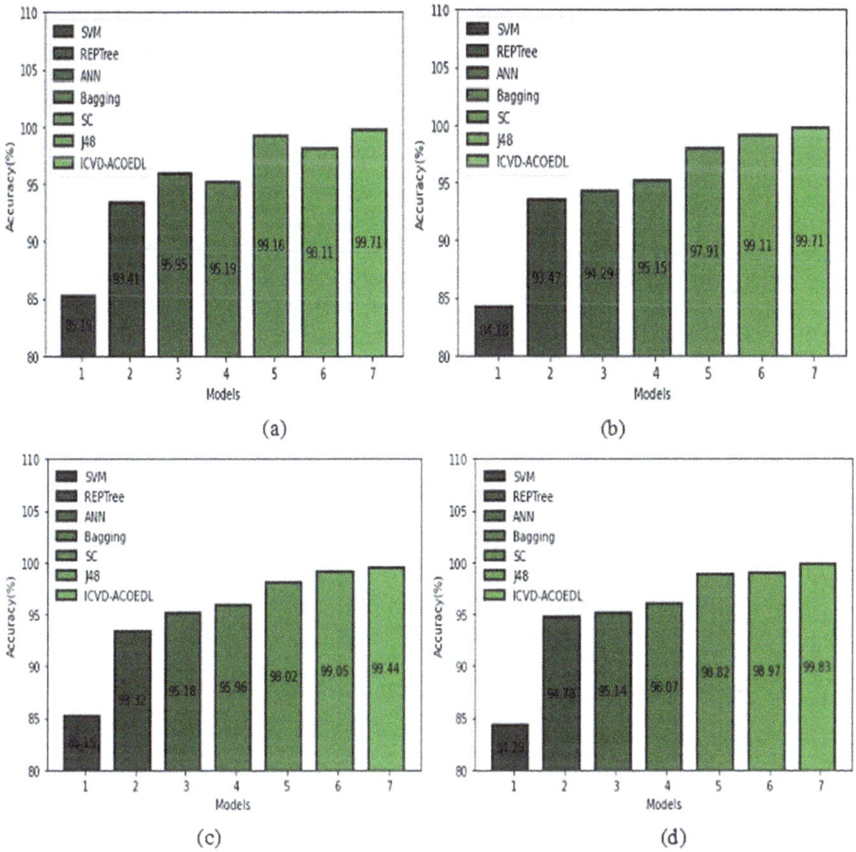

FIGURE 8.8 Accuracy analysis of the ACVD-ACOIDL approach with existing algorithms: (a) accuracy, (b) precision, (c) recall, and (d) F-score.

of 99.83%. These results confirm the improved CVD classification performance of the ACVD-ACOIDL method, which outperforms other methods in F1 scoring.

8.5 CONCLUSION

This study presents a pristine ACVD-ACOIDL method for the accurate detection of CVD, applying FS and hyperparameter tuning methods. The method begins with the preprocessing of medical data with minimum and maximum scalars, and then ACO. The DLINN classifier is used for CVD classification and Bayesian optimization is used for its hyperparameter optimization. Improving the accuracy of CVD detection is the main objective of this combined approach. Experimental results show a significant improvement over previous methods, with 99.71% improved accuracy, and an improved ACVD-ACOIDL method on the benchmark medical dataset. Future research may see the inclusion of data clustering and outlier detection methods for the ACVD-ACOIDL method, leading to reliable and accurate classification results in CVD diagnosis.

REFERENCES

[1] L. D. Weberling, D. Lossnitzer, N. Frey, and F. André, "Coronary computed tomography vs. cardiac magnetic resonance imaging in the evaluation of coronary artery disease," *Diagnostics*, vol. 13, no. 1, p. 125, Dec. 2022.

[2] P. Wang, Z. Lin, X. Yan, Z. Chen, M. Ding, Y. Song, and L. Meng, "A wearable ECG monitor for deep learning based real-time cardiovascular disease detection,' Electrical Engineering and Systems Science Signal Processing, 2022. *arXiv:2201.10083*

[3] M. C. Badescu, O. V. Badulescu, L. I. Butnariu, I. B. Bojan, M. C. Vladeanu, N. Dima, C. E. Vlad, L. G. Foia, M. Ciocoiu, and C. Rezus, "Cardiovascular risk factors in patients with congenital hemophilia: A focus on hypertension," *Diagnostics*, vol. 12, no. 12, p. 2937, Nov. 2022.

[4] M. Swathy and K. Saruladha, "A comparative study of classification and prediction of cardio-vascular diseases (CVD) using machine learning and deep learning techniques," *ICT Exp.*, vol. 8, no. 1, pp. 109–116, Mar. 2022.

[5] M. A. Eid, K. Mehta, J. A. Barnes, Z. Wanken, J. A. Columbo, D. H. Stone, P. Goodney, and M. M. Smith, "The global burden of peripheral artery disease," *J. Vascular Surg.*, vol. 77, no. 4, pp. 1119–1126, Apr. 2023.

[6] N. Culliford-Semmens, E. Tilton, N. Wilson, J. Stirling, R. Doughty, T. Gentles, B. Peat, E. Dimalapang, and R. Webb, "Echocardiography for latent rheumatic heart disease in first degree relatives of children with acute rheumatic fever: Implications for active case finding in family members," *eClinicalMedicine*, vol. 37, Jul. 2021, Art. no. 100935.

[7] R. O. Escárcega, M. J. Lipinski, M. García-Carrasco, C. Mendoza-Pinto, J. L. Galvez-Romero, and R. Cervera, "Inflammation and atherosclerosis: Cardiovascular evaluation in patients with autoimmune diseases," *Autoimmunity Rev.*, vol. 17, no. 7, pp. 703–708, Jul. 2018.

[8] C. Chen, C. Qin, H. Qiu, G. Tarroni, J. Duan, W. Bai, and D. Rueckert,"Deep learning for cardiac image segmentation: A review," *Front. Cardiovasc. Med.*, vol. 7, p. 25, Mar. 2020.

[9] Y. Ma, M. U. Hassan, D. Niu, and L. Wang, "The segmentation of glandular cavity based on K-means and mathematical morphology," in *Proceedings of4th International Conference on Systems and Informatics. (ICSAI)*Nov. 2017, pp. 1287–1291.

[10] Y. A. Z. A. Fajri, W. Wiharto, and E. Suryani, "Hybrid model feature selection with the bee swarm optimization method and Q-learning on the diagnosis of coronary heart disease," *Information*, vol. 14, no. 1, p. 15, Dec. 2022.

[11] C. Kim, G. Lee, H. Oh, G. Jeong, S. W. Kim, E. J. Chun, Y.-H. Kim, J.-G. Lee, and D. H. Yang, "A deep learning–based automatic analysisof cardiovascular borders on chest radiographs of valvular heart disease: Development/external validation," *Eur. Radiol.*, vol. 32, no. 3, pp. 1558–1569, Mar. 2022.

[12] B. Kolukisa and B. Bakir-Gungor, "Ensemble feature selection and classification methods for machine learning-based coronary artery disease diagnosis," *Comput. Standards Interfaces*, vol. 84, Mar. 2023, Art. no. 103706.

[13] M. K. Malnajjar and S. S. Abu-Naser, "Heart sounds analysis and classification for cardiovascular diseases diagnosis using deep learning," 2022. edu.ps/xmlui/handle/123456789/3534

[14] P. K. Shrivastava, M. Sharma, P. Sharma, and A. Kumar, "HCBiLSTM: A hybrid model for predicting heart disease using CNN and BiLSTM algorithms," *Meas., Sensors*, vol. 25, Feb. 2023, Art. no. 100657.

[15] M. A. Qureshi, K. N. Qureshi, G. Jeon, and F. Piccialli, "Deep learningbasedambient assisted living for self-management of cardiovascularconditions," *Neural Comput. Appl.*, vol. 34, no. 13, pp. 10449–10467, Jul. 2022.

[16] V. Chang, V. R. Bhavani, A. Q. Xu, and M. Hossain, "An artificial intelligence model for heart disease detection using machine learning algorithms," *Healthcare Anal.*, vol. 2, Nov. 2022, Art. no. 100016.

[17] P. Mathur, S. Srivastava, X. Xu, and J. L. Mehta, "Artificial intelligence, machine learning, and cardiovascular disease," *Clin. Med. Insights, Cardiol.*, vol. 14, Jan. 2020, Art. no. 117954682092740.

[18] S. Hong, Y. Zhou, J. Shang, C. Xiao, and J. Sun, "Opportunities and challenges of deep learning methods for electrocardiogram data: A systematic review," *Comput. Biol. Med.*, vol. 122, Jul. 2020, Art. no. 103801.

[19] S. Suganyadevi, V. Seethalakshmi, and K. Balasamy, "A review on deep learning in medical image analysis," *Int. J. Multimedia Inf. Retr.*, vol. 11, no. 1, pp. 19–38, Mar. 2022.

[20] M. U. Hassan, S. Alaliyat, and I. A. Hameed, "Image generation models from scene graphs and layouts: A comparative analysis," *J. King Saud Univ.-Comput. Inf. Sci.*, vol. 35, no. 5, May 2023, Art.no. 101543.

[21] O. Ghorbanzadeh, T. Blaschke, K. Gholamnia, S. Meena, D. Tiede, and J. Aryal, "Evaluation of different machine learning methods and deeplearning convolutional neural networks for landslide detection," *Remote Sensing*, MDPI, vol. 11, no. 2, p. 196, Jan. 2019.

[22] Y. Ma, J. Zhang, D. Niu, M. U. Hassan, and X. Zhao, "An unsupervised approach for 3D medical image registration," in Proc. 2019 7th Int. Conf. Inf. Technol., IoT Smart City, 2019, pp. 259–263.

[23] K. K. L. Wong, G. Fortino, and D. Abbott, "Deep learning-based cardiovascular image diagnosis: A promising challenge," *Future Gener. Comput. Syst.*, vol. 110, pp. 802–811, Sep. 2020.

[24] M. Chen, Y. Hao, K. Hwang, L. Wang, and L. Wang, "Disease prediction by machine learning over big data from healthcare communities," *IEEE Access*, vol. 5, pp. 8869–8879, 2017.

[25] K. Matsushita, N. Ding, M. Kou, X. Hu, M. Chen, Y. Gao, Y. Honda, D. Zhao, D. Dowdy, Y. Mok, J. Ishigami, and L. J. Appel, "The relationship of COVID-19 severity with cardiovascular disease and its traditional risk factors: A systematic review and meta-analysis," *Global Heart*, vol. 15, no. 1, p. 64, Sep. 2020.

[26] K. C. Siontis, P. A. Noseworthy, Z. I. Attia, and P. A. Friedman, "Artificial intelligence-enhanced electrocardiography in cardiovascular disease management," *Nat. Rev. Cardiol.*, vol. 18, no. 7, pp. 465–478, Jul. 2021.

[27] W. A. W. A. Bakar, N. L. N. B. Josdi, M. B. Man, and M. A. B. Zuhairi, "A review: Heart disease prediction in machine learning & deep learning," in Proceedings of signal processing and its applications, 19thIEEE international colloquium. *(CSPA)*, Mar. 2023, pp. 150–155.

[28] I. S. Brites, L. M. Silva, J. L. Barbosa, S. J. Rigo, S. D. Correia, and V. R. Leithardt, "Machine learning and IoT applied to cardiovascular diseases identification through heart sounds: A literature review," in Proc. Int. Conf. Inf. Technol. Syst. Cham, Switzerland: Springer, Feb. 2022, pp. 356–388.

[29] U. Nagavelli, D. Samanta, and P. Chakraborty, "Machine learning technology-based heart disease detection models," *J. Healthcare Eng.*, vol. 2022, pp. 1–9, Feb. 2022.

[30] P. Arpaia, R. Cuocolo, F. Donnarumma, A. Esposito, N. Moccaldi, A. Natalizio, and R. Prevete, "Conceptual design of a machine learning based wearable soft sensor for non-invasive cardiovascular risk assessment," *Measurement*, vol. 169, Feb. 2021, Art. no. 108551.

[31] R. T. Selvi and I. Muthulakshmi, "An optimal artificial neural network based big data application for heart disease diagnosis and classification model," *J. Ambient Intell. Humanized Comput.*, vol. 12, no. 6, pp. 6129–6139, Jun. 2021.

[32] M. M. Ali, B. K. Paul, K. Ahmed, F. M. Bui, J. M. W. Quinn, and M. A. Moni, "Heart disease prediction using supervised machine learning algorithms: Performance analysis and comparison," *Computers in Biology and Medicine.*, vol. 136, Sep. 2021, Art. no. 104672.

[33] M. Ganesan and N. Sivakumar, "IoT based heart disease prediction and diagnosis model for healthcare using machine learning models," in Proc. IEEE Int. Conf. Syst., Comput., Autom. Netw. (ICSCAN), Mar. 2019, pp. 1–5.

[34] J. P. Li, A. U. Haq, S. U. Din, J. Khan, A. Khan, and A. Saboor,"Heart disease identification method using machine learning classificationin e-healthcare," *IEEE Access*, vol. 8, pp. 107562–107582, 2020.

[35] R. Atallah and A. Al-Mousa, "Heart disease detection using machine learning majority voting ensemble method," in Proc. 2nd Int. Conference on New Trends in Computer Science" (ICTCS), Oct. 2019, pp. 1–6.

[36] M. Noale, F. Limongi, and S. Maggi, "Epidemiology of cardiovascular diseases in the elderly," Advances in Experimental Medicine and Biology, Frailty *and Cardiovascular Diseases: Research into an Elderly Population*, 2020, pp. 29–38.

[37] M. Athanasiou, K. Sfrintzeri, K. Zarkogianni, A. C. Thanopoulou, and K. S. Nikita, "An explainable XGBoost-based approach towards assessing the risk of cardiovascular disease in patients with type 2 diabetes mellitus," in Proceedings of the IEEE 20th International Conference on Bioinformatics and Bioengineering (BIBE), Oct. 2020, pp. 859–864.

[38] P. H. Charlton, P. A. Kyriacou, J. Mant, V. Marozas, P. Chowienczyk, and J. Alastruey, "Wearable photoplethysmography for cardiovascular monitoring," *Proc. IEEE*, vol. 110, no. 3, pp. 355–381, Mar. 2022.

[39] D. Chieng and P. M. Kistler, "Coffee and tea on cardiovascular disease (CVD) prevention," *Trends Cardiovascular Med.*, vol. 32, no. 7, pp. 399–405, Oct. 2022.

[40] L.-C. Tao, J.-N. Xu, T.-T.Wang, F. Hua, and J.-J. Li, "Triglyceride-glucose index as a marker in cardiovascular diseases: Landscape and limitations,"*Cardiovasc. Diabetol.*, vol. 21, no. 1, pp. 1–17, Dec. 2022.

[41] G. Battineni, G. G. Sagaro, N. Chintalapudi, and F. Amenta, "The benefits of telemedicine in personalized prevention of cardiovascular diseases(CVD): A systematic review," *J. Personalized Med.*, vol. 11, no. 7, p. 658, Jul. 2021.

[42] H. E. Bays, P. R. Taub, E. Epstein, E. D. Michos, R. A. Ferraro, A. L. Bailey, H. M. Kelli, K. C. Ferdinand, M. R. Echols, H. Weintraub, and J. Bostrom,"Ten things to know about ten cardiovascular disease risk factors," *Amer. J. Preventive Cardiol.*, vol. 5, Mar. 2021, Art. no. 100149.

[43] V. V. Dickson, J. Jun, and G. D. Melkus, "A mixed methods study describing the self-care practices in an older working population with cardiovascular disease (CVD): Balancing work, life and health," *Heart Lung*, vol. 50, no. 3, pp. 447–454, May 2021.

[44] G. K. Ellis, J. A. Robinson, and G. B. Crawford, "When symptoms of disease overlap with symptoms of depression," *Austral. Family Phys.*, vol. 35, no. 8, pp. 647–649, 2006.

[45] N. F. A. Alhadeethy, A. M. Zeki, and A. Shah, "Deep learning model for predicting and detecting overlapping symptoms of cardiovascular diseases in hospitals of UAE," *Turkish J. Comput. Math.Educ. (TURCOMAT)*, vol. 12, no. 14, pp. 5212–5224, 2021.

[46] C.-S. Hsu, S.-H. Wen, J.-S. Hung, T.-T. Liu, C.-H. Yi, W.-Y. Lei, F. Pace, and C.-L. Chen, "Overlap of dyspepsia in patients with gastro esophageal reflux disease: Impact of clinical, metabolic, and psychosocial characteristics,"*Digestive Dis. Sci.*, vol. 62, no. 4, pp. 994–1001, Apr. 2017.

[47] A. Chaddha, E. A. Robinson, E. Kline-Rogers, T. Alexandris-Souphis, and M. Rubenfire, "Mental health and cardiovascular disease," *Amer. J. Med.*, vol. 129, no. 11, pp. 1145–1148, 2016.

[48] G. M. Goodwin, "Depression and associated physical diseases and symptoms," *Dialogues Clin. Neurosci.*, vol. 8, no. 2, pp. 259–265, Jun. 2006.

[49] A. Daoulah, A. Elfarnawany, T. Al Garni, A. S. Hersi, M. Alshehri, W. Almahmeed, N. Yousif, R. Abuelatta, A. Alasmari, and N. E. Elsheikh-Mohamed, "Outcomes of myocardial revascularization in diabetic patients with left main coronary artery disease: A multicenter observational study from three Gulf countries," *Cardiovasc. Revascularization Med.*, vol. 46, pp. 52–61, Jan. 2023.

[50] B. Muthu, S. Cb, P. M. Kumar, S. N. Kadry, C.-H. Hsu, O. Sanjuan, and R. G. Crespo, "A framework for extractive text summarization based on deep learning modified neural network classifier," *ACM Trans. Asian Low-Resource Lang. Inf. Process.*, vol. 20, no. 3, pp. 1–20, May 2021.

[51] G. Atteia, A. Alhussan, and N. Samee, "BO-ALLCNN: Bayesianbased optimized CNN for acute lymphoblastic leukemia detection in microscopic blood smear images," *Sensors*, vol. 22, no. 15, p. 5520, Jul. 2022.

[52] M. Siddhartha. Heart disease dataset (Comprehensive) statlog + Cleveland + Hungary dataset. Available: www.kaggle.com/datasets/sid321axn/heart-statlog-clevelandhungary-final. [Accessed May 22, 2023].

[53] N. Mary, B. Khan, A. A. Asiri, F. Muhammad, S. Alqhtani, K. M. Mehdar, H. T. Halwani, T. Aleyani, and K. A. Alshamrani, "Investigating of classification algorithms for heart disease risk prediction," *J. Intell. Med. Healthcare*, vol. 1, no. 1, pp. 11–31, 2022.

[54] A. Kumar Dubey, K. Choudhary, and R. Sharma, "Predicting heart disease based on influential features with machine learning," *Intell. Autom. Soft Comput.*, vol. 30, no. 3, pp. 929–943, 2021.

9 Utilizing Explainable Artificial Intelligence for Parkinson's Disease Diagnosis through the Analysis of Spiral and Wave Drawings with Integrated Data Augmentation

S. Murugaveni, Harisudha Kuresan, N. Sri Sai Charan Reddy, Perala Manoj, and Gaddam Rohit

9.1 INTRODUCTION

According to statistics published by "parkinsonsnewstoday.com", seven to ten million individuals worldwide suffer from Parkinson's disease (PD), with a frequency that varies from 41 cases per 100,000 in the fourth decade of life to more than 1,900 cases per 100,000 in those 80 years of age and beyond. Region, age, sex, and other variables all affect the incidence and prevalence of PD. After Alzheimer's disease, PD is the second-most prevalent neurodegenerative illness.

PD is a neurodegenerative condition that evolves slowly over time. In order to slow down the evolution of the illness and avoid the major consequences usually observed in its late stages, it may be useful to treat people presenting early indications of PD. Deficiency in dopamine can lead to impairments in the body's motor function [1]. Neurons in the area called the substantia nigra pars compacta produce the biological substance dopamine. This compound plays a crucial role in controlling motor functions. PD is an uncommon neurologic disorder characterized by motor symptoms. These symptoms encompass hand, head, and leg tremors, swelling of the body, stiffness in muscles, issues with posture and balance, and challenges with the

DOI: 10.1201/9781003484233-9

movement of humans [2,3]. Drawing complex shapes like spirals and waves calls for deft hand-eye coordination and fine motor control. Examining the accuracy of PD patients' drawn figures is one way for doctors to evaluate their motor skills and spot any discrepancies or variances in performance [4]. Both the Unified PD Rating Scale (UPDRS) and Hoehn and Yahr (HY) measure the severity of PD at various stages. The fluctuation in these scores over the years reflects the advancement of the disease [5]. It's crucial to emphasize that detecting the disease in the early stage can significantly improve the patient's quality of life.

At present, diagnosing PD relies on clinical evaluations, which are labor-intensive and require a significant number of human specialists. Therefore, there's a need for automated early detection of PD in the healthcare sector [6]. PD affects the basal ganglia and cortex in the brain, leading to a condition known as bradykinesia that progresses to micrographia. PD frequently gets mistaken for other conditions due to the similarity in symptoms. These conditions include multiple system atrophy (MSA), progressive supranuclear palsy (PSP), and Huntington's disease [7]. Investigations into deep transfer learning methods applied to spiral and wave sketches have validated their effectiveness in distinguishing individuals with PD from healthy individuals. Deep learning is a great tool for processing massive datasets since its models improve with training. However, within the corpus of current literature, a deep neural classifier is often described as a "black box" method. Researchers are unable to learn the specifics of the relationship between input and output due to the opaque nature of the process. Because of its widespread use in many fields, including medicine, interpretability is of the utmost importance. Our main objective is to improve the interpretability of the proposed PD prediction model by integrating the local interpretable model-agnostic explanation (LIME) and Shapley additive explanations (SHAP) into the image classification process. This study examines the early detection of PD utilizing hand drawing and spiral datasets collected from PD patients. VGG19 is merged with an attention mechanism and explainable artificial intelligence (XAI).

9.2 RELATED WORK

In this modern era, artificial intelligence (AI) in healthcare has grown in popularity. An extensive amount of research was done in the past on the early diagnosis of PD. For instance, handwriting has emerged as a potential biomarker for early PD diagnosis in recent years. This is due to the fact that handwriting may be used to evaluate a person's cognitive and motor abilities, and handwriting's graphical features can identify the ambiguity of strokes caused by tremor movements.

A variety of machine learning methods have been utilized to distinguish between individuals with PD and those without. Drotar et al. [8] used support vector machines (SVMs) in numerous handwriting tasks and achieved an accuracy of 81.3% using the PaHaW database. This database includes data from 37 individuals with PD and 38 healthy individuals [9]. Handwriting samples were gathered through seven different tasks, which included writing a syllable, a word, or a sentence. In their research, Pereira et al. [10] employed advanced deep learning methods, specifically utilizing a convolutional neural network (CNN). Their focus was on distinguishing various characteristics within handwritten samples sourced from a hand drawing PD dataset, consisting of 74 individuals with PD and 18 individuals without the condition. Das et al. [11] introduced a predictive model designed for the early detection of PD through the application of diverse classification techniques. Ultimately, their findings revealed that neural networks surpassed other classifiers, achieving an impressive accuracy of 92.2% in the classification process.

Predicting the onset of PD via digitized spiral drawings is a potential biomarker, as stated by Meghakamble et al. [12]. After mathematically processing the feature-engineered dataset, they used four machine learning classifiers and produced results with an accuracy of 91% and an area under the curve (AUC) of 98.1%. Saravanan et al. [4] integrated the VGG and Inception v3 algorithms to improve the classification process, assessing visual features of handwriting for the identification of PD. Their approach resulted in a notable achievement, attaining an accuracy of 98.5% in the classification process. By utilizing a multi-layer perceptron (MLP) for categorization and assessing motor symptoms using kinematic data, they demonstrated the validity of these tests.

One effective method for analyzing movement tremors in disorders affecting motor abilities is digitized spiral analysis (Danna et al. 2019). A great degree of dexterity and motor coordination are necessary for spiral sketching. It's regarded as a sympathetic motor assessment. The UPDRS-III is the most widely accepted and widely used grading system for PD.

PD affects a person's ability to walk, write, speak, and coordinate their movements, among other motor functions. Given that PD is classified as a neurodegenerative motor condition, numerous quantitative measures of motor decline and non-motor biomarkers have been proposed by researchers. Diagnosing and monitoring PD is costly and time-consuming, in addition to the discomfort of the patient going to the clinic for a physical examination [12].

A group of cumulative characteristic significance techniques, which comprises the six earlier approaches, is identified using the SHAP framework, which also demonstrates that there exists one approach in this group that satisfies desired criteria. The cohesive theme that SHAP creates across the literature is a positive indication that general guidelines for interpreting models can guide the creation of new techniques. Another XAI technique called LIME makes use of a local estimation of the framework to offer comprehensible and interpretable insights into the variables that are most significant and pertinent to the model's predictions. LIME investigates and assesses the local faithfulness of a forecast by examining its surrounding area.

Clinical invasive procedures are only available at an early stage and carry a high risk due to resource scarcity in developing nations. In the past, PD was assessed using conventional non-invasive examinations, like the spiral drawing pen paper test and handwriting test. These drawings must be gathered, preserved, and analyzed by humans, which takes time and is prejudiced. Digitizing (digital) tablets, which are being used in biological research, make it easier to obtain drawing samples. Compared to the pen and paper method, the usage of graphics tablets enables academics to create a broad range of picture analysis and processing approaches.

9.3 METHODOLOGY

9.3.1 Dataset Description

A spiral and wave drawing made by a healthy individual resembles typical spiral and wave shapes almost exactly. However, because of their sluggish motor movements and impaired hand-brain coordination, people with PD draw spirals and waves that greatly vary from ideal shapes and seem deformed. Downloaded from Kaggle, the drawing dataset contains the spiral and wave drawing samples of 102 participants: 51 with PD and 51 in good condition. There are two types of photos in the author's dataset [13], and 102 samples are arranged in spirals and waves.

9.3.2 Data Preprocessing and Augmentation

The study's image collection underwent scaling. The spiral sketch images were scaled to 224 pixels in width and 224 pixels in height, while the wave sketch images were resized to 224 pixels in width and 224 pixels in height. It is evident from the images gathered for the study that they were deficient in brightness, contrast, and general clarity. Therefore, histogram equalization was used to accomplish contrast augmentation and correction over all the photos. In order to get ready for training, every image underwent a static policy-based augmentation. Since the dataset contained comparatively few images, applying CNN, a deep learning algorithm, became difficult. In order to increase the dataset's variety and include some synthetic examples in the training dataset, image augmentations were done. Tables 9.1 shows the different image augmentation parameters that were used for the training data for spiral and wave sketching,

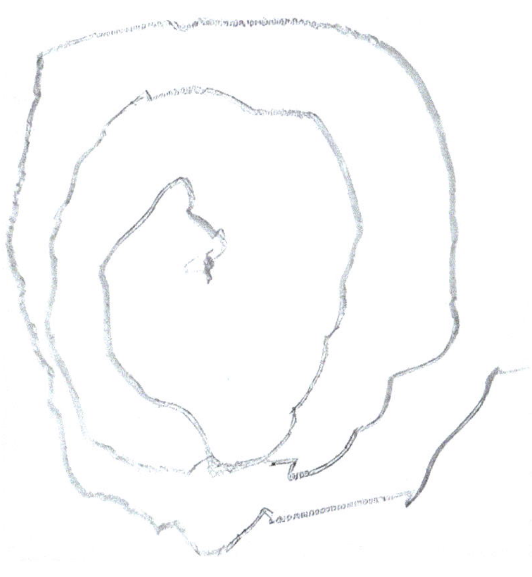

FIGURE 9.1 Spiral drawing – PD sample.

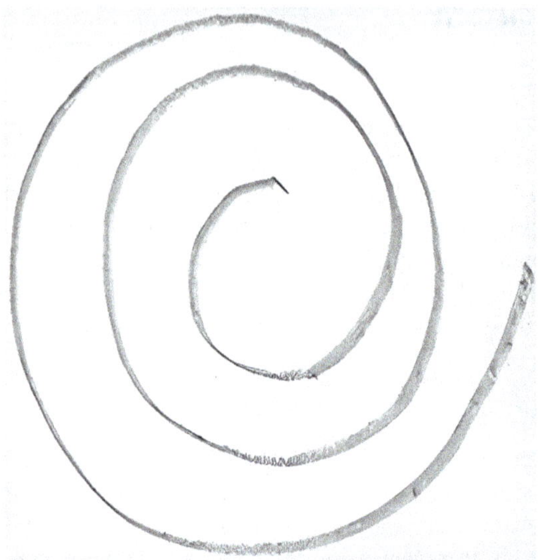

FIGURE 9.2 Healthy sample.

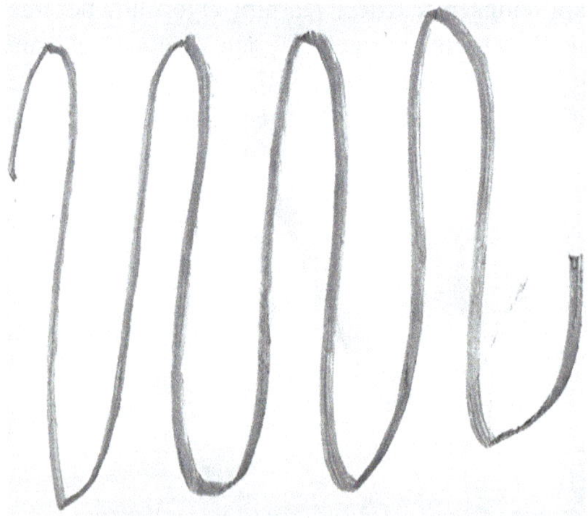

FIGURE 9.3 Wave drawing – healthy sample.

respectively. Furthermore, the histogram-equalized and enhanced pictures from the wave and spiral drawings in the training dataset are shown in Figures 9.3 and 9.4.

There was a 70/30 split between the training and validation sets.

9.3.3 Proposed Model

The introduction of deep learning and subsequent advancements in machine intelligence have caused a paradigm change across all industries. More precisely, the

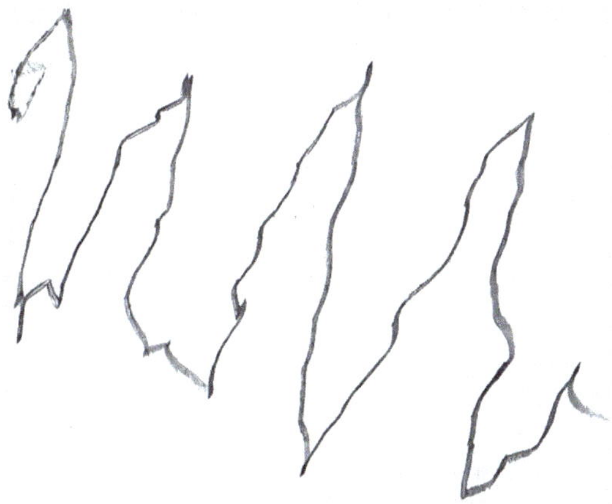

FIGURE 9.4 Parkinson sample.

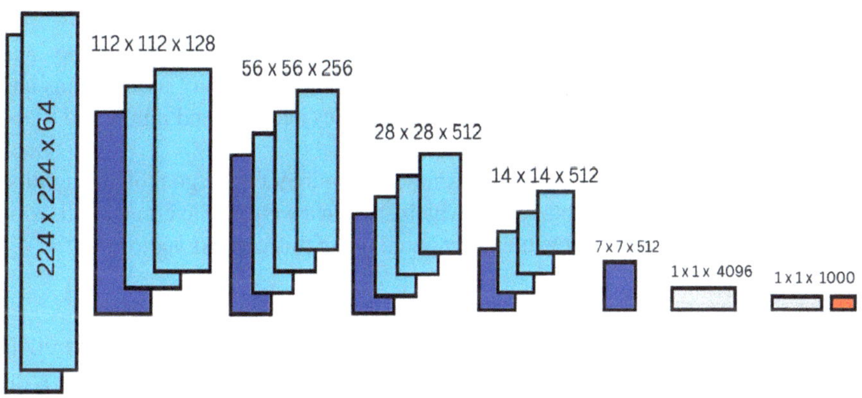

FIGURE 9.5 VGG19 architecture.

development of deep learning and advanced computer-aided detection systems has effectively led to more accurate and exact diagnosis in the healthcare industry. When it comes to PD, several biomarkers must be examined in order to determine a patient's clinical state. PD is known to induce a number of deficits, including dispersed motor flexibility and hand tremors, which make it harder to write and sketch. As a result, assessing writing and drawing skills might be seen as a critical indicator for identifying PD and tracking severity. Several deep learning models, like VGG19, Inception v3, and Vision Transformers, are trained on the dataset.

9.3.3.1 VGG19

The Visual Geometry Group at Oxford University created VGG, a group that created AlexNet, which was released in 2012 and improved on traditional CNNs. Deep convolutional neural layers are used by VGG to boost accuracy, and it builds on some of the concepts from its predecessors, as shown in Figure 9.5. There are 19 layers in the

VGG19 variation of the VGG model (16 convolution layers, 3 fully linked layers, 5 max pool layers, and 1 softmax layer).

This network was given an RGB image with a fixed size of (224 × 224), indicating that the matrix structure was (224, 224, 3). The mean RGB value for each pixel, calculated throughout the whole training set, was removed in the single preprocessing step. Using kernels with a stride of one pixel and a size of (3 × 3), they were able to cover the whole image. Spatial padding was used to preserve the spatial resolution of the picture. Stride 2 was used across 2 × 2 pixel windows for max pooling. In order to increase nonlinearity, speed up calculation, and boost model classification, the rectified linear unit (ReLU) was utilized. Earlier models relied on sigmoid or tanh functions. The ReLU proved to be more effective than these three fully linked layers. The implementation includes a softmax function as the last layer, a layer with 1000 channels for a 1000-way ILSVRC classification, and two 4096-sized layers as the first two.

9.3.3.2 Attention

Attention was initially suggested as an extension of recurrent neural networks. Following the release of the Transformer model, attention gained popularity and was swiftly included into other deep learning models for a range of applications and activities, including recommender systems, time series datasets, and image and video processing.

An overview of the attention model is shown in Figure 9.6. The goal of all attention models is to produce the context vector, which is often a weighted average of all value vectors. The prediction output is then computed using this context vector.

9.3.3.3 Proposed Model (VGG19 with an Attention Mechanism)

In this work, an investigation was conducted on how well VGG19 Net fared in the Large-Scale Visual Recognition competition from 2014. Figure 9.7 shows the suggested design of VGG19 with an attention mechanism. Using VGG19 Net and attention modules, this proposed method develops a unique deep transfer fusion learning model for PD classification. Spiral and wave drawings were used by VGG19

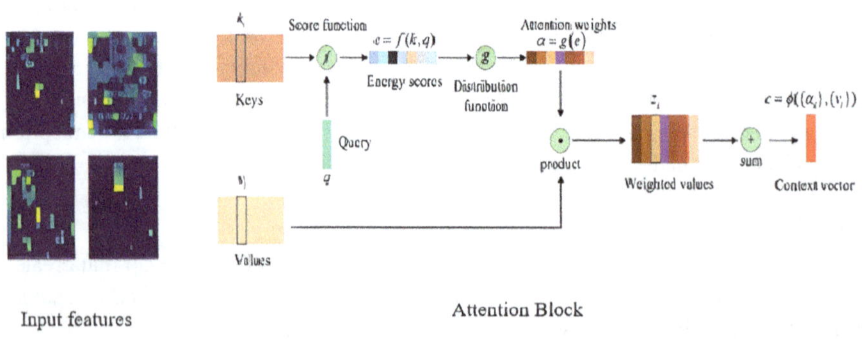

FIGURE 9.6 Attention mechanism.

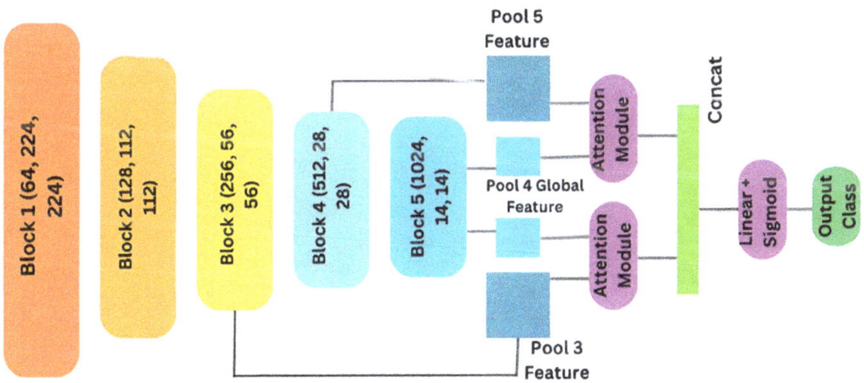

FIGURE 9.7 Architecture of fusion of VGG19 and an attention mechanism.

TABLE 9.1
Comparison of various deep learning techniques

Models	Accuracy	Precision	Recall	F1 score
VGG19	83.8	79.6	80.66	80.19
VGG19-attention (proposed model)	97.5	96.34	94.04	95.18

Net to extract basic features and the high-dimensional features were extracted using attention modules. To minimize overfitting, deep transfer learning models are favored from scratch with a small dataset to discriminate PD patients from healthy individuals.

9.4 RESULTS AND DISCUSSION

The classifiers developed in this study are VGG19 without attention and VGG19 with an attention mechanism. The fusion of VGG19 and an attention mechanism achieved strong results in detecting PD from spiral and wave sketches. VGG19 with an attention mechanism demonstrated an accuracy of 97.5%, recall rate of 96%, precision rate of 97.5%, and overall F1 score of 96.94%. VGG19 without attention had an accuracy of 83.8%. The corresponding plots for various parameters are shown in Figures 9.8 (a)–(c), 9.9 (a)–(d), 9.10, and 9.11.

9.5 MODEL INTERPRETABILITY USING LIME AND SHAP

Machine learning model predictions are explained using LIME and SHAP interpretability approaches. By locally estimating a black box model with a simplified one, and to help with PD prediction and to identify the pixels that cause misclassification, LIME mainly focuses on clarifying the super pixels of spiral and wave patterns

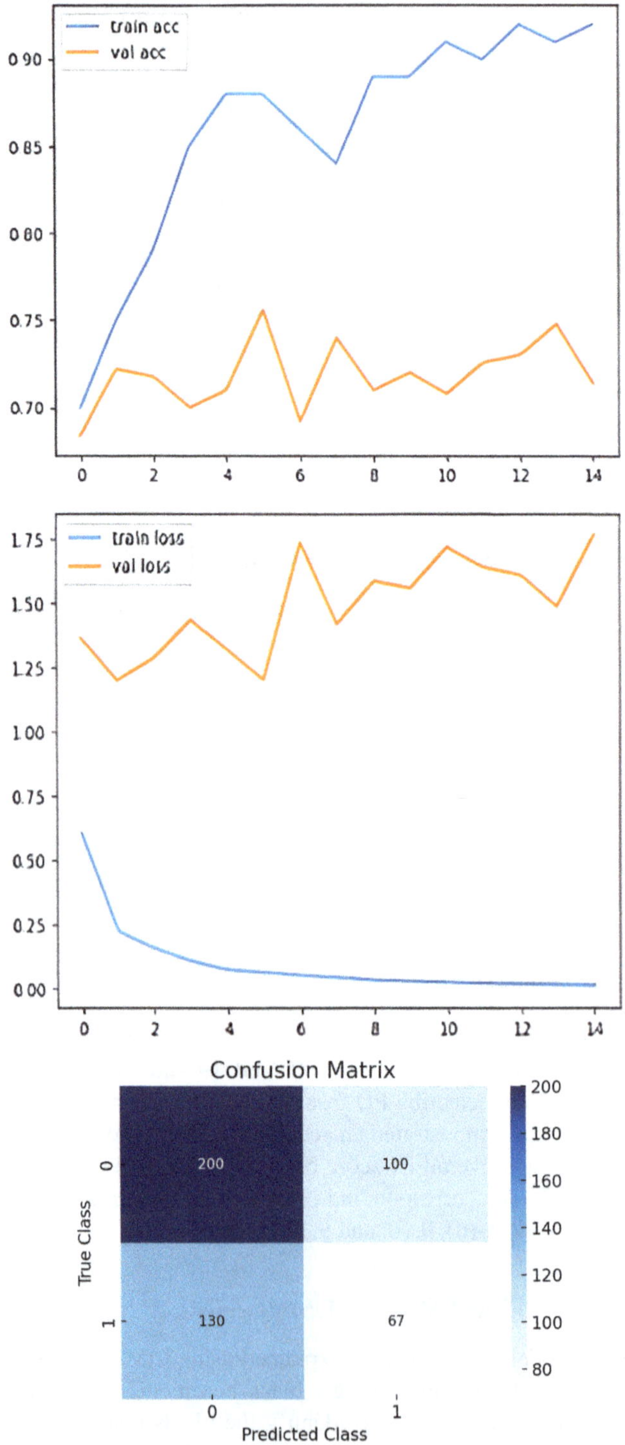

FIGURE 9.8 (a) VGG19 accuracy plot. (b) Loss curves. (c) Confusion matrix.

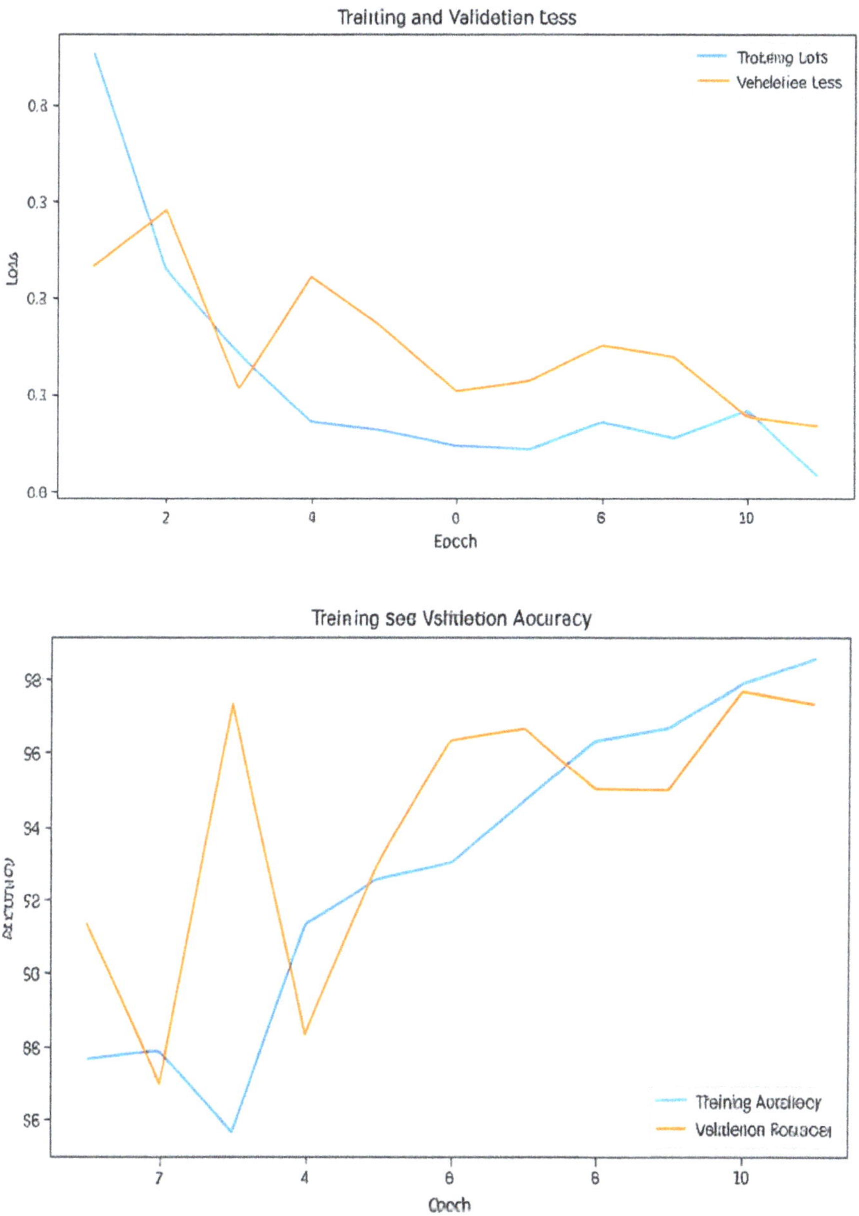

FIGURE 9.9 (a) VGG19 with attention – loss curve. (b) Accuracy plot. (c) ROC curve. (d) Confusion matrix.

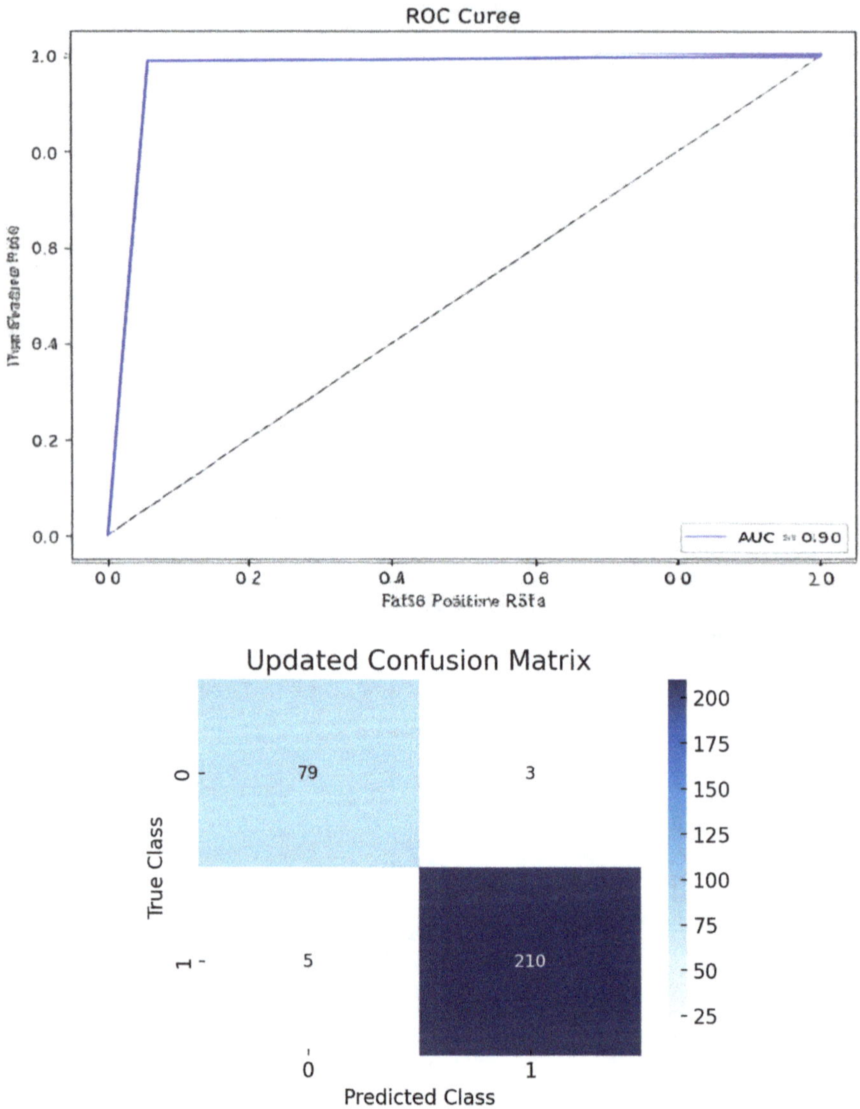

FIGURE 9.9 (Continued)

as shown in Figures 9.12 (a)–(c). LIME offers explanations that are related to the problem, making it easier to grasp specific predictions. Conversely, SHAP provides game-theoretic global interpretations that yield precise and consistent explanations for every prediction. Both approaches seek to increase the transparency of complicated models and the understandability of their conclusions.

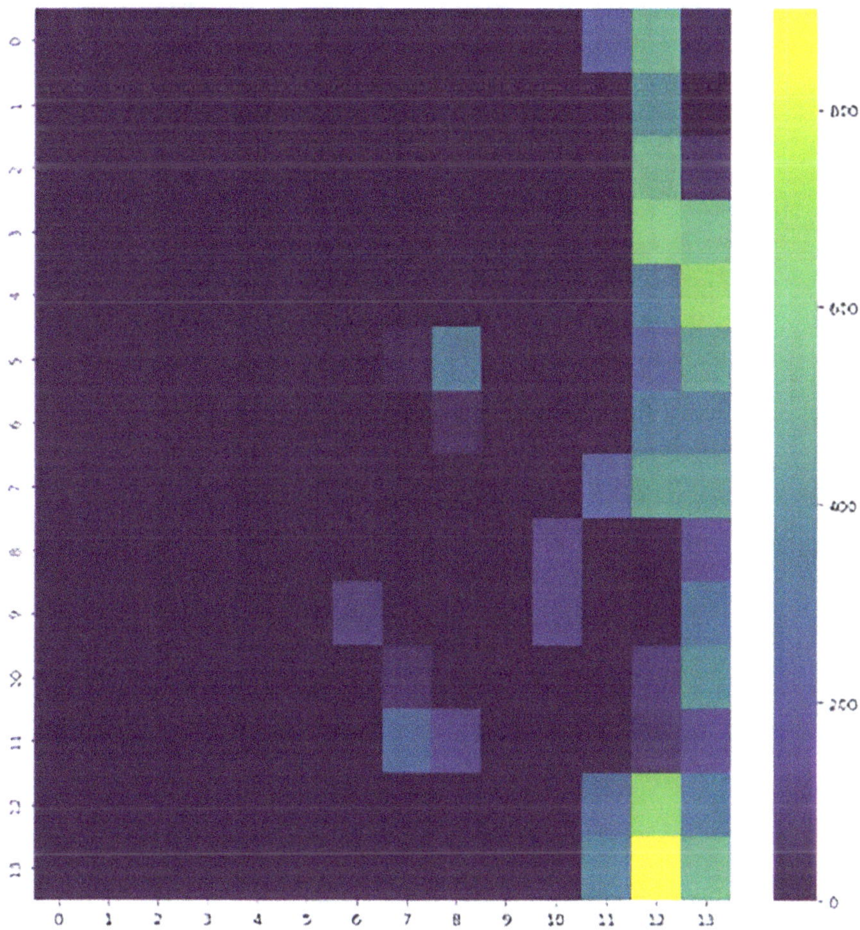

FIGURE 9.10 Feature map.

9.6 CONCLUSION

The goal of this research was to diagnose PD in its early stages by creating a modified deep learning model that combines the advantages of two deep transfer learning models. With an attention mechanism enabled, VGG19 achieved an overall F1 score of 96.94%, recall rate of 96%, accuracy rate of 97.5%, and precision rate of 97.5%. The experimental results lead us to conclude that spirals are more informative than waves. Additionally, the model developed on a combination of both drawings can be improved by adding variability in the dataset. We validated our model's predictions using LIME and SHAP, demonstrating their improved performance in diagnosing PD. Researchers and practitioners in the field of deep transfer learning and XAI may benefit from our study's findings when developing reliable diagnostic classifiers for PD.

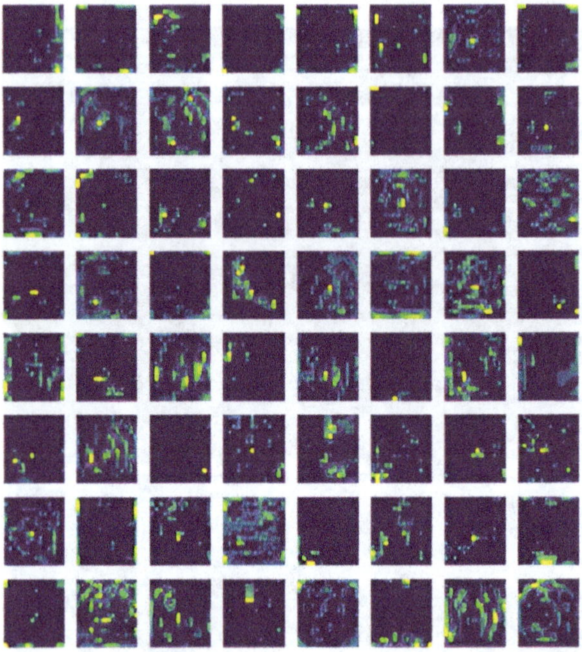

FIGURE 9.11 Features extracted by VGG19.

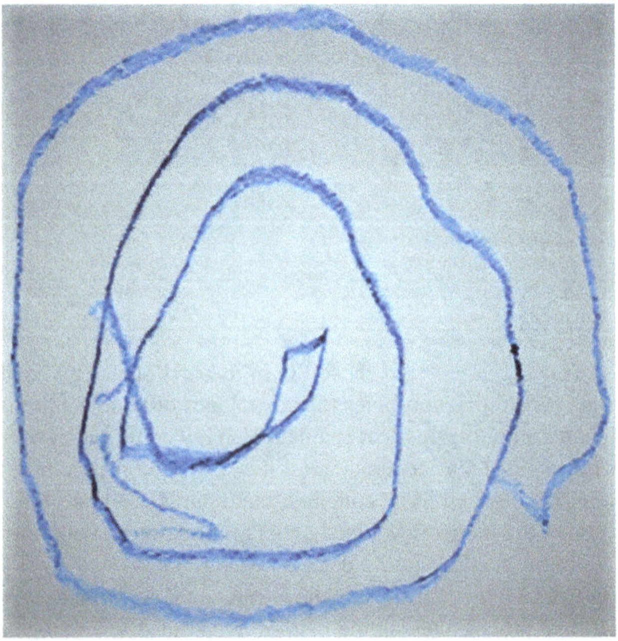

FIGURE 9.12 (a) Model predicted output (PD). (b) Super pixel. (c) SHAP explanation on the PD predicted model (VGG19 + attention).

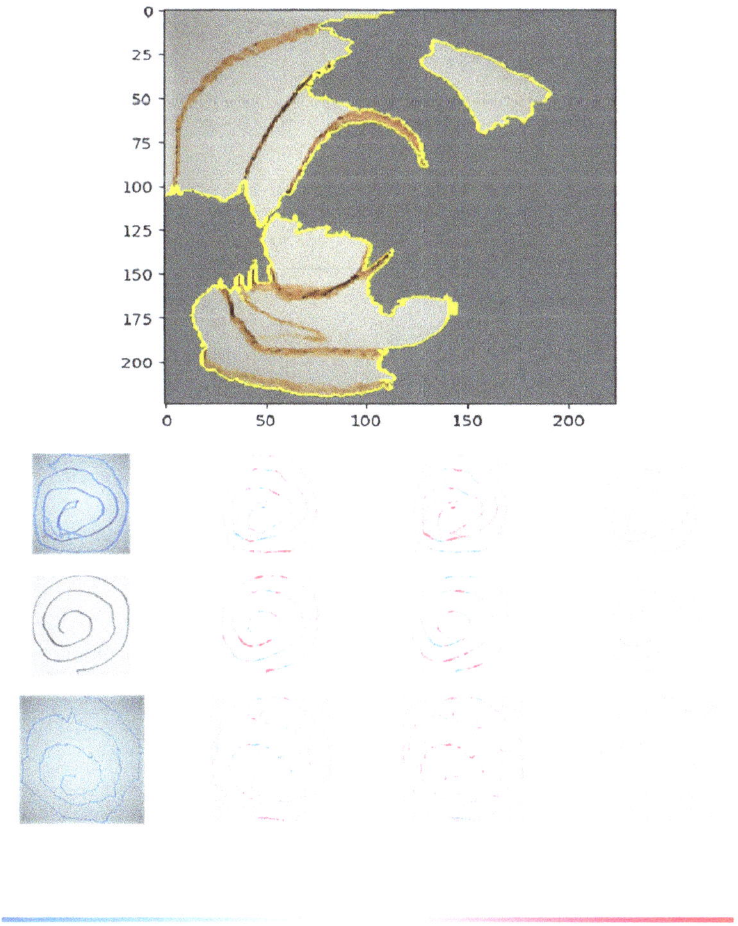

FIGURE 9.12 (Continued)

REFERENCES

[1] Shinde, Sumeet, et al. "Predictive markers for Parkinson's disease using deep neural nets on neuromelanin sensitive MRI." *NeuroImage: Clinical* 22 (2019): 101748.

[2] Kuresan, Harisudha, Dhanalakshmi Samiappan, and Sam Masunda. "Fusion of WPT and MFCC feature extraction in Parkinson's disease diagnosis." *Technology and Health Care* 27.4 (2019): 363–372.

[3] Chou, Chinmei, et al. "Using machine learning methods to detect physical conditions with postural balance." *Journal of Ambient Intelligence and Humanized Computing* (2020): 1–7. Volume 14, pages 14499–14505,

[4] Saravanan, S., et al. "Explainable Artificial Intelligence (EXAI) models for early prediction of Parkinson's disease based on spiral and wave drawings." *IEEE Access* (2023). Volume: 11, **Page(s):** 68366 - 68378

[5] Huo, Weiguang, et al. "A heterogeneous sensing suite for multisymptom quantification of Parkinson's disease." *IEEE Transactions on Neural Systems and Rehabilitation Engineering* 28.6 (2020): 1397–1406.
[6] Razzak, Imran, Iqra Kamran, and Saeeda Naz. "Deep analysis of handwritten notes for early diagnosis of neurological disorders." *2020 International Joint Conference on Neural Networks (IJCNN)*. IEEE, 2020.
[7] Veer, Karan, and S. K. Pahuja. "Gender based assessment of gait rhythms during dual-task in Parkinson's disease and its early detection." *Biomedical Signal Processing and Control* 72 (2022): 103346.
[8] Drotár, Peter, et al. "Decision support framework for Parkinson's disease based on novel handwriting markers." *IEEE Transactions on Neural Systems and Rehabilitation Engineering* 23.3 (2014): 508–516.
[9] El-Sayed, Rania Salah. "A hybrid CNN-LSTM deep learning model for classification of the Parkinson disease." *IAENG International Journal of Applied Mathematics* 53.4 (2023). Volume 53, Issue 4:
[10] Pereira, Clayton R., et al. "Handwritten dynamics assessment through convolutional neural networks: An application to Parkinson's disease identification." *Artificial Intelligence in Medicine* 87 (2018): 67–77.
[11] Caron, Mathilde, et al. "Emerging properties in self-supervised vision transformers." *Proceedings of the IEEE/CVF International Conference on Computer Vision.* 2021.
[12] Kamble, Megha, Prashant Shrivastava, and Megha Jain. "Digitized spiral drawing classification for Parkinson's disease diagnosis." *Measurement: Sensors* 16 (2021): 100047.
[13] Naseer, Amina, et al. "Refining Parkinson's neurological disorder identification through deep transfer learning." *Neural Computing and Applications* 32 (2020): 839–854.

10 Review of Medical Sensors for Healthcare Monitoring Systems Using Machine Learning Algorithms

M. K. Srilekha, S. Uma Maheswari, N. R. Shanker, and J. Gayathri

10.1 INTRODUCTION

The lifestyles of people have changed significantly in recent times. Lifestyle changes lead to diseases. Fatty liver disease is one of the diseases that arises due to lifestyle modification and it has become the most oppressive liver ailment. Although fatty liver disease is harmless, without early diagnosis, it develops into inflammatory cell infiltration and necrosis. This condition leads to fibrosis, which can further develop into cirrhosis, finally leading to hepatocellular carcinoma. A histopathological examination through liver puncture is the gold standard to detect fatty liver disease. Another test called a biopsy is the gold standard method for non-alcoholic fatty liver disease (NAFLD) [1]. However, histopathological examination through liver puncture and biopsy are invasive, i.e., only small portions of the liver are observed [2]. Additionally, it is associated with possible complications such as bile leakage, bleeding, and infection. Magnetic resonance imaging (MRI) and computed tomography (CT) detect NAFLD. CT makes use of ionizing radiation for imaging [3]. NAFLD is related to biochemical dysfunction and hepatocellular fat content. Traditional ultrasound imaging exhibits an understanding in the diagnosis of fatty liver disease, whereas MRI, CT, and imaging techniques are found to have limitations in the analysis of NAFLD. Thus, research must be done to identify non-interfering technology for the diagnosis of fatty liver disease. A wireless body area network (WBAN) represents a group of upcoming and substantial network models that provide continuous healthcare monitoring [4]. WBAN measures body parameters such as glucose levels in the blood, cholesterol, and infectious agents. Eventually, data are gathered and transmitted to the cloud for analysis. The minimal storage in nano-sensors requires the design of energy-efficient standards (e.g., data collection schemes) for such networks.

DOI: 10.1201/9781003484233-10

10.2 RELATED WORK

WBANs are used for healthcare solutions. Wireless sensor networks (WSNs) are commonly brought together on a band or vest, which the patient must wear. However, sensors are attached to a part of the patient's skin. The patient's real-time data are then transmitted to a hospital, where doctors observe the patient's vital parameters. Based on the medical history and complaints of the patient, imminent treatment and medication guidelines are conveyed to the paramedic. WBAN assists doctors in collecting the patient's health information, so necessary treatment is initialized to the patient during hospitalization [5]. Thus, compact, light, small, and transportable sensors are seen to be influencing present-day healthcare and slowly correcting age-old impediments. Body micro-sensor points have significantly accelerated healthcare choices. WBANs have been constrained in the practical use of sensor nodes. The micro-component sensors of a WBAN are insufficient for providing widespread healthcare solutions. They have failed to offer cellular-level precision and accuracy in the measurement of vital signs. Comprehensive healthcare technologies using these types of wireless sensors have been found to be inconvenient due to the pain felt by the patient when these micro-components are pierced into the skin. On the other hand, the latest advancements in nanotechnology have resulted in a possible solution to the above-mentioned limitations through micro-scale WBAN, which is based on healthcare solutions.

Furthermore, nanotechnology allows medical device fabrication at the nano scale of 1–100 nm. Nano-devices are seen as a group of molecules, which is able to activate actuation, simple sensing, and computation tasks [6]. These nano-devices are linked, through a wireless biological nano-sensor network. The sensors communicate with a stationary or moving nano-scale data acquisition unit. In contrast to conventional WSNs, nano-networks communicate between sensor nodes mechanically, electromagnetically, or molecularly. However, common forms of communication within nano-networks are through electromagnetic waves using nano-transceivers and nano-antennas for the transmission of high-frequency signals [7]. However, the complexity involved in the fabrication of nano-transceiver units is slightly challenging and combines several nano-scale nodes into a nano-device. The output power of the nano-transceiver is not reliable for a two-direction communication channel. Moreover, communication across the nano-devices needs a physical connection between the transmitter and receiver modules. Furthermore, molecular communication across nano-devices involves communication inside the human body. This form of message communication is encrypted in molecules with necessary inter-molecular parameters, such as polarization or relative element position. The combination of transmitter and receiver units on nano-devices are feasible due to the small size. Another critical difference between traditional and biological nano-sensor networks is the speed at which data are transferred. In traditional nano-sensor networks, signals are transmitted at the speed of light, whereas in the latter case, information transmission is dependent on the communication mode.

The effect of the electromagnetic signal on the human body is also a potential issue. Spurious noise accompanied with communication requires special attention for segregation and separation.

One of the direct applications of wireless biological nano-sensor networks is health monitoring. Sensors offer cellular-level precision. For instance, a biological nano-sensor node can measure the pH at different sites within an individual cell. Additionally, these sensors facilitate oxygen and cholesterol measurement, identification of cancer cells, and hormonal disturbances.

10.3 APPLICATIONS IN DISEASE CARE

10.3.1 Intrabody Nano-Scale Optical Communication

In [8], in vivo wireless nanosensor networks (iWNSNs) were presented for nano-device communication with the human body, and allowed for in vivo analysis and diagnosis. iWNSNs monitor the human body on subcellular and cellular levels. To understand this technology within the human body, the transmission of electromagnetic waves is required to be modeled by considering the aspect of the dynamics of the cells at the nano level. Various simulations have been performed, but this technology is seen to be lacking dynamism, modularity, and velocity. A simulation using the Python programming language was proposed to improve the optofluid communication medium by considering the characteristics of light interactions within the human body. This includes a two-dimensional matrix in which each entry presents a tiny area of a biological part with a dielectric constant based on the electromagnetic characteristics of the substance. A vector is computed for every element of the matrix that includes the amplitude, phase, and optical wave being transmitted at a particular point in the area. This simulation is further limited to the analysis of photon propagation in blood vessels. The proposed base includes medium modeling and paves the way for the development of in vivo wireless communication.

10.3.2 Skin-based Nano-networks

A tetrahertz (THz) device is used to measure the optical parameter of human skin tissue [9]. Skin samples are made from artificial types of materials. A particular procedure is used to culture the second layer: the dermis. However, type 1 collagen makes up the majority of the dermis layer in this stratum. The majority of artificial skin is made of commercially available collagen. Type 1 collagen is initially added to the medium to create the base solution. Fibroblast cells are added last and a 1 molar NaOH solution is added to maintain a constant pH. The The Queen Mary University of London (QMUL) system is used to assess the collected human skin and cultivated collagen. Initially, synthetic sample skin is put in a polystyrene sample holder. The polystyrene material is used as a window. Due to transparency in the THz range, polystyrene was chosen as the material for the window. The usual range of THz time-domain spectroscopy at QMUL is 0.1–4 THz, allowing for a more thorough spectral investigation. The low-temperature gallium arsenide (LT-GaAs) photoconductive antenna is a THz transmitter with an approximate gap size of 0.5 mm and bias voltage of 200 V. This characteristic makes it easier to position the laser beam. As an electro-optic detector, a 2 mm-thick ZnTe crystal guarantees a sufficient interaction length between the THz wave in the crystal and the probe beam. The skin is divided into different layers: dermis, epidermis, and subcutis or hypodermis. The stratum corneum is the outermost layer and is made up of dead cells. The next layer, namely the epidermis, serves as a chemical and diffusion barrier separating us from the outside environment. The second layer, namely the dermis, is made up of a variety of connective tissues that include reticulum, collagen, elastin, and protein. This layer is the thickest of the three layers, ranging in thickness from 1.5 to 4 mm. The layer is made up of large cells and structures, such as sweat glands, hair follicles, and blood and lymph vessels. The third layer, namely the subcutis, also known as the hypodermis, is composed of collagen and fat. A generalized model is created and simulated using detailed data. Several models, such as homogeneous, flat, and stratified, are used in this study.

10.3.3 Cuffless Blood Pressure Measurement for NAFLD

In [10], the author implemented a continuous, non-interfering, cuff-less ambulant blood pressure (BP) monitoring system. The purpose of the BP monitoring system is to assess wave velocity. Wave velocity is inversely proportional to the pulse transit time. This system is widely based on optophysiological and electrical measurements made in the chest region. Moreover, continuous BP and other physiological data can be measured with a device called IsenseU-BP+. The purpose of this system is to report findings from the initial clinical assessment of large patient groups. The purpose of the study is to determine IsenseU-BP+ utilized to measure high-quality signals in order to calculate the pulse transit time (PTT). A total of 18 patients with NAFLD underwent 23 runs of the test regimen. Measurements are taken while the subject was supine, as well as while pedaling indoors. Subsequently, using validated reference sensors, variations in BP were detected and compared with variations in PTT. In the resting state, IsenseU-BP+ recorded high-quality signals from the patients. Regardless of age, body type, or body mass index, 17 out of 18 patients had numerically acceptable quality signals. However, the lack of exact reference locations on the human body made evaluation during indoor riding challenging.

When the patient is lying down on his or her back, IsenseU-BP+ measures PTT without affecting signal quality. However, because BP readings are inaccurate, measurement during physical activity, such as indoor cycling, is restricted. Therefore, a number of clinics and hospitals would greatly benefit from real-time, non-invasive BP monitoring. Although these systems are now regarded as the gold standard for hypertension, they may have drawbacks that the approach suggested here could mitigate.

10.3.4 Self-Powered Health and Environmental Monitoring

The NSF Advanced Self-Powered Systems of Integrated Sensors and Technologies (ASSIST) center's most recent developments are presented in [11]. The center's development examines the main challenges faced by wearable health systems by investigating several technologies that guarantee durability, a long battery life, and a high user comfort level. Meanwhile, much robust and medically tested sensor information from multimodal sensing has resulted in various architecture data streams. The ASSIST center has foresight in using nanotechnology to create wearable, wireless, self-powered, and miniature sensing devices that can be used to track personal cleanliness and wellness. With the use of these tools, medical professionals and patients may contribute to a fundamental change in the quality of care. State-of-the-art developments for highly effective nano-structured energy cultivators and storage capacitors are presented in this chapter. The key problem in utilizing state-of-the-art technologies is combining them into a single device that may revolutionize group health services, from producing nano-scale raw materials to constructing body-worn structures.

Linear oscillators in the body motion sensor are mainly used to monitor vibrations that are very close to their natural frequencies. These frequencies are not very good at picking up vibrations that are outside of this extremely limited band. In order to increase the tiny quantity of energy from mechanical motion, the motion acquiring method combines precise mechanical design that gathers energy from the moving body and transmits it to a piezoelectric material. Using piezoelectric sheets in conjunction with an electrical circuit to generate energy is an effective method of transferring mechanical energy to electrical energy. Figure 10.1 depicts this schematically. Stated differently, more mechanical harvesters are edge-loaded cantilevers, with the resonance frequency adjusted to correspond with the structure's movement.

It is possible to generate high-end outputs by simultaneously varying each component of the system, as is being done in the ASSIST Center. Many strategies to enhance the weak energy from body motion are being experimented with. The creation of low-frequency, somewhat broad resonance scavengers is one of the approaches. This causes an end-loaded cantilever to partially strain the piezoelectric material, increasing the generation of energy. It is also possible to create devices with resonance frequencies between 7 and 10 Hz by properly designing the hinges and end mass. In essence, this calls for the deposition of lead zirconate titanate (PZT) films onto metal foils with sizable coefficients of thermal expansion. By removing ferroelectric polarization from the film's plane, dielectric permittivity decreases and the piezoelectric coefficient rises. In addition, the mechanical stability of the metal substrates is better than that of brittle passive elastomeric layers, such silicon nitride and silicon (Si). The film can be produced for a wide range of harvester designs, such as the hinged design

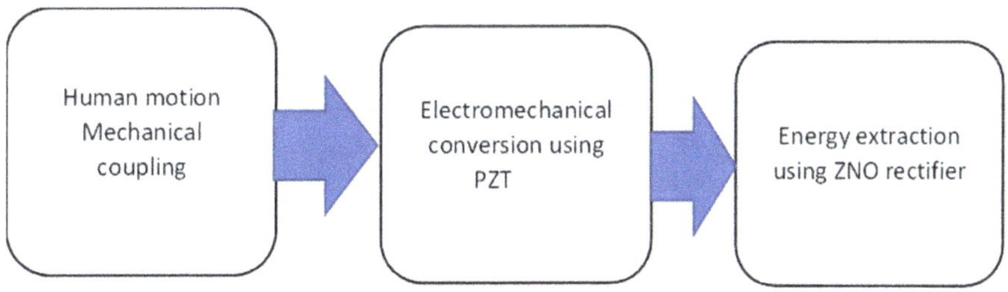

FIGURE 10.1 Body motion sensor.

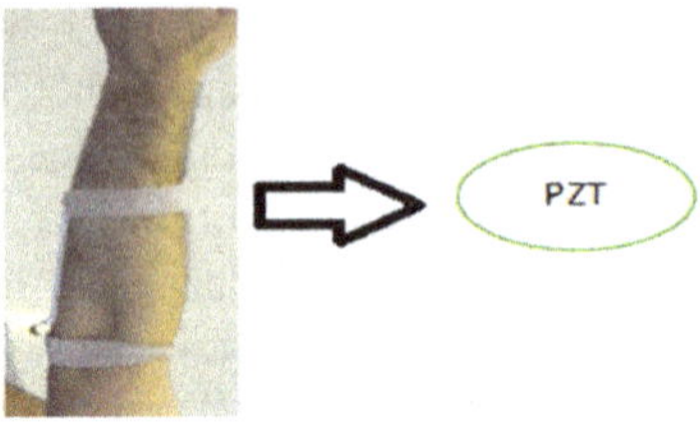

FIGURE 10.2 Piezoelectric sensor on the elbow.

previously discussed, and for harvesters that are joint-based. Figure 10.2 shows how piezoelectric film on nickel foil is utilized for energy signal detection when a person's elbow is moved.

Kapton tape is a thin layer of orange material that is located around the elbow and encloses PZT film that is based on nickel. When the harvester straightens its elbow, the space between the attachment points reduces. Consequently, this puts stress on the PZT and generates force with every elbow movement. The mechanical harvester extracts an electrical signal from the PZT and stores it for later use. To enable storage in batteries or supercapacitors, these outputs need to be adjusted. Diodes with a relatively high voltage are also used by different rectifiers to "turn on." Additionally, the piezoelectric film generates very low voltages (0.2–0.3 V), which are much lower than the threshold that serves as a gauge for how much power is "lost" from the system. It is possible to manipulate the voltage produced by the diode to almost zero volts to extract the highest power from the harvester. To conserve a significant amount of energy, fast switching between the two voltage levels can also be done. The strategy in this instance involves integrating electronics onto mechanical energy harvesting equipment to enable high-speed switching and observation of the harvester output's zero crossing point. ZnO thin-film transistors (TFTs) are used to accomplish this objective. As a result, electronics can theoretically be integrated directly onto the mechanical energy harvester. Stable TFTs are necessary since they result in high gain amplifiers. A piezoelectric energy harvester typically produces very low voltages. Thus, traditional diode-based rectification systems may result in energy losses. Therefore, if power matching and power combining tactics are used, they cause issues. Integrated electronics raise the energy harvester's possible output. Furthermore, ASSIST has been demonstrated as a combination of ZnO TFT and PZT micro electromechanical devices without affecting the operation of any component. Twin gate ZnO TFTs in an enhancement/depletion mode arrangement provide a gain of > 100 in a basic inverter. This solution is critical for providing low voltage, TFT-based rectification for the piezoelectric energy harvester. Active rectification has been used for the mechanical energy harvester to overcome issues associated with the higher knee voltage (0.3 V) of the Ge diode.

For this reason, twin gate ZnO TFTs with ZnO layers that range in thickness from 10 to 50 nm were created. This enables us to reduce the voltage value to almost zero by using the gate at the top of the TFT. Additionally, it enables low power operations for the amplifier by utilizing the depletion loads. The expected range of the alternating current output for a lead zirconate titanate human body kinetic energy harvester is from 100 millivolts to 5 volts. The full-wave active rectifier may be directly mounted on the PZT harvester and can operate with load resistance of up to 10 kW.

10.3.5 Ultra-Low Power Electronics

The capacity to interface with sensors, perform computations to extract valuable information by aggregating data, store data, utilize power harvesting technologies, and manage and communicate wirelessly are the most important features of wearable and flexible systems. However, wearable systems use commercial off-the-shelf components integrated into a printed circuit board (PCB). The most obvious drawback of this method is that most commercial-off-the-shelf (COTS) chips draw excessive amounts of power when run nonstop without heavy-duty cycling. Recent studies show that electronics incorporated into a system on chip (SoC) can make it smaller, cheaper, and more energy-efficient. One chip contains the full bio-electric wireless sensor, for instance, thanks to the SoC. When the SoC measures an electrocardiogram (ECG), extracts the heart rate, and transmits the heart rate data via radio waves, it only uses 19 W. Additionally, it can function without the need of an internal or external battery by harnessing the energy from body heat through the use of a thermoelectric generator (TEG). The development of flexible, self-powered wearable sensors is greatly encouraged by these kinds of SoCs. Because of the amazing advancements in flexible and wearable electronics based on a nanowire (NW), silver NWs, as depicted in Figure 10.3, are used for health-related purposes [12]. This technology's most notable feature is its capacity to adapt to the curved shape of the human body and to change in accordance with motions. Stretchable electronics have made numerous exciting developments because of a new technique called micro-fabricated ribbons. The unequaled ductility of these ribbons is caused by pre-strain induced buckling. Utilizing a similar approach, SiNWs find widespread application in stretchy electronics [13]. SiNWs have been moved to a polydimethylsiloxane (PDMS) substrate that had been previously stretched. When the substrate is released, the SiNW microribbons bend into a wavy or three-dimensional (3D) coiled structure. Compared to the wavy shape, the 3D coiled shape is more ductile. For instance, the AgNW network has been embedded beneath the elastomer PDMS substrate surface to create AgNW conductors. It is possible to print AgNWs in a variety of designs and shapes. The

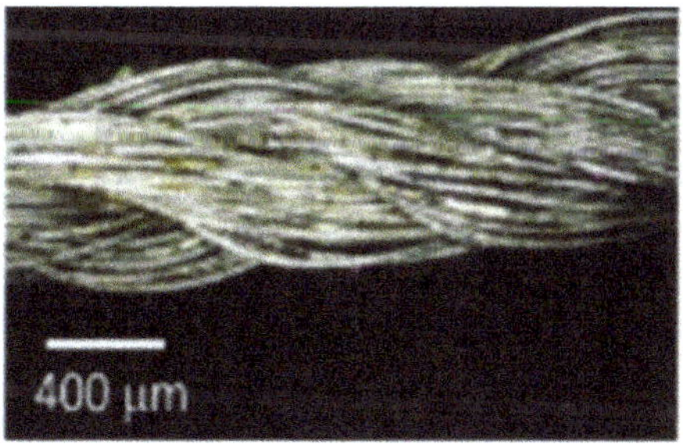

FIGURE 10.3 Silver nanowire.

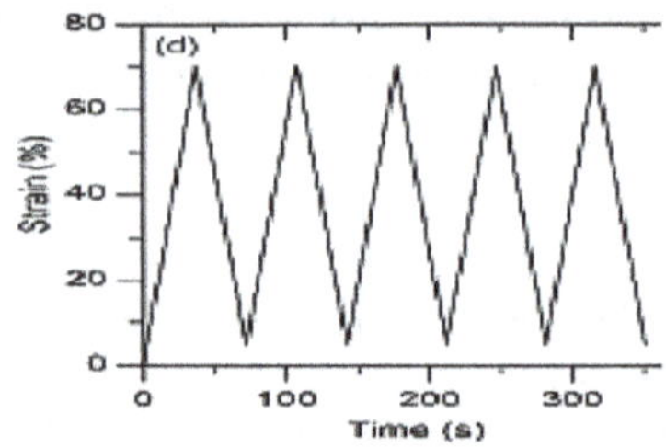

FIGURE 10.4 Electric performance of the AgNW conductor.

AgNW/PDMS composite exhibits superior ductility (> 50% strain with steady conductivity) and high conductivity (> 5000 S/cm).

Figure 10.3 illustrates the mechanism behind the high ductility of AgNW conductors and their dynamic performance in relation to strain. These extremely ductile conductors have the potential to be worn as conformal electrodes for bioelectronic sensing applications. Because there are fewer body movements with AgNW dry electrodes for ECG, they perform better than traditional wet Ag/AgCl electrodes. It is important to note that these AgNW electrodes are appropriate for long-term use because they do not employ the electrolytic gel layer. A capacitive sensor can be created by sandwiching two of these conductors between a dielectric layer. Figure 10.4 shows the performance of silver NW.

A variety of sensors are employed in daily life. The information is sent to phone apps so that users can access things like their BP, sugar levels, and medicines. It assists in responding promptly to prevent any risks to one's life or health.

10.3.6 Heart Care Monitoring System

IBANs (placed BANs) are a particular subclass described in [14], where the nodes are sensors that are placed as implants within the human body. A few sensors on the IBAN are in communication with the control unit. These surgical implants have the ability to either supplement or completely replace any compromised brain connections, and they may even be able to be controlled outside.

Minimizing energy consumption is crucial for tiny implanted devices. This requires using suitable antennas and ensuring relatively short transmission ranges, usually less than a meter but up to a few meters, while considering the special circumstances of signal propagation via bodily tissues.

Figure 10.5 illustrates artery-disseminated nano-sensors that gather data on chemical particles and biological processes. The most numerous type of node in a nanonetwork is a nano-sensor. The nano-sensor reads data from the blood and the data is transmitted. Several nano-routers support nano-sensors in different domains inside the circulatory system. These routers get data to the nano-interface and gather data that is supplied by nano-sensors. The system's operation is greatly influenced by the node density and nano-device communication range, as these factors affect the way data are delivered to the health monitoring system. The mode encompasses software

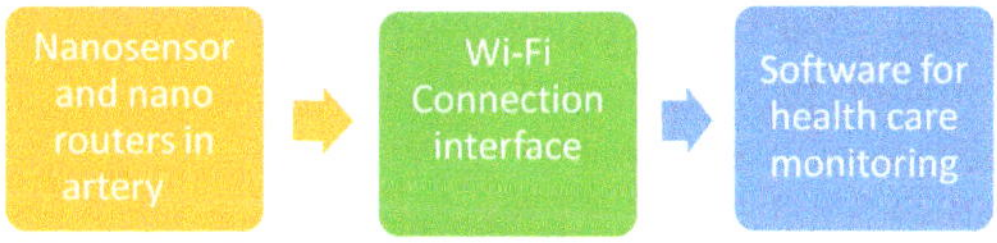

FIGURE 10.5 Internet of Nano Things for heart monitoring.

implementations on WNSN devices, in time on-off keying (TS-OOK) modulation, a basic access protocol to MAC, a flooding algorithm-based routing mechanism, a general model of message production and processing, and an interface to an external network. The functions of the node model are consistent with the actual nano-node design.

10.3.7 Vital Sign Monitoring System

In [15], environmental sensing devices for wearable health are discussed. The Internet of Nano Things as it functions inside the telemedicine service chain is presented in this study. It comprises an examination of different methods for gathering, handling, and disseminating medical data that are published internationally. Suggestions for the development of the specified problems are provided, and the research and development status of nano-sensor networks and telemedicine standards are analyzed.

It is possible to apply telemedicine in contemporary war theater settings with success. Test results from a nano-sensor network operating in the human circulatory system corroborate the studies. Possible information loss and medical information delivery delays occur at nano-interfaces at BAN and wireless area network (WAN) interface points.

The progress of civilization, including social and technical advancements, will change people's perspectives on the world and optimize the use of its resources [16]. Patients with serious illnesses need specialized care that requires continuous, non-invasive monitoring. These monitoring systems use sensors attached within the human body to gather data on the patient's physiological state. Then, they send the gathered data to specialized medical equipment using Wi-Fi, 3G, and long-term evolution (LTE) technologies. After the data are processed, the information is sent to medical professionals in the form of traits or alarms, enabling them to electronically prescribe medication or deliver medication remotely. By lowering the cost of advanced technologies and providing continuous monitoring, automation enhances the quality of medical care. It reduces the necessity for medical staff to actively participate in data gathering, analysis, and prescription delivery. Various sensors are used for continuous healthcare monitoring. Additionally, information can be sent to phone apps so users can check their body temperature, BP, or sugar level. By enabling prompt action, serious risks to one's life or health can be avoided. The doctor is responsible for gathering and analyzing every vital indicator that the sensors have measured. A light-emitting diode (LED), liquid-crystal display (LCD), and buzzer serving as a status indicator are also included in the system. This technology is also integrated into a mobile application that shows the user's position and vital sign measurement, and notifies the healthcare professional if an anomaly is found. The Arduino Nano microcontroller processes sensor input to provide users with both visual and aural feedback. Three distinct vital sign measures are chosen via a push button and the power supply is a 9-volt power adaptor. The results are shown on an LCD screen and an LED turns on in accordance with the range of vital sign readings to alert the user anytime an anomaly is found. The LED is also utilized to show the device's standby mode. The Android-based mobile application additionally displays the outcome of real-time vital sign measurement. This is connected to the system through the HC-05 Bluetooth module. Additionally, the mobile application can automatically send a notice message anytime an anomaly is found. The ProSim 8 Vital Signs Simulator is a tool for precise calibration and measurement.

10.3.8 Information Technology for Health and Environment

In [17], the authors describe tracking the recovery of long-term lesions. They developed a sensing wound pad using integrated fluorescence-coupled biosensors for non-invasive wound monitoring. This technology is expected to find utility in a wide range of industries, including the rapidly expanding media and healthcare sectors. This working prototype uses fluorescence readings for sensing and displaying the pH value of the wound. A variety of users and applications can benefit from such a sensor. Patients can use it for self-evaluation at home, while clinicians can use it in clinics to assess the pH progression of chronic wounds precisely. To create a sensing patch, the scientists modified a commercial wound pad that contained fluorescent molecules. The redesigned pad included spots made of hydrogel or textile fibers that contained the fluorescent molecules. The pH of skin model underneath affects the intensity of the spots' fluorescence. The increased number of parameters being monitored and the sensors' sensitivity to body motion is responsible for the unpredictable high rates of false alarm in newborn monitoring. Newborn care utilizes a computer vision approach to calculate the heart rate and respiration rate without physical touch, aiming to minimize incorrect alarm triggers. Personalized medicine using therapeutic medication monitoring. This project aims to reduce healthcare costs by developing a technology platform that enables personalized treatment via therapeutic drug monitoring. The ISyPeM II project has explored new sensor technology, software, and hardware data processing approaches, and a drug release mechanism using a silicon membrane. An integrated approach to therapeutic drug monitoring combines prescription decision assistance, interoperability in complex data-sharing scenarios, and innovative point-of-care compatible testing.

10.3.9 Micro Biochip to Monitor Cancer

The research paper [18] details the procedure for identifying cancer antigen CA 125 from a small biofluid sample. The biochip in a microfluidic channel is connected to a sensor platform that detects cancer antigen in biofluid passing through the channel. The sensing platform is constructed in the layer to enhance the detection signal and the immobilization of the antibody on the nano-circuit. Antigen-antibody interaction occurs when biofluid flows across the immobilized antibody in the micro-channel. The sensing circuit capacitance readings are altered. The concentration of the targeted cancer antigen in the biofluid sample is shown by the change in capacitance. To test the biochip's functioning, 55 ug/ml of CA125 antigens at a pH of 7.4 was employed in this experiment. Comparing the capacitance following antigen-antibody interaction to bare electrodes revealed a shift of 679.62 pF. The convenient use of a small bio-chip allows for the immediate evaluation of a cancer biomarker from a blood sample, enhancing cancer management via better disease monitoring. The micro bio-chip features surface-treated micro-channels that ensure blood sample flow without requiring an external device. Nano electrodes on the micro-channels' surface function as a capacitance sensing mechanism to identify cancer antigen-antibody complex formation. The biochip contains a spiral micro-channel with dimensions of 200 um in width and 107 um in depth. An Si wafer mold is used in a soft lithography process to create the microchannels on the PDMS after the channels are etched. A thorough reactive ion etching procedure combined with photolithography is used to manufacture the Si wafer featuring micro-channels.

10.3.10 Pressure Sensor for Electronic Skin

A monolithic 3D-printed pressure sensor with reliable and sensitive sensing performance was presented in [19]. A 3D-printed water-soluble template is filled with an elastomer prepolymer to create the porous structured dielectric. The porosity can be adjusted to adjust sensing performance. The bottom and top electrodes of the 3D-printed conductive thermoplastic are integrated [20]. Air has a lower dielectric constant than PDMS, which results in lesser porosity in the PDMS layer and a lower initial capacitance value. The porosity of the porous structure PDMS layer boosts the pressure sensor's sensitivity. Porosity increases due to the pressure sensor's sensitivity, which reduces stiffness. Larger capacitance is achieved with the same pressure input. Furthermore, an increase in capacitance can be attained by raising the dielectric constant through the closure of pores under external pressure.

10.3.11 Medical Sensor for Sleep Apnea

One of the main sleep diseases that is underdiagnosed is obstructive sleep apnea (OSA) [21]. This is a contributing factor to several dangerous cardiovascular conditions, such as stroke. Medical equipment for long-term ambulatory monitoring of OSA is lacking. Presently available methods are expensive, invasive, heavy, and unsuitable for long-term ambulatory monitoring. In this study, a wearable, precise, and energy efficient device for long-term continuous monitoring of OSA was proposed. This is an embedded system for the Internet of Things, and closes the distance between professional supervision and at-home healthcare. The method is predicated on utilizing a single channel ECG signal to monitor the patient. It computes the sleep apnea score in an efficient time domain manner, while adhering to strict resource limits of embedded devices. This method can classify data from a publicly accessible database (PhysioNet

Apnea-ECG) with an accuracy of 88.2%. This method offers patient-specific online analysis that considers each patient's unique profile. The continuous OSA screening method can reach a battery life of 46 days, while maintaining accuracy and energy efficiency. INYU is a wearable gadget that uses less energy and records a single lead ECG using a 24-bit analog to a digital converter. It uses a frequency range of 250 Hz to 16 kHz for operation. Impedance pneumography is used to measure the ECG using electrodes made of silver chloride. An ultra-low power 32-bit microprocessor with 32 MHz as its maximum frequency of operation is used. The microprocessor characteristics include 384 KB flash storage and 48 kB of RAM. This device may operate as a fully independent device for continuous recording due to its internal capabilities and communication possibilities. When a base station becomes accessible, it uploads the recorded and analyzed data. For instance, a smartphone that complies with Bluetooth Low Energy standards is utilized for this function. The smartphone then sends the online data to a remote medical center so that a doctor can manually review it or present it on screen.

10.3.12 Nano-Communication in Big Data Analytics

The large data produced by nano-sensors and nano-communication networks for upcoming medical and biomedical applications is discussed in this research [22]. The aim is to develop advanced healthcare systems that use 4P principles – predictive, preventive, personalized, and participatory – to assist in medical diagnosis, monitoring, and treatment. Utilizing practical intelligence and learning capabilities in conjunction with traditional medical and health data can enhance decision-making efficiency through the analytical potential of the vast amount of data collected in these networks. Additionally, a big data analytics methodology for obtaining insights from large amounts of healthcare data is used. Futuristic smart healthcare needs this to address connected issues and take advantage of potential future application prospects. Numerous industries, including the military, biomedical, environmental, industrial, agricultural, and smart office management, use nano-sensors extensively. Advancements in nanotechnology have sped up the progress of nano-sensor development, leading to the ultimate creation of a network of millions of linked devices at the nano-scale. This network would generate vast quantities of data, requiring the implementation of advanced participatory, preventive, customized, and predictive healthcare infrastructure. By analyzing data to enable early diagnosis, the vast volume of data gathered from the framework can lead to a decrease in healthcare costs. Perceived by patients, the ongoing evaluation of the biomarkers acquired through IoBN has the potential to completely prevent or identify the early beginning of fatal diseases, beyond current technological capabilities. The challenges of collecting extensive and diverse health data over a prolonged period stem from the interaction of big data analytics with nanotechnology. By collecting data from several sensor arrays and scrutinizing the extensive amount of data, clinical research is certain to achieve new levels of success. The primary characteristics of big data in the healthcare system setting was discussed. Table 10.1 shows the distribution of sensors on the human body.

TABLE 10.1
On-body sensors

On-body sensor	Position of sensor	Sensor type
Head	Hat	EEG
Upper limb	Arm, wrist, finger	Heart rate, accelerometer
Chest	Patches, pockets, necklace, strap	Respiration rate, heart rate
Waist, hip, back	Belt, pocket, bag	Gyroscope
Lower limb	Pocket, leg, thigh	EMG, accelerometer
Foot	Shoes, ankle, insole	Gyroscope, pressure

10.4 SENSOR SCREEN PRINTING

The modification of nano-ink into fabric using a stenciled mesh is part of the screen printing process. In addition, the nanomaterial ink is processed inside the mesh, which fills in the spaces that were previously empty. A force that acts in a downward direction brings the mesh into contact with the substrate. The mesh can be pulled vertically, resulting in a filament due to the cohesive force. This filament then leads to the deposition of the substrate. During the last step, the ink is applied to the substrate and then spread vertically into the filament structure.

The stokes equation in cylindrical polar coordinates offers an analytical framework for studying ink flow and elucidates the process of ink transfer in screen printing:

$$\Psi = \mathrm{rVT}(\phi, \alpha) \tag{1}$$

where the symbol 'r' denotes the radius and 'ϕ' represents the phase angle. The symbol 'Ψ' represents the ink's motion in relation to the squeegee and 'V' indicates the squeegee's velocity as defined in Eq. (1). The Taylor function is represented by $T(\phi, \alpha)$, where α is the angle of the squeegee. The flow velocity for screen printing remains constant at 30 mm/s for the whole procedure. It is advisable to maintain the print speed at 60 mm/s. The squeegee exerts a pressure of 10 kg and has a hardness of 70 durometers on shore 'A'. The squeegee is positioned at a 45-degree angle. The cured material has a thickness of about 5–10 m. The printing margin is 0 mm and two strokes are employed in this operation. Table 10.2 displays the screen printing technique used in creating the sensor.

10.5 MACHINE LEARNING AND ALGORITHMS IN SIGNAL PROCESSING

Machine learning (ML) includes several analyses, including association, clustering, regression, and classification. These studies include a few methods, such as logistic regression, simple linear regression, naive Bayes, and support vector machines. Regression analysis is employed here because house price prediction is the prediction of a continuous value, and regression is used to predict continuous variables

TABLE 10.2
Screen printing techniques for sensor fabrication sensors

S No.	References	Problem statement	Methodology
		Sensors – Screen Printing – Research Article	
1.	Riemer (1989) [23]	Fundamentals of the screen printing technique	The basics of screen printing are discussed and an analytical model of screen printing technique is introduced.
2.	Zavanelli *et al.* (2021) [24]	Screen printing technique using conductive ink nanomaterials	Screen printing involves combining fluid dynamics, ideal ink characteristics, nanomaterials, binders, solvents, and rheological agents to create inks. Conductive ink is used for detecting and conducting items.
3.	Naghdi *et al.* (2022) [25]	Color changing nano-sensor based on the GONH2 nanosheet and bromophenol blue	A novel colorimetric nano-sensor is developed and monitors minced fish package freshness based on a bromophenol blue dye pH level indicator with the GONH2 nanosheet.
4.	Hieu *et al.* (2020) [26]	Zinc telluride-coated zinc oxide nanorods and hydrogen sulfide nano-sensor controlled by a PN circuit	Zinc telluride in hydrogen sulphide gas sensing using ZnO nanorods is discussed. Sensor performance in the zinc telluride coating nano-transducer achieves a high response and offers high temperature stability at 200°C
5.	Wang *et al.* (2010) [27]	Wireless system on a chip designed for interfacing biomedical signals in body sensor networks	Displaying a mixed signal silicon chip is needed for a wearable and implanted body sensor network. The blocks are a low-power analog sensor interface for pH and temperature, multiplexer, 8-bit microprocessor, RF section, and wireless transmitter.

[34]. Regression analysis uses various statistical methods to describe the connection between a dependent variable (target variable) and an independent variable (predictor variable) by including one or more independent variables.

ML challenges are categorized as

- Supervised ML
- Unsupervised ML
- Reinforcement learning

TABLE 10.3
Screen printing techniques for sensor fabrication sensors

S No.	References	Problem statement	Methodology
Transforms/Machine Learning in Signal Processing – Research Article			
1.	Frankston (2015) [28]	Application Program Interface Things Speak	Interconnection of computers to local networks to form a worldwide Internet. The Web application is used by computers to enable people to work in the same room or around the world.
2.	Chen *et al.* (2014) [29]	Algorithm for blind signal separation for temporal prediction and differential search	A blind signal separation algorithm for differential search is proposed for a high amount problem in the blind signal separation algorithm on bio-inspired optimization. The temporal predictability of the signal is used as the main function.
3.	Subasi *et al.* (2020) [30]	Surface electromyography signal classification using Tunable Q wavelet transform, bagging and boosting for hand movement recognition	Surface EMG (sEMG) plays a vital role in prosthetic hands. The sEMG signal is denoised and feature extraction is done using TQWT. The obtained feature is extracted and fed as an input to classifiers. Bagging and boosting ensemble classifiers have different performance measures.
4.	Birge *et al.* (2001) [31]	Model selection through Gaussian regression	Gaussian regression is based on the penalization of least square criteria viewed as a generalization of Mallows' Cp (statistics for a particular set of regressors) to choose the list of models.
5.	Shahin *et al.* (2020) [32]	Classification of rapid cardiovascular images using combined deep characteristics and long short-term memory	A deep learning method is utilized to categorize ECG perspectives for the purpose of determining their physiological placement. The features of the spatial CNN are taken from each frame in echo motion. Neutrosophic temporal motion characteristics are derived from echo motion activity. The spatial and neutrosophic temporal CNN characteristics are combined using a method that involves concatenating the features.

Deep learning is the branch of ML that uses a multilayered neural network, called a deep neural network, to replicate the intricate decision-making capability of the human brain [35]. Table 10.3 examines several ML methods.

TABLE 10.4
Wireless communication standards

Wireless communication	Protocol standard	Frequency	Distance	Data rate	Modulation	Power
Bluetooth	IEEE 802.15.1	2.4 GHz	10 m	< 1 Mbps	Frequency hop spread spectrum	1–100 mW
ZigBee	IEEE 802.15.4	915 MHz - 2.4 GHz	10–75 m	40 kbps 250 kbps	DSSS	Very low
NFC	ISO	13.56 Mhz	20 cm	424 kbps	ASK	Very low
UWB	IEEE 802.15.3	3.1–10.6 GHz	30 m	100–1024 Mbps	OFDM	<= 1 mW
Wi-Fi	IEEE802.11 a/b/g	2.4Ghz	< 100 m	11 Mbps	OFDM DSSS	60–70 mW

10.6 WIRELESS COMMUNICATION STANDARDS FOR HEALTHCARE MONITORING SYSTEMS

Short-range wireless communication is used. Wireless communication utilizes technology standards such as Wi-Fi, Bluetooth, NFC, UWB, RFID, and ZigBee. Table 10.4 enumerates the attributes of these standards. In terms of power usage, UWB is beneficial because it uses less power than other standards. For wireless short-range communication, UWB offers a high data rate at a reasonable cost. Several wireless communication standards and their specifications for healthcare monitoring systems are displayed in Table 10.4.

10.7. CURRENT RESEARCH ON HEALTHCARE MONITORING SYSTEMS

The wearable systems chosen are listed in Table 10.5 along with hardware, sensors, type of communication, physiological parameters measured, application, and its advantages. This review is focused on nano-sensor wearable devices. Table 10.5 summarizes the various healthcare monitoring systems.

10.8 DESIGN OBJECTIVES

The aim of remote monitoring is useful to physicians because it allows them to access patient data without attending the patient in person.

The objectives involved in designing wearable healthcare system are as follows:

1. A low-cost microcontroller makes it simple to construct the healthcare system.
2. A lightweight and low-power system.
3. Power-efficient communication over extended distances.

TABLE 10.5
Healthcare monitoring system

Literature	Physiological parameter	Sensor	Communication module	Hardware description	Application	Advantages
Intra body nano-scale optical communication [33]	Cell	Light	Optofluid model	Simulation	Intra-body communication	Light propagation in larger biological tissues
Skin-based nano-networks	Human skin (collagen)	Polystyrene window	Nano-communication	THz system at QMUL	Tetrahertz wave propagation in human skin	Electromagnetic channel modeling at THz for a body-centric nano-network
Non-invasive cuffless BP measurement	BP	PPG sensor	Bluetooth	32-bit ARM Cortex M3 microcontroller	Hypertension and cardiovascular application	Cuffless BP measurement
Wearable health and environmental sensing	BP. heart rate, body motion	Flexible electrode, PZT, silver nanowire	Bluetooth	ARM microcontroller	Sensing modalities for physiological and environmental sensing	High efficiency Low-power computation
Internet of Nano Things	BP, sugar level, body temperature	Nano-sensor	Wi-Fi	Nano-microcontroller	Nano-sensor network functioning in the human circulatory system	Less delay

(continued)

TABLE 10.5 (Continued)
Healthcare monitoring system

Literature	Physiological parameter	Sensor	Communication module	Hardware description	Application	Advantages
Vital sign monitoring using Android	Heart rate, body temperature, blood oxygen saturation	Pulse oximeter sensor, ECG sensor, temperature sensor	Bluetooth	Arduino Nano	Device assembled for home monitoring application	Accuracy in result
Micro biochip to monitor cancer	Cancer	Micro biochip using (polydimethyl siloxane), gold nano integrated electrode	Bluetooth	Micro controller	Cancer monitoring and diagnosis	Biochip with sensing platform to detect cancer antigen
Pressure sensor for application in electronic skin	Electronic skin	3D-printed pressure sensor	-	-	Skin monitoring	Stable noise-free and perfectly reversible signal
Online sleep apnea	Cardiac monitoring	INYU sensor	Bluetooth	ARM Cortex M3	Sleep apnea detection	Good battery life time
Role of RF communication big data analytics perspective	ECG, lung cancer	Graphene sensor, bio nano-sensor	Nano molecular communication	Nano-microcontroller	Nano-communication for healthcare monitoring	Privacy, security

4. To collect information from a nano-sensor, transfer it to a microcontroller, and then notify the physician. Through online analysis, the physician makes additional diagnoses and treatments based on the patient's data.

10.9 PROPOSED ARCHITECTURE

The system comprises a sensing module, microcontroller module, and wireless communication module. The system comprises a nano-sensor connected to a microprocessor. The nano-sensor is used for detecting fatty liver. Zigbee functions as a wireless module that offers an integrated solution. The nano-sensor is used for signal detection.

The microcontroller unit processes the signal and saves the patient's physiological characteristics, which are subsequently displayed on the doctor's computer. The data is sent straight to the doctor's computer screen through the internet using the Zigbee module.

The patient's body is linked to the nano-sensor. The signal detected by the nano-sensor is transmitted to the microcontroller as an analog signal. The analog signal that is supplied as an input from the sensor is converted to digital form by the microcontroller analog-to-digital converter (ADC). After processing the data, the microcontroller sends them via the Zigbee module. The information is then shown on the doctor's screen. The patient can receive the right medication from the doctor or caregiver after analyzing such data.

Figure 10.6 shows the proposed system architecture, where data are wirelessly transmitted to the recipient by the nano-sensor. They are sent to the doctor's PC via an Arduino connection for processing. The information is then shown on the doctor's screen. The patient can receive the right medication from a doctor or caregiver after that data is analyzed.

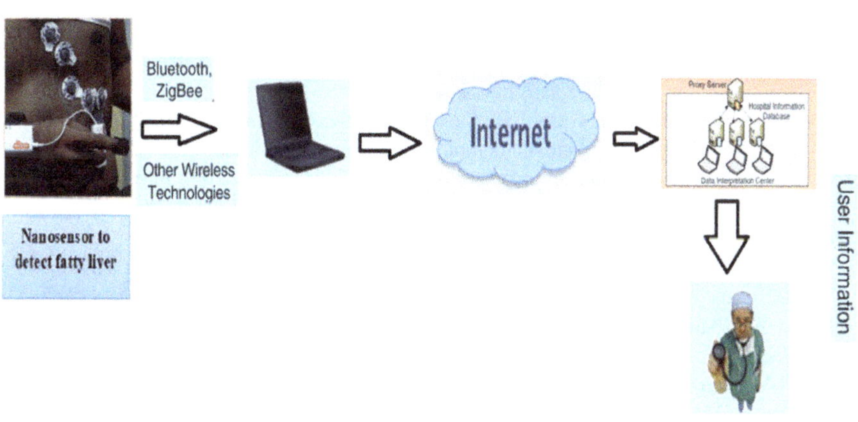

FIGURE 10.6 Healthcare system for NAFLD.

10.10 CONCLUSION

This review discusses research on nano-sensors used in healthcare monitoring systems to provide an in-depth understanding of different nano-sensors used in commercial systems. Identifying wearable sensors may enhance their functioning and increase quality of life. This article discusses several kinds of sensors and their usage in a healthcare monitoring system. Interfaces on a smartphone and remote location enable the user and the supervising person to monitor the patient's health by providing real-time and historical physiological data.

REFERENCES

[1] Nalbantoglu I, Brunt EM. Role of liver biopsy in nonalcoholic fatty liver disease. *World Journal of Gastroenterology: WJG*. 2014 Jul 7;20(27):9026.

[2] Dirwal AR, Hamzah KJ, Aljabory HA, Mohammed QA. Histopathological study of features invaded of hepatocellular carcinoma in liver parenchyma. *Biochemical and Cellular Archives*. 2019 Oct 1;19(1):1925–8.

[3] Li Q, Dhyani M, Grajo JR, Sirlin C, Samir AE. Current status of imaging in non-alcoholic fatty liver disease. *World Journal of Hepatology*. 2018 Aug 8;10(8):530.

[4] Al Barazanchi I, Hashim W, Alkahtani AA, Abbas HH, Abdulshaheed HR. Overview of WBAN from literature survey to application implementation. In *2021 8th International Conference on Electrical Engineering, Computer Science and Informatics (EECSI)*, 2021 Oct 20 (pp. 16–21). IEEE.

[5] Rathee D, Rangi S, Chakarvarti SK, Singh VR. Recent trends in Wireless Body Area Network (WBAN) research and cognition based adaptive WBAN architecture for healthcare. *Health and Technology*. 2014 Sep;4:239–44.

[6] Nasrollahzadeh M, Sajadi SM, Sajjadi M, Issaabadi Z. An introduction to nanotechnology. *Interface Science and Technology* 2019 Jan 1 (Vol. 28, pp. 1–27).

[7] Lu Y, Ni R, Zhu Q. Wireless communication in nanonetworks: Current status, prospect and challenges. *IEEE Transactions on Molecular, Biological and Multi-Scale Communications*. 2020 Jun 22;6(2):71–80.

[8] Elayan H, Shubair RM, Jornet JM. Bio-electromagnetic the propagation modeling for in-vivo wireless nanosensor networks. In *2017 11th European Conference on Antennas and Propagation (EuCAP)*, 2017 Mar 19 (pp. 426–430). IEEE.

[9] Chopra N, Yang K, Abbasi QH, Qaraqe KA, Philpott M, Alomainy A. THz time-domain spectroscopy of human skin tissue for in-body nanonetworks. *IEEE Transactions on Terahertz Science and Technology*. 2016 Aug 31;6(6):803–9.

[10] Seeberg TM, Orr JG, Opsahl H, Austad HO, Roed MH, Dalgard SH, Houghton D, Jones DE, Strisland F. A novel method for continuous, noninvasive, cuff-less measurement of blood pressure: Evaluation in patients with nonalcoholic fatty liver disease. *IEEE Transactions on Biomedical Engineering*. 2016 Sep 12;64(7):1469–78.

[11] Misra V, Bozkurt A, Calhoun B, Jackson T, Jur JS, Lach J, Lee B, Muth J, Oralkan Ö, Öztürk M, Trolier-McKinstry S. Flexible technologies for self-powered wearable health and environmental sensing. *Proceedings of the IEEE*. 2015 Apr;103(4):665–81.

[12] Li W, Zhang H, Shi S, Xu J, Qin X, He Q, Yang K, Dai W, Liu G, Zhou Q, Yu H. Recent progress in silver nanowire networks for flexible organic electronics. *Journal of Materials Chemistry C*. 2020;8(14):4636–74.

[13] Sun B, Xu R, Han X, Xu J, Hong W, Xu Y, Fu Z, Zhu H, Sun X, Wang J, Cui P. Ultra-high temperature tolerant flexible transparent electrode with embedded silver

nanowires bundle micromesh for electrical heater. *npj Flexible Electronics*. 2022 Jun 20;6(1):48.

[14] Jarmakiewicz J, Parobczak K, Maślanka K. On the Internet of Nano Things in healthcare network. In *2016 International Conference on Military Communications and Information Systems (ICMCIS)*, 2016 May 23 (pp. 1–6). IEEE.

[15] Misra V, Bozkurt A, Calhoun B, Jackson T, Jur JS, Lach J, Lee B, Muth J, Oralkan Ö, Öztürk M, Trolier-McKinstry S. Flexible technologies for self-powered wearable health and environmental sensing. *Proceedings of the IEEE*. 2015 Apr;103(4):665–81.

[16] Haghi M, Danyali S, Ayasseh S, Wang J, Aazami R, Deserno TM. Wearable devices in health monitoring from the environmental towards multiple domains: A survey. *Sensors*. 2021 Mar 18;21(6):2130.

[17] Mayor P, Rajman M, De Micheli G. Nano-Tera. ch: Information technology for health, environment, and energy. *IEEE Design & Test*. 2017 Sep 29;34(6):109–18.

[18] Nunna BB, Mandal D, Zhuang S, Lee ES. A standalone micro biochip to monitor the cancer progression by measuring cancer antigens as a point-of-care (POC) device for enhanced cancer management. In *2017 IEEE Healthcare Innovations and Point of Care Technologies (HI-POCT)*, 2017 Nov 6 (pp. 212–215). IEEE.

[19] Yoon J, Choi B, Lee Y, Han J, Lee J, Park J, Kim Y, Kim DM, Kim DH, Kang MH, Kim S. Monolithically 3D-printed pressure sensors for application in electronic skin and healthcare monitoring. In *2017 IEEE International Electron Devices Meeting (IEDM)*, 2017 Dec 2 (pp. 40–2). IEEE.

[20] Roy S, Deo KA, Lee HP, Soukar J, Namkoong M, Tian L, Jaiswal A, Gaharwar AK. 3D printed electronic skin for strain, pressure and temperature sensing. *Advanced Functional Materials*. 2024 Jan 9:2313575.

[21] Surrel G, Aminifar A, Rincón F, Murali S, Atienza D. Online obstructive sleep apnea detection on medical wearable sensors. *IEEE Transactions on Biomedical Circuits and Systems*. 2018 May 7;12(4):762–73.

[22] Galal A, Hesselbach X. Nano-networks communication architecture: Modeling and functions. *Nano Communication Networks*. 2018 Sep 1;17:45–62.

[23] Riemer DE. The theoretical fundamentals of the screen printing process. *Microelectronics International*. 1989 Jan 1;6(1):8–17.

[24] Zavanelli N, Yeo WH. Advances in screen printing of conductive nanomaterials for stretchable electronics. *ACS Omega*. 2021 Mar 31;6(14):9344–51.

[25] Naghdi S, Rezaei M, Bahramifar N, Kuswandi B. Preparation and characterization of intelligent color-changing nanosensor based on bromophenol blue and GONH2 nanosheet for freshness evaluation of minced Caspian sprat (Clupeonella cultriventris caspia) stored at 4° C. *Chemical Papers*. 2022 May;76(5):3133–46.

[26] Hieu NM, Hien TT, Chinh ND, Quang ND, Hung NM, Van Phuoc C, Lee SM, Jeong JR, Kim C, Kim D. ZnTe-coated ZnO nanorods: Hydrogen sulfide nano-sensor purely controlled by pn junction. *Materials & Design*. 2020 Jun 1;191:108628.

[27] Wang L, Yang GZ, Huang J, Zhang J, Yu L, Nie Z, Cumming DR. A wireless biomedical signal interface system-on-chip for body sensor networks. *IEEE Transactions on Biomedical Circuits and Systems*. 2010 Mar 15;4(2):112–7.

[28] Frankston B. # APIFirst: How things speak to each other [Bits Versus Electrons]. *IEEE Consumer Electronics Magazine*. 2015 Jul 15;4(3):86–9.

[29] Zhang H, Wang G, Cai P, Wu Z, Ding S. A fast blind source separation algorithm based on the temporal structure of signals. *Neurocomputing*. 2014 Sep 2;139:261–71.

[30] Hammad M, Iliyasu AM, Subasi A, Ho ES, Abd El-Latif AA. A multitier deep learning model for arrhythmia detection. *IEEE Transactions on Instrumentation and Measurement*. 2020 Oct 26;70:1–9.

[31] Birgé L. Model selection for Gaussian regression with random design. *Bernoulli*. 2004 Dec;10(6):1039–51.

[32] Shahin AI, Almotairi S. An accurate and fast cardio-views classification system based on fused deep features and LSTM. *IEEE Access*. 2020 Jul 20;8:135184–94.

[33] Johari P, Jornet JM. Nanoscale optical wireless channel model for intra-body communications: Geometrical, time, and frequency domain analyses. *IEEE Transactions on Communications*. 2017 Dec 27;66(4):1579–93.

[34] Bhasin H, Bhatia S. Application of genetic algorithms in machine learning. *IJCSIT*. 2011;2(5):2412–5.

[35] Basheer S, Bhatia S, Sakri SB. Computational modeling of dementia prediction using deep neural network: analysis on OASIS dataset. *IEEE Access*. 2021 Mar 17;9:42449–62.

11 Breast Cancer Classification Using Machine Learning

A Study

S. Muthumari, J. Suganthi, B. Nagarajan, and M. Mageshwari

11.1 INTRODUCTION

Cancer is the second leading factor of global human mortality, accounting for more than 10 million deaths. It is the major cause of around 70% of deaths in developing and underdeveloped countries. Among the different sorts of malignancy, breast cancer accounts for about 6.4% of the mortality rate. Breast cancer is caused by genetic history, obesity, hormonal changes or imbalance, radiation therapy, or even reproductive factors. According to a World Health Organization (WHO) report, globally, 1,000,000 women are newly determined to have malignancy of the breast consistently every year. Among them, the survival rate is about 50% due to delayed diagnosis [1]. Breast cancer is caused by the abnormal mutation of cancerous cells or reckless division of the cells. The expansion of malignant tumors to proximate neighboring cells could lead to metastization or spread toward other parts of the body. Benign masses cannot expand to other tissues. Due to the absence of symptoms, the early detection of breast cancer is difficult. Accurate diagnosis has the ability to differentiate between benign and malignant tumors.

The development of a programmed calculation that works within the forecast, acknowledgment, and characterization is effectively done with the use of machine learning (ML) apparatus. The major steps in the ML are data collection, model selection, and training and testing the model [2]. ML is applied in the field of the growth of malignancy of the breast analysis for the classification of tumor and malignancy, prediction of the gene sequence responsible for the cancer, and determination of prognosis. Bayak, Kirci, and Ensari [3] analyzed the support vector machine (SVM) and artificial neural network (ANN) for predicting the breast cancer diagnosis. Asri et al. [4] juxtaposed ML algorithms to predict the difficulty level of breast cancer and diagnostic approaches. SVM has achieved the maximum accuracy value with the lowest error rate. Bazazeh and Shubair [5] conducted a similar investigation of ML algorithms for identifying and diagnosing breast cancer. Ahmad et al. [6] applied these algorithms to investigating the recurrence rate of breast cancer. Bektas and Babur [7] observed the

DOI: 10.1201/9781003484233-11

prognosis of breast cancer with this algorithm. Chen et al. [8] applied the SVM algorithm to the Wisconsin Diagnostic Breast Cancer (WDBC) dataset.

11.2 MACHINE LEARNING

ML is a sub-field of artificial intelligence (AI) that is widely used in biomedical research and diagnosis, especially in terms of the effectiveness of its approach in the classification and prediction of breast cancer. AI assists us with extricating data from the premise of past encounters and distinguishes a hard-to-see design from an enormous and loud dataset.

Over the years, ML algorithms have been applied to envision the recurrence of breast cancer. ML methods are classified as black box and white box techniques. The former works based on information boost and yield responses with zero information on their inner methods, which will always remain unclear from the user's perspective. The latter permits the assessment and clarification of their interior guidelines, and the results may be derived analytically and the outcomes might be obtained scientifically from a given arrangement of sources of information [9].

11.3 BREAST CANCER CLASSIFICATION (BCC)

Breast cancer is classified on the basis of nine characteristics as follows: 1. single epithelial cell size; 2. uniformity of cell shape; 3. uniformity of cell size; 4. marginal adhesion; 5. clump thickness; 6. normal nuclei; 7. bland chromatin; and 8. bare nucleoli [10]:

1. Single epithelial cell size – Enlarged epithelial cells are signs of malignancy.
2. Uniformity of cell size – Calculate the consistency and sample size.
3. Consistency of cell size – Measure the cell shapes and differentiate minute differences.
4. Marginal adhesion – Cancer malignancy spread all over the organ and normal cells are linked to each other.
5. Clump thickness – Consider the layered structure.
6. Normal nuclei – There are many nuclei in the disease cells, unlike the normal cells.
7. Bland chromatin – It explains the texture of the nucleus. In disease cells, it has a uniform shape. In tumors, chromatin seems to be coarser.
8. Bare nucleoli – Cores are not highlighted by cytoplasm.

11.4 MACHINE LEARNING TECHNIQUES

1. ANN
2. SVM and least squares SVM
3. Self-organizing map (SOM)
4. Association rule learning (ARL)
5. Naive Bayes
6. Isotonic separation

7. Random forest
8. *K*-nearest neighbor (KNN)
9. Linear discriminant analysis
10. Restricted Boltzmann machines (RBMs)
11. *K*-means algorithm
12. Decision tree
13. Logistic regression (LR)
14. Bootstrap aggregating (bagging) techniques
15. Boosting procedure
16. Genetic algorithm (GA)

11.4.1 Decision Tree (DT)

DTs operate based on the divide and conquer methodology. They are used for classification and regression analysis. Here, a partition is divided into two methods.

Numerical partition: According to the discrete values, this partition is generated.

Nominal partition: The nominal partition is generated on the basis of splitting the tree depending on attributes values.

Every node's average error is minimized using a general approach:

$$I(S) = \sum_{j=0}^{n} P_j f(P_j, P_j^2, P_j^3, \ldots\ldots P_j^C)$$

where n denotes the number of partitions, P_j^C is the proportion of elements of class C falling into node j, P_j is the probability of falling into node j, and f is a function of impurity.

DTs can be characterized by the recursive parceling of the information space from the root hub to numerous branch hubs, wherein the root hub is the first of the choice tree, from which the active edges make different sub-hubs. Hubs with active edges are known as inward hubs, while hubs with approaching edges are called leaves, to such an extent that each leaf is assigned to a class. Two or more sub-spaces are divided from the sub-spaces by the inner hubs according to the conditional trial in information highlight esteems. In general, a solitary component is relegated in each inside hub, though the element space is partitioned dependent on the element esteems. For ceaseless highlights, each cordial edge of the hub addresses a specific reach. In the DT, an information vector is calculated by controlling all the nodes from the root to the child, as a consequence of mutations tried using some other approach.

The most mainstream DT approaches are the Iterative Dichotomiser (ID3) algorithm [11], C4.5 and C5.0 [6], and classification and regression tree (CART) algorithm [12], which constructs the tree utilizing entropy-based measures as a tree partitioning criterion. The information gain or gain ratio is a frequently used entropy-based resource. Information gain finds the attribute that provides significant information when used as a splitting criterion. The addition ratio finds the number

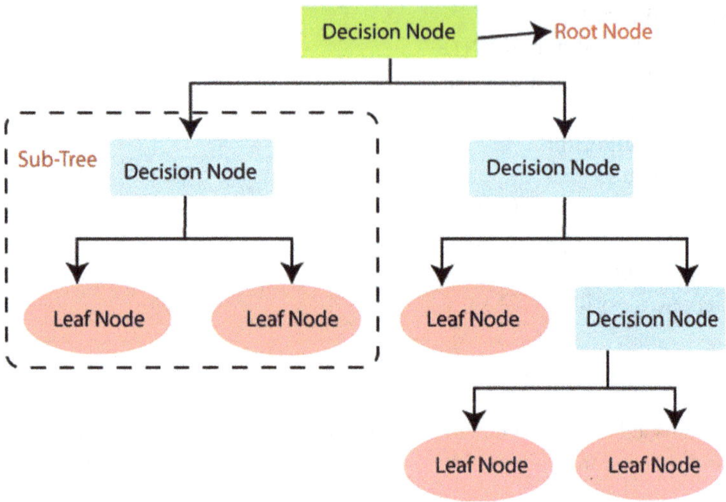

FIGURE 11.1 Decision tree.

and size of branches in the choice tree when the quality is picked to be utilized as the partitioning rule [13]. C4.5 was further extended as C5.0, which offers upgrades like speed, memory utilization, pruning, and weighting plans [9]. As DTs can handle both constant and remote qualities, that is, mixed variables, the rules generated by them are easily interpreted and understood in terms of healthcare contexts, DTs seem to be computationally efficient in the context of BC recurrence. Figure 11.1 shows the DT.

To understand the DT operation in the breast cancer recurrence scenario, a certain number of patients and two classes, repeat and non-repeat, are considered. Each patient is described by various aspects. To build a classification tree, the DT algorithms initially determine the patient attribute that serves as the root of the tree, based on the attribute selection measure. For every limb of the attribute, the most instructive attribute follows the same logic. Then, the final tree is found to be complete. A majority voting scheme is employed when specimens belonging to different classes are located on the same branch. The leaf of the tree constitutes the most regular class. After the DT is constructed, the test samples that are neglected during tree building are used for evaluation. For classifying those instances, the tree traverses from the root to the final leaf, guided by the instance values at each step .

11.4.2 Logistic Regression (LR)

The interrelated variables, that is, a group of independent variables and dichotomous dependent variables, are described by a mathematical method called LR that calculates a group of uncovered parameters using a maximum feasibility method [9]. LR interferes with a probabilistic view of categorization and is not used for regression. It uses a logistic function that relates a point to a range [0,1] in multidimensional feature space, which can be recognized as a membership probability with the

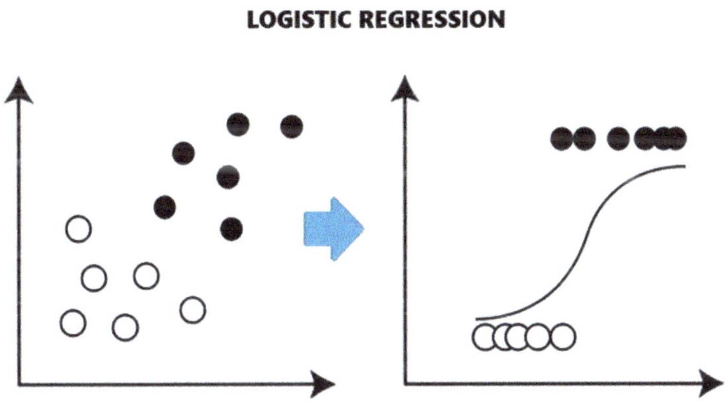

FIGURE 11.2 Logistic regression.

help of a threshold. Finally, LR gives the class probability for the considered vectors. Class issuance is done based on the selected threshold. The benefit is that it clearly shows how the outputs are justified by the inputs through the final generated equation. Figure 11.2 illustrates LR.

When LR is concerned with the breast cancer recurrence scenario, 1 is given to repetitive events and 0 is given to non-recurrence events. To regulate the patient's recurrence, LR fits a logistic function to the training data, while defining the probabilistic function mapping an input to the recurrence probability. The probability of a recurrence event lies in the interval ranging from 0 to 1. This could be translated as a binary class assignment indicating non-recurrence as 0 and recurrence as 1, with the application of a decision threshold.

11.4.3 Support Vector Machine (SVM)

Vladimir Vapnik [14] introduced SVMs for finding the adaptive decision hyperplane that enables the maximization of the disconnected edge between the data points of distinct classes [15]. The adaptive hyperplane is defined by the middle region of the separation margin. The data points that lie proximate to the hyperplane are referred to as support vectors. Consider a two-class scenario, in which patients are characterized by tumor size and age. Several decision boundaries could be defined for separating the recurrence and non-recurrence classes. In SVM, the maximization of the decision boundary margin is assured by the optimization criteria. Hence, the decision boundary is remotely located from both classes. In a nonlinear recurrence problem, a kernel function is employed in SVMs to convert data points into a higher-dimensional space, aiding in the differentiation between two categories: those with recurrence and those without. Within the initial input space, the class of recurrent data points is positioned within a circle, whereas the class of non-recurrent data points is positioned outside the circle. It proves unfeasible to establish a linear boundary within the input space. SVM solves this problem through the mapping of the data points in the higher-dimensional space by adding new features.

11.4.4 Least Squares Support Vector Machine (LS-SVM)

LS-SVM is a reduction of the SVM model, as shown in Figure 11.3. It has a least squares loss function and equality constraints, and a dual solution can be found by solving a linear system instead of a quadratic programming problem. It maps the data into a high-dimensional feature space [16].

11.4.5 Boosting

A boosting procedure was introduced that is similar to bagging. A subset of '*n*' training examples is taken randomly without replacement from the initial training set such that *n* is less than the total number of training examples '*N*' (the training subset is Z1). Z1 is used for training C1, a weak classifier. Later, Z2,a training subset (with $N > n$) is created such that Z2 contains half of the samples misclassified by the weak classifier C1, and a second weak classifier C2 is trained. All training samples from the initial training set NN, for which the weak classifiers C1C_1 and C2C_2 are ultimately trained to oppose the third weak classifier C3C_3, are considered.

A voting scheme for the weak classifiers C1, C2, and C3 (Kumar, 2012) is used to obtain the final classifier.

The renowned boosting algorithm called adaptive boosting (AdaBoost) was established and selects the training subsets based on a weighting scheme. The weights of the correctly classified samples are reduced, while the weights of the misclassified samples are increased. The probability of the classified samples being chosen in the next stage is determined by the weights. Hence, there is a high probability of the misclassified samples being learned again. A specific weight is assigned to each classifier

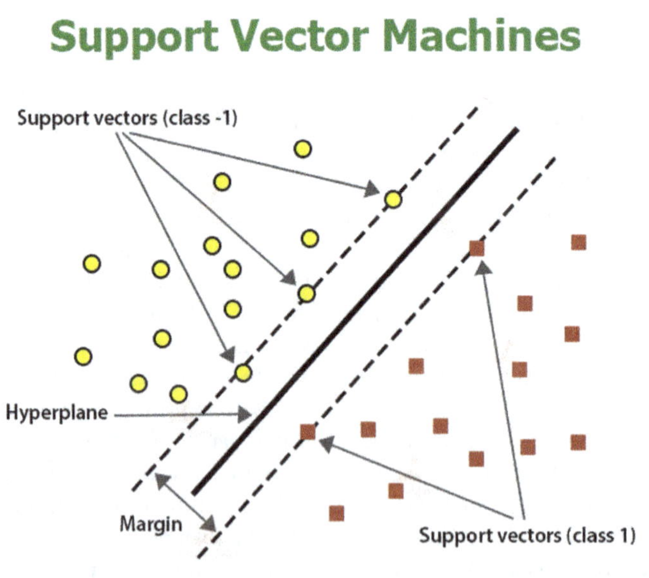

FIGURE 11.3 SVM classification.

according to its training in the set. The linear combinations of the M classifiers that contribute with the connected weight define the final classifier [15].

AdaBoost is known as a meta-algorithm that is used to improve production together with other learning techniques. It focuses on sequentially applying weak classifiers for a classification problem. Henceforth, the algorithm is applied on the modified data repeatedly.

Friedman et al. [17] formulated LogitBoost, which fits an LR model by means of Newton steps to find the parameter estimation [9].

The application of the boosting technique for the breast cancer recurrence scenario is similar to the bagging technique, except for the selection of the classifier as a weak one and variation in the training data for each classifier. A total of 50% of the wrongly labeled patients from ensemble C1 are included in the training data of ensemble C2. Finally, the patients are classified as per the bagging procedure.

11.4.6 Naive Bayes (NB)

The naive Bayes classifier considers the patterns of each class by means of a probability distribution to make decisions, while assuming the presence of a probabilistic correlation among the features and class [18]. Bayesian classification regulates the probability of pattern 'X' belonging to a class C_i, where $P(C_i|X)$ is referred to as the posteriori probability. While assuming the classification problem with two posteriori probabilities $P(C_1|X)$ and $P(C_2|X)$, the naive Bayes rule says that

- If $P(C_1|X) > P(C_2|X)$, then pattern X belongs to class C_1.
- If $P(C_1|X) < P(C_2|X)$, then pattern X belongs to class C_2.

If both posteriori probabilities are equal, then the choice is arbitrary. As per the fact that the naive Bayes approach uses probability rules, it inherits statistical strength. Additionally, it allows the inclusion of researcher experience in the modeling process of the classifiers. It is easily understood as it is a white box method.

Let us consider two classes: recurrence and non-recurrence, a single attribute with positive and negative values, and a test instance with a positive attribute value. To determine recurrence for the patient, naive Bayes has to predict the posteriori probability values. The posteriori probability represents the conditional class probability of the positive attribute case, while observing the repeating and non-repeating events in the tutoring data. The final posteriori probability of the recurrence and non-recurrence events is obtained from the direct multiplication of the precedence and possibilities. Thus, the naive Bayes approach classifies the victim on the basis of the posterior probability values. For example, if the posteriori probability of the recurrence class is greater than the non-recurrence class, then the patient is categorized as a repetitive case.

11.4.7 Association Rule Learning (ARL)

The correlation of variables in a file [19] is exposed by ARL by treating all variables as categorical, which is not applicable when dealing with numerical data. The regulation contains two major things: support and confidence. The former finds out the population percentage that sticks to a unique rule and the latter is the unit of assurance related to each of the uncovered rules. The final rules returned are easy enough for users to accept. Due to the vast data exploration, ARL is highly advantageous [17]. ARL is used for the discovery of the interesting relationship between the attributes associated with the recurrence of breast cancer. The objective of association rule mining is to establish the recurrent acceptances of the items in the dataset. In this case, the values of the attributes in the dataset seem to frequently appear together.

11.4.8 Isotonic Separation

Isotonic separation is a linear programming model devised in [16]. It complies with the principles of isotonic consistency that assumes a sequential relationship of all the points located in the space, described by $S1 = \{(x, y): C_x > C_y\}$, where C_x and C_y denote the coordinate vectors representing the attribute values of '*x*' and '*y*', in all dimensions. Therefore, the feature space comprises (x, y) pairs of sequential data points such that the two-classification problem is considered as follows:

- If the attribute value '*x*' is classified as associated with the class **β**1, then '*y*' should be classified as belonging to class **β**1 and vice versa.
- If the attribute value '*y*' is classified as associated with the class **β**2, then '*x*' should be classified as belonging to class **β**2.

In the recurrence scenario, if certain patients have recurrent registered attribute values and if others exhibit similar values, then they are also treated as recurrent. The misclassification cost is accounted for in the isotonic separation in which a penalty is applied for each misclassified data point. The misclassification of the recurrent patient as non-recurring and non-recurring patient as recurrent receives a penalty. Hence, the total cost incurred for the misclassification is minimized. The total cost involves the number of misclassified recurrent and non-recurrent patients.

11.4.9 Random Forest

The random forest method, shown in Figure 11.4, is used for its clarity relating to instruction, tuning, and operational discharge [18]. Random forest is an ensemble classifier, comprising multiple DTs that are trained independently on a random data subset. A forest that is the ensemble of the DTs is created by using the bagging method. For each tree node, the random selection of '*x*' number of features out of the total input features '*X*' (assuming $x \ll X$) is performed. The node is divided by the best splitting of '*x*' features. The most voted class is finally picked by the forest, over the tree nodes, by taking the mean value of all the trees. Random forest algorithms work similar to individual DTs. The differences are as follows:

i. Random option of the instruction data and input traits.
ii. Creation of the forest is performed according to the classification results generated by multiple individual trees.

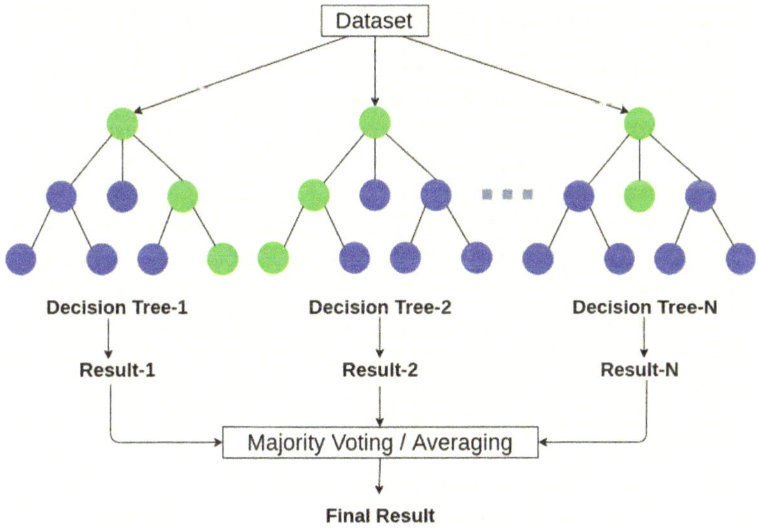

FIGURE 11.4 Random forest.

In the training phase, the numbers of individual DT prototypes are brought about through the random division of the file. Then, the testing of the load data is performed by considering every sole DT. This is done to determine the class of a patient. The assignment of the concluding class is decided using majority polling.

11.4.10 *K*-Nearest Neighbor (KNN)

KNN comes under supervised learning in which the nearest neighbors K in a spot are selected through the minimization of similarity measures, such as the Euclidean distance and Mahalanobis distance between the points [8]. The KNN algorithm computes the distance to labeled samples for determining the class of unlabeled samples. Then, the k nearest neighbors and corresponding tags are determined. The unlabeled sample is categorized using majority polling or by a weighted majority. The distance to all data points (training patients) included in the breast cancer recurrence dataset is computed for determining the assignment of a class to the data points. Either the majority polling or weighted strategy is applied for choosing the class to which the data point is a part, in accordance with the task of assigning a class to the 'k' closest patients. KNN is a non-parametric approach used for regression and classification analysis. The input comprises k classes in the dataset, which is a small and positive integer. The input data are allotted to the class that is higher among its k nearest neighbors. If the value is $k = 2$, then the input data are assigned to a class of two nearest neighbors since the dataset contains only two classes. The classes are cancerous tumor and non-cancerous tumor. The Euclidean distance is used to measure the distance between two data points.

11.4.11 Artificial Neural Network (ANN)

These are computational frameworks involving the functioning of human brain simulation with three layers: the input, output, and processing layer (or unseen layer) (Minsky & Papert, 1969). The data are received by the input layer, the result is communicated via the output layer, and the hidden layer is in charge of data processing and the calculation of results.

ANNs have the ability to capture nonlinearities and complex interactions between factors. Trained on a number of prognostic factors, neural networks have been reported to improve the accuracy of survival prediction. In patients with breast cancer, earlier studies have reported promising results for neural network models [20].

While considering breast cancer recurrence, two features, such as tumor size and age, describe the patients. The main objective is to determine the recurrences for the patient. In this scenario, the ANN approach could contemplate two loads and yields in the input and output layers respectively. There is a need to specify the configuration of the hidden layers, its stimulation task, and the initial masses of the synapses. During ANN instruction, the hidden layers could sequentially learn the synapses' masses that result in highly accurate classification results. Hence, the topmost grid of the masses increased by the two features could be achieved by ANN for the accurate prediction of recurrence and non-recurrence. It is vital to observe that the ANNs do not yield a single class allotment for classification problems. Instead, ANN outputs a probable answer for each class. After the instruction phase is complete, the ANN prototype classifies the patients based on the final matrix of weights.

11.4.12 SOM

SOMs are a class of artificial network that indicates all data in a map, generally with low dimensions. In the training phase, the input samples are used by SOMs to build the map, by positioning every node next to the node with the most equal weights, which is termed the best matching unit (BMU) [21]. The weights of the BMUs and adjacent nodes are adapted iteratively with each other whenever a new instruction set is applied to the SOM [22]. In the mapping stage, the classification of the test input vectors is performed on the basis of the space of the input vectors with available nodes.

For SOM, the instruction stage is completely unconventional from the class allotment. As SOMs are data-driven, patient data alone is needed for building the SOM map. The weights of the maps are adjusted until the placement of each patient near to its most equal neighbor somehow for input data clustering. After completing map generation and weight determination, the class most often allotted to a neuron suits its label. This grant assigns trial patients based on their proximity to existing clusters .

11.4.13 *K*-Means

This algorithm is based on partitioned clustering and is widely used for its efficiency, easy instrumentation, and victory over a diverse scope in image processing. Initially, the required clusters, K, have to be specified to set up centroids randomly. All points' k centroids are taken into account, and every point is allotted to its closer centroids. The mean vectors of each cluster are calculated from new centroids, which are modified through each step of the algorithm. New centroids for each point are taken into account to calculate new distances, which keeps being repeated [23].

11.4.14 Bagging Techniques

Bagging makes use of bootstrap samples for training many classifiers in order to combine them to attain the final classification. Generally, a bootstrap sample is formed from randomly selecting (with replacement) from an *m*-size training set. From *n* bootstrap samples, *n* classifiers C_1, C_2, C_3..., C_n are built [22] and different instruction sets are used by everyone. At the end, classifier C_b is built using all the C_n classifiers and also combining them using majority voting.

Bagging can be directly applied to the breast cancer recurrence dataset. Various bootstrap samples are acquired from the dataset so that for a specific classifier, each sample serves as training data. The intended patients for testing are categorized through a selected set of classifiers. When the results of every classifier are weighed up, the majority persistent class for a patient is established as its absolute class project. For example, if a patient is classified as C1 = recurrence, C2 = non-recurrence, and C3 = recurrence, by the above conditions, the patient is determined to belong to the recurrence class.

11.4.15 Linear Discriminant Analysis (LDA)

LDA, a linear transformation technique, is employed in the pre-processing phase in order to reduce the dataset size, that is, to avoid overfitting and reduce the computational cost of classification. At the same time, it is further employed separately for categorization, derived from the searching theory to combine attributes linearly, which permits maximization distinction. Recently, the between-class and within-class variance ratio has increased by the escalation criterion of LDA. LDA, also known as Fisher discriminant analysis (FDA), was initially designed to handle only two classes [22]. However, over the following decade, the LDA framework was extended to accommodate multiple classes.

11.4.16 Restricted Boltzmann Machines (RBM)

RBM machines exhibit a key characteristic: they are restricted to having connections only between adjacent layers. RBMs are considered probabilistic neural networks, where their units, resembling neurons, are activated based on a probabilistic component. [1]. In general, a layer of inputs or visible units, along with hidden units, are available. All the hidden units are connected with every visible unit. As stated earlier, the hidden units are no longer connected with each other and visible units are not connected to each other.

In addition to being a unique feature of learners, it is also used for grouping in algorithms such as supervised and black-box methods [20]. In the classification phase, RBMs are considered as a framework for the combined distribution between the neuron layer and visible layer of inputs. The probability distribution of the class '*x*' belonging to class '*y*' is computed to determine the most probable class label based on the joint probability [21].

11.4.17 Genetic Algorithm (GA)

Drawing inspiration from Darwin's theory of evolution, GAs apply the principle of the 'survival of the fittest' to identify the optimal solution from a population of individual candidates [23]. Robustness governs the quick fix that is to be maintained and solutions that are to be discarded.

While predicting breast cancer recurrence, the GA is used as an optimization technique for ANNs. Starting with an initial population of randomly generated ANNs, a fitness function is defined to serve as a classifier for the iterative process. Each ANN is estimated during each generation. ANNs with best fitness values go to the upcoming propagation. In addition, the current ANNs are produced through merging distinct ANNs with good outcomes. Mutations happen using the layout of the unknown layers from distinct ANNs. Therefore, the number of individuals in the population remains constant . The same process is redone continuously until the best ANN is selected or a rich amount of age groups is attained.

11.5 CONCLUSION

Different techniques for BCC using ML are plainly exposed in this chapter. Apart from this, there are many techniques emerging day by day in ML. ML provides a wide variety of techniques for solving cancer-related complications

REFERENCES

1. Delen, D., Walker, G., & Kadam, A. (2005). Predicting breast cancer survivability: A comparison of three data mining methods. *Artificial Intelligence in Medicine*, *34*(2), 113–127.
2. Aaltonen, L. A., Salovaara, R., Kristo, P., Canzian, F., Hemminki, A., Peltomäki, P., Chadwick, R. B., Kääriäinen, H., Eskelinen, M., & Järvinen, H. (1998). Incidence of hereditary nonpolyposis colorectal cancer and the feasibility of molecular screening for the disease. *New England Journal of Medicine*, *338*(21), 1481–1487.
3. Ahmad, L. G., Eshlaghy, A., Poorebrahimi, A., Ebrahimi, M., & Razavi, A. (2013). Using three machine learning techniques for predicting breast cancer recurrence. *Journal of Health and Medical Informatics*, *4*(124), 3.
4. Altman, N. S. (1992). An introduction to kernel and nearest-neighbor nonparametric regression. *The American Statistician*, *46*(3), 175–185.
5. Agrawal, R., Tomasz Imieliński, & Swami, A. (1993). Mining association rules between sets of items in large databases. In *Proceedings of the 1993 ACM SIGMOD International Conference on Management of Data* (pp. 207–216).
6. Ayer, T., Alagoz, O., Chhatwal, J., Shavlik, J. W., Kahn Jr, C. E., & Burnside, E. S. (2010). Breast cancer risk estimation with artificial neural networks revisited: Discrimination and calibration. *Cancer*, *116*(14), 3310–3321.
7. Amrane, M., Oukid, S., Gagaoua, I., & Ensari, T. (2018). Breast cancer classification using machine learning. In *2018 Electric Electronics, Computer Science, Biomedical Engineerings' Meeting (EBBT)*.
8. Boser, B. E., Guyon, I. M., & Vapnik, V. N. (1992). A training algorithm for optimal margin classifiers. In *Proceedings of the Fifth Annual Workshop on Computational Learning Theory*.

9. Belciug, S., Salem, A.-B., Gorunescu, F., & Gorunescu, M. (2010). Clustering-based approach for detecting breast cancer recurrence. In *2010 10th International Conference on Intelligent Systems Design and Applications*.
10. Bektaş, B., & Babur, S. (2016). Machine learning based performance development for diagnosis of breast cancer. In *2016 Medical Technologies National Congress (TIPTEKNO)*.
11. Asri, H., Mousannif, H., Al Moatassime, H., & Noel, T. (2016). Using machine learning algorithms for breast cancer risk prediction and diagnosis. *Procedia Computer Science, 83*, 1064–1069.
12. Bayrak, E. A., Kırcı, P., & Ensari, T. (2019). Comparison of machine learning methods for breast cancer diagnosis. In *2019 Scientific Meeting on Electrical-Electronics & Biomedical Engineering and Computer Science (EBBT)*.
13. Bazazeh, D., & Shubair, R. (2016). Comparative study of machine learning algorithms for breast cancer detection and diagnosis. In *2016 5th international conference on electronic devices, systems and applications (ICEDSA)*.
14. Breiman, L. (2001). Random forests. *Machine learning, 45*(1), 5–32.
15. Breiman, L., Friedman, J., Stone, C. J., & Olshen, R. A. (1984). *Classification and regression trees*. CRC Press.
16. Brijain, M., Patel, R., Kushik, M., & Rana, K. (2014). *A survey on decision tree algorithm for classification*.
17. Chaurasia, V., & Pal, S. (2014). Data mining techniques: To predict and resolve breast cancer survivability. *International Journal of Computer Science and Mobile Computing IJCSMC, 3*(1), 10–22.
18. Molina, C., Prados-Suarez, B., Prados, D. R. M., & Pena, Y. C. (2013). Improving hospital decision making with interpretable associations over datacubes. *Studies in Health Technology and Informatics, 197*, 91–95.
19. Chandrasekaran, R., Young, U . R., Varghese, S. J., & Hong, S. (2005). Isotonic separation. *INFORMS Journal on Computing, 17*(4), 462–474.
20. Chen, H.-L., Yang, B., Liu, J., & Liu, D.-Y. (2011). A support vector machine classifier with rough set-based feature selection for breast cancer diagnosis. *Expert Systems with Applications, 38*(7), 9014–9022.
21. Chen, Y., Sun, J., Huang, L.-C., Xu, H., & Zhao, Z. (2015). Classification of cancer primary sites using machine learning and somatic mutations. *BioMed Research International, 2015*.
22. Efron, B., & Tibshirani, R. J. (1994). *An introduction to the bootstrap*. CRC Press.
23. Fischer, A., & Igel, C. (2012). An introduction to restricted Boltzmann machines. In *Iberoamerican Congress on Pattern Recognition*.

12 Secure Compressive Sensing in Medical Imaging Using Fractional-Order Hyperchaotic Systems

S. Kayalvizhi and S. Malarvizhi

12.1 INTRODUCTION

In the last 20 years, information technology has become essential to the medical field, greatly improving the availability, traceability, and fluidity of data through advances in electronic health records (EHRs), biomedical databases, and public health systems. However, the rapid growth of healthcare-related data has introduced significant challenges in data management, storage, and processing. These challenges can be categorized as follows:

Large Scale: The digitalization of healthcare, including the widespread adoption of hospital information systems and wearable health devices, has resulted in an immense increase in medical data volume.

Rapid Generation: Medical devices, particularly wearables, continuously collect data that require prompt processing to respond to emergencies effectively.

Various Structures: Healthcare data come in diverse formats, including structured, semi-structured, and unstructured data from clinical exams, treatments, and monitoring devices, encompassing text, images, audio, and video.

The efficient transmission of the substantial data generated by these sources necessitates data reduction techniques that do not compromise signal quality. The Shannon or Nyquist sampling theorem is applied by conventional image and video capture systems, which need sampling rates that are at least two times the highest frequency of the signal. Nevertheless, following the Nyquist rate leads to an unfeasibly huge number of samples in high-data-rate scenarios like image or video processing. Compressive sensing (CS) offers an innovative solution, enabling signals to be sampled at rates significantly below the Nyquist threshold while still allowing for

DOI: 10.1201/9781003484233-12

accurate reconstruction of the original signal from fewer measurements [1, 2]. This approach addresses the need for data reduction and enhances security, as the raw data, when unintelligible, require specific reconstruction algorithms, adding a layer of encryption. Additionally, integrating CS with cryptographic methods can further improve data security in medical imaging applications.

According to the Nyquist–Shannon sampling theorem, the sample rate needs to be at least twice the bandwidth in order to accurately record the signal. Nonetheless, a signal can be reconstructed from fewer samples if it is sparse in its domain or any transform domain. CS uses a measurement matrix that is incoherent with the sparse transform vector to combine the operations of capture and compression. The restricted isometry property (RIP) needs to be met in order for the reconstruction to be correct. Using random Gaussian matrices is a popular method for creating a measurement matrix.

One of the core challenges in the CS context is having a proper sensing matrix that satisfies RIP. A common approach is to build the measurement matrix from the random Gaussian matrix. There is totally unpredictable behavior in nonlinear dynamic systems, so-called deterministic chaos. The following features are presented in chaotic systems: extreme sensitivity to initial values and parameters, pseudorandomness, and unpredictability[3]. Frunze provided a method by using the tent map to construct a measurement matrix [4]. Lei developed a measurement matrix called the logistic map with a chaotic series [5]. Kafedziski studied chaotic sequences generated by various chaotic systems [6, 7]. In recent decades, the hyperchaotic system has attracted fast-growing interest. It is typically a chaotic system that includes multiple positive Lyapunov exponents, meaning that the dynamic is continuously distributed in several different directions. Due to their enhanced instability and complexity compared to traditional chaotic systems, hyperchaotic systems offer significant advantages, prompting their widespread application in image encryption [8–10]. Norouzi et al. introduced a system utilizing sequences generated by a hyperchaotic system to effectively diffuse an image, yielding favorable outcomes [8]. A new image encryption algorithm was developed by Wang and Zhang based on the genetic and Lorenz hyperchaotic methods [9].

Most researchers use fundamental-order chaotic image encryption methods. Hyperchaotic fractional-order systems have been observed to have increased nonlinearity and degrees because of the complex geometric representation [11, 12]. For the encryption of color images, Wang et al. applied the Lorenz hyperchaotic fractional-order system [13]. The three-dimensional (3D) Lorenz fractional-order system and Chen chaotic structures were used by Wu et al. and Zhao et al. [14], respectively.

Inspired by the aforementioned studies, in this chapter, we delve into the theoretical development of measurement matrices utilizing three distinct four-dimensional (4D) fractional hyperchaotic sequences. Additionally, we evaluate the efficacy of these matrices in terms of image reconstruction quality. We consider fractional-order hyperchaotic (FOHC) systems [15–18] for the investigation. The experimental results show that FOHC sequences enhance encryption along with the CS of images.

The remainder of the chapter is structured as follows: 12.2. CS basics, 12.3 block CS (BCS), 12.4. FOHC systems, 12.5. generation of the measurement matrix, 12.6. experimental analysis, and 12.7. conclusion.

12.2 COMPRESSIVE SENSING

CS introduces a novel approach to simultaneous sampling and signal compression [1,2]. A one-dimensional (1D) sparse signal x of length N can be represented as follows in terms of CS theory:

$$x = \sum_{i=1}^{L} S_i \Psi_i = S\Psi \tag{1}$$

where S as an $L \times 1$ column vector of weighting coefficients. An orthonormal basis of size $N \times N$ is given by $\boldsymbol{s}_i = \boldsymbol{x}, \boldsymbol{\Psi}_i$ and $\Psi = \{\Psi_1, \Psi_2 \cdots \Psi_N\}$. The signal P is designed to be K sparse [2]. Reconstruction can only be successful if there is incoherency between the bias and measurement matrix. The estimation form y is then given by

$$y = \Phi x = \Phi \Psi S = \Theta S \tag{2}$$

where y is a vector of dimension $M \times 1$ and Θ is a matrix of type $\Phi \times \Psi$. RIPs should be met for accurate reconstruction [1].

12.3 BLOCK COMPRESSIVE SENSING

Gan [19] proposed a simple yet effective compressive block method for sensing images, where CS is applied to each block separately. The image is divided into smaller blocks, which reduces the size of the measurement matrix as it is dependent on the dimensions of the image data. Consequently, this approach decreases computational complexity and storage requirements. Let x_k be a 1D vector representing the kth block of the input image $\boldsymbol{x}$. The output is then given by

$$y_k = \Phi_b x_k \tag{3}$$

where Φ_b is a $Q_b \times b^2$-th measurement matrix that satisfies the orthonormality condition, where $Q_b = \left[\frac{Q}{N} b^2\right]$.

Linear reconstruction in BCS can introduce artifacts and noise due to blocking effects. To mitigate these issues, the BCS-smoothed projected Landweber (SPL) reconstruction approach is employed [19]. The initial estimation is denoted by x^0. The recovered signal is obtained from the initial estimate through subsequent calculations and thresholding. The estimation of the projected Landweber (PL) algorithm at the $(f+1)$th iteration is given by [20]

$$\breve{\breve{x}}(f) = \breve{x}^{(f)} + \frac{1}{r}\Psi\Phi^{T}\left(y - \Phi\Psi^{-1}\breve{x}^{(f)}\right) \tag{4}$$

$$\breve{x}^{(f+1)} = \begin{cases} \breve{\breve{x}}(f), \left|\breve{\breve{x}}(f)\right| \geq \gamma^{(k)} \\ 0, \quad else \end{cases} \tag{5}$$

In this context, r is the scale, and each iteration threshold is $\gamma(f)$. To prevent blocking artifacts, Wiener filtering is incorporated into the basic reconstruction system of the PL algorithm, adjusting the threshold at each iteration. This approach improves image accuracy by ensuring smoothness [21]. The reconstructed image in the $(f + 1)$th iteration, denoted by $x(f + 1)$, is as follows:

$$x^{(f+1)} = SmoothedPL\left(x^{(f)}, y, \Phi_b, \Psi, \lambda\right)$$

$$\breve{x}^{(f)} = W\left(x^{(f)}\right)$$

$$foreach\ block\ j$$

$$\breve{\breve{x}}(f = \hat{x}_j^{(f)} + \Phi_b^T\left(y - \Phi_b\breve{x}_j^{(f)}\right)$$

$$\breve{\breve{x}}(f) = Th\left(\breve{x}^{(f)}, \lambda\right)$$

$$\bar{x}^{(f)} = \Psi^{-1}\hat{\hat{x}}^{(f)}$$

$$x_j^{(f+1)} = \bar{x}_j^{(f)} + \Phi_b^T\left(y - \Phi_b\bar{x}_j^{(f)}\right)$$

$$H^{(f+1)} = \frac{1}{\sqrt{L}}x^{(f+1)} - \breve{x}_{\not{2}}^{(f)}$$

$$\text{terminate when } \left|H^{(f+1)} - H^{(f)}\right| < 10^{-4}$$

$$x = x^{(f+1)}$$

$$initial\ value\ x^{(0)} = \Phi^T y$$

where W(•) represents an adaptive 3 × 3 Wiener filter and Th(•) denotes a threshold operation defined as

$$Threshold(\xi,\lambda) = \frac{\left(\sqrt{\xi^2+\xi_p^2} - \lambda\frac{\sqrt{3}\sigma^{(i)}}{\sigma_\xi}\right)_+}{\sqrt{\xi^2+\xi_p^2}}.\xi \tag{6}$$

where

$$(g)_+ = \begin{cases} 0, & if\ g < 0 \\ g, & else \end{cases}$$

where ξ, ξ_p are the coefficient of the transform and its parent coefficient, respectively. In the proposed approach, the contourlet transform (CT) [22] is utilized, followed by image reconstruction using BCS-SPL-CT.

12.4 FRACTIONAL-ORDER HYPERCHAOTIC SYSTEMS

To illustrate how measuring matrices generated by various hyperchaotic systems enhance the security and restoration quality of CS images, this section employs three 4D fractional hyperchaotic systems.

12.4.1 Fractional-Order Chen Hyperchaotic System

A new hyperchaotic Chen system that was developed from the original Chen system was presented by Li et al. [15]. It has the following characteristics:

$$\frac{d^{q1}x_1}{dt^{q1}} = \beta(x_2 - x_1) + x_4$$

$$\frac{d^{q2}x_2}{dt^{q2}} = \gamma x_1 - x_1x_2 + \lambda x_2$$

$$\frac{d^{q3}x_3}{dt^{q3}} = x_1x_2 - \alpha x_3$$

$$\frac{d^{q4}x_4}{dt^{q4}} = x_2x_3 + rx_4 \tag{7}$$

The system exhibits hyperchaotic behavior with initial values of (2, 2, 1, −1). This behavior is also observed when parameters are adjusted to $\beta = 35$, $\gamma = 7$, $\alpha = 3$, $r = 0.5$, $\lambda = 12$, and $q^i = 0.96$. Here, the control system parameters are β, α, γ, λ, r, and q. Figure 12.1 displays the simulation's output.

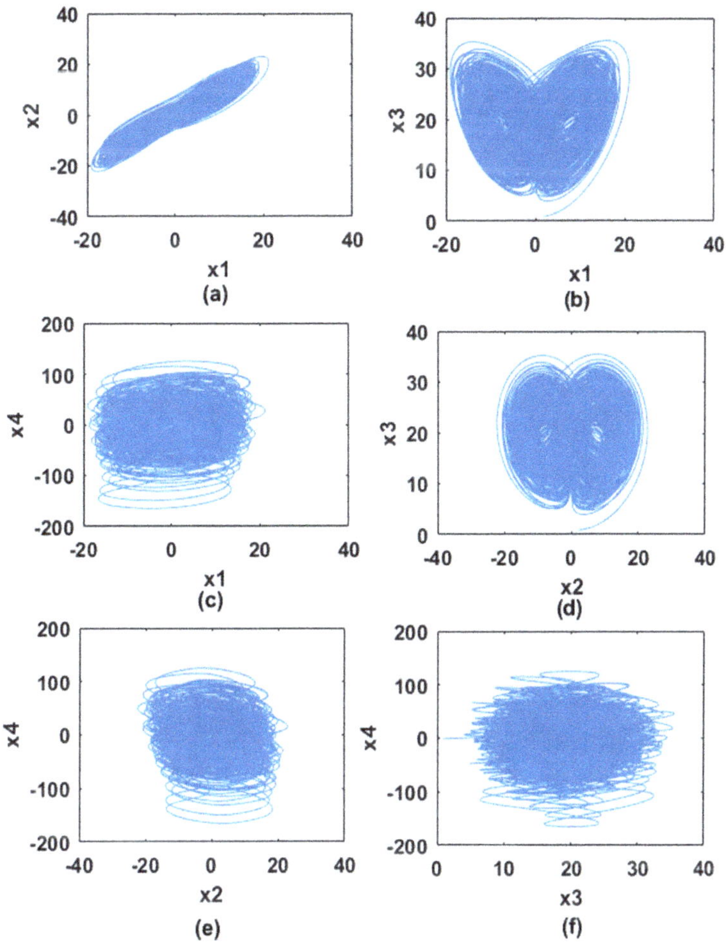

FIGURE 12.1 FOHCC system.

12.4.2 Fractional-Order Lorenz Hyperchaotic System

The 4D fractional-order Lorenz system was created by Wang and Song [17] and is explained as follows:

$$\frac{d^{q1}x_1}{dt^{q1}} = a\left(x_2 - x_1\right) + x_4$$

$$\frac{d^{q2}x_2}{dt^{q2}} = cx_1 - x_2 - x_1x_3$$

$$\frac{d^{q3}x_3}{dt^{q3}} = x_1x_2 - bx_3$$

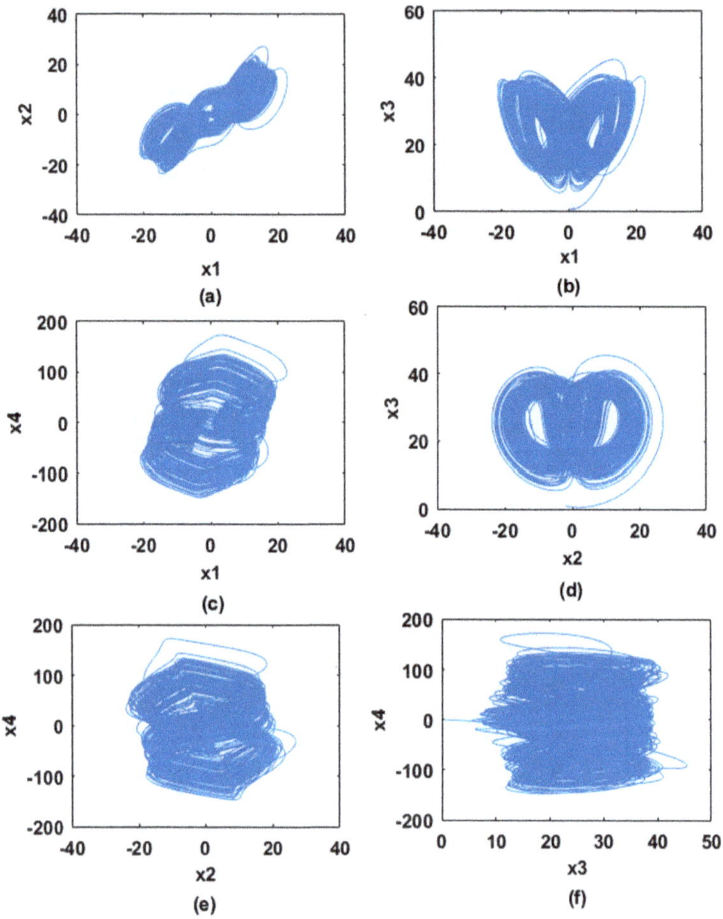

FIGURE 12.2 FOHCL system.

$$\frac{d^{q4}x_4}{dt^{q4}} = -x_2x_3 + rx_4 \tag{8}$$

The system exhibits hyperchaotic behavior with initial values of (2, −2, 1, −1), and $q^i = 0.98$ ($i = 1, 2, 3, 4$), $b = 8/3$, $a = 10$, $r = -1$, and $c = 28$, as in Figure 12.2.

12.4.3 Fractional-Order Lü Hyperchaotic System

A new hyperchaotic system based on the Lü method was developed by Chen et al. (18) in 2006 and is given by

$$\frac{d^{q1}x_1}{dt^{q1}} = a\left(x_2 - x_1\right) + x_4$$

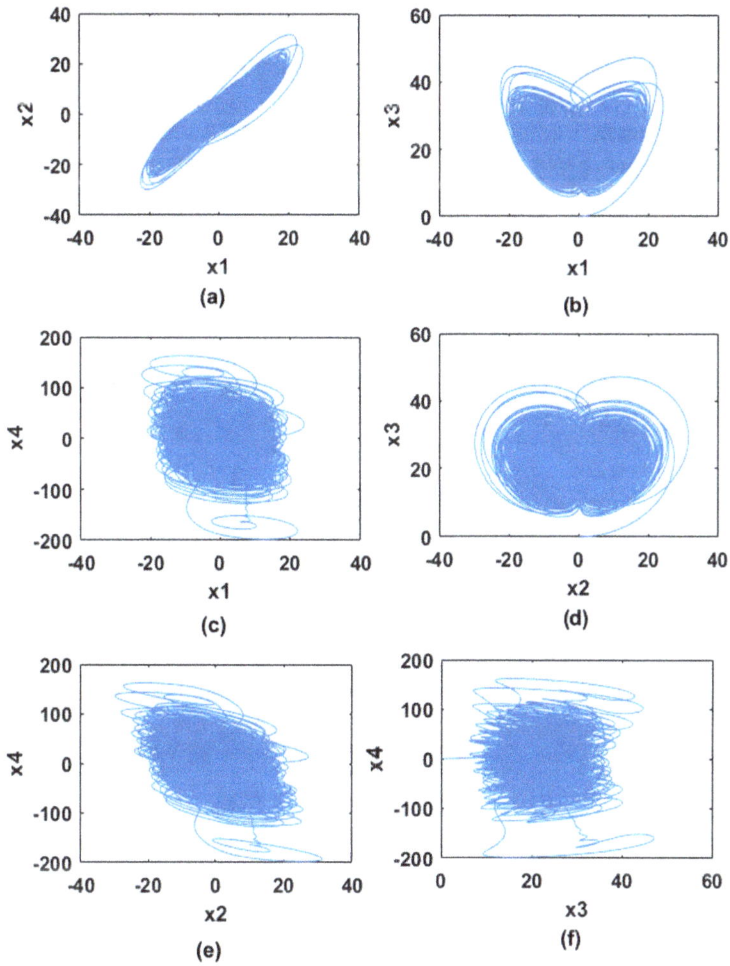

FIGURE 12.3 FOHCLU system.

$$\frac{d^{q2}x_2}{dt^{q2}} = -x_1x_3 + cx_2$$

$$\frac{d^{q3}x_3}{dt^{q3}} = x_1x_2 - bx_3$$

$$\frac{d^{q4}x_4}{dt^{q4}} = x_1x_3 + dx_4 \tag{9}$$

where a, b, and c are system constants and d is the control parameter. This system exhibits hyperchaotic behavior with $a = 36$, $b = 3$, $c = 20$, $q_i = 0.95$, and $d = 1.30$, and initial values (0.1, 0.1, 0.1, 0.2), as shown in Figure 12.3.

12.5 GENERATION OF THE MEASUREMENT MATRIX

To generate measurement matrices, FOHC sequences are utilized. The hyperchaotic system is predicted N_0 times to enhance stability and mitigate the adverse effects of pseudo-randomness. The system iterates M × L times. Four state values are generated and stored during each iteration i as $\{x_1^i, x_2^i, x_3^i, x_4^i\}$. The values generate two different key values in each iteration:

$$\left(s_j^a\right)^i = \text{mod}\,ulo\left\{ floor\left[\left(\left(\left|x_j^i\right| - floor\left(\left|x_j^i\right|\right)\right)\times 10^{15}\right)/10^8\right], 256\right\},\ j = 1,2,3,4 \quad (10)$$

$$\left(s_j^b\right)^i = \text{mod}\,ulo\left(floor\left(\text{mod}\,ulo\left\{\left[\left(\left|x_j^i\right| - floor\left(\left|x_j^i\right|\right)\right)\times 10^{15}\right], 10^8\right\}\right), 256\right),$$
$$j = 1,2,3,4 \quad (11)$$

The vector s^i is formed by concatenating Eqs. (10) and (11) as given below:

$$s^i = \left[\left(s_1^a\right)^i, \left(s_2^a\right)^i, \left(s_3^a\right)^i, \left(s_4^a\right)^i, \left(s_1^b\right)^i, \left(s_2^b\right)^i, \left(s_3^b\right)^i, \left(s_4^b\right)^i\right] \quad (12)$$

The s^i values are compiled into sequence q, $q = [s_1, s_2 \ldots, s_{m\times n}]$ for each iteration. q^j, $j \in [1,8mn]$ can indicate a sequence q. The measurement matrix M × N is obtained through MN number of successive elements in the hyperchaotic fractional-order sequences q.

12.6 EXPERIMENTAL RESULTS

This section aims at providing an experimental investigation into the application and examination of the accuracy of the reconstruction and encryption process by the measurement matrices produced by each hyperchaotic fractional system for the CS of digital images.

We employ the BCS-SPL-DDWT algorithm for image reconstruction and conduct detailed simulations using three different measurement matrices. For the experimental analysis, two medical digital images, each with a resolution of 512 × 512, are used.

S. No	Test Image	
1	Image CT 1	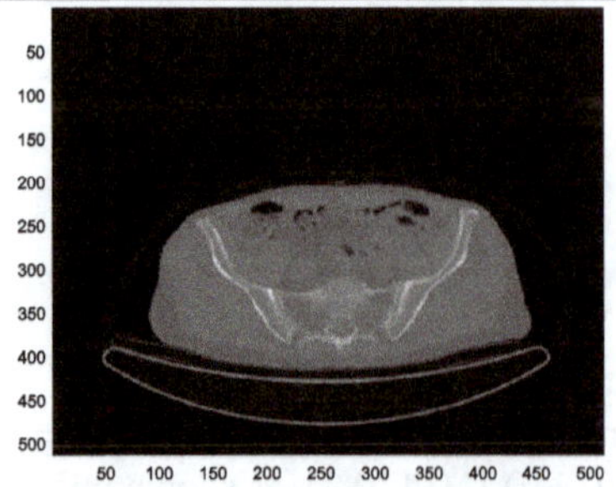

S. No	Test Image	
2	Image CT 2	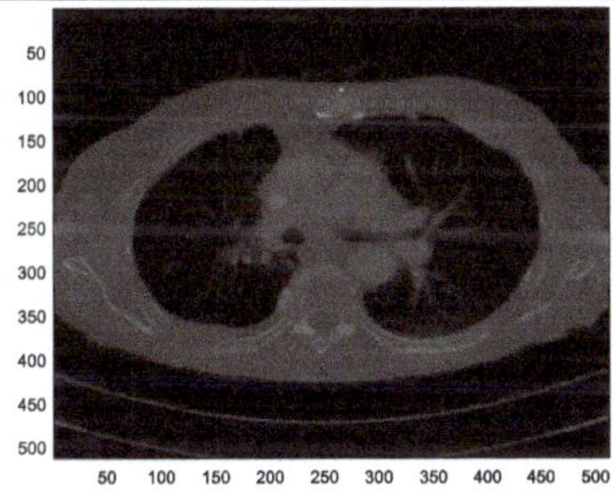

TABLE 12.1
Correlations for the FOHC Chen system

Image	Correlation	Input image	Rate of measurement		
			0.5	0.3	0.1
Image CT 1	Hor	0.9943	0.0003	0.0040	0.0013
	Ver	0.9848	0.0023	0.0020	0.0018
	Dia	0.9805	0.0009	0.0063	0.0021
Image CT 2	Hor	0.9959	0.0029	0.0090	0.0006
	Ver	0.9909	0.0007	0.0014	0.0095
	Dia	0.9878	0.0006	0.0051	0.0065

TABLE 12.2
Correlations for the FOHCL system

Image	Correlation	Input image	Rate of measurement		
			0.5	0.3	0.1
Image CT 1	Hor	0.9943	0.00007	0.0019	0.0083
	Ver	0.9848	0.0028	0.0006	0.0034
	Dia	0.9805	0.0008	0.0018	0.0040
Image CT 2	Hor	0.9959	0.0035	0.0023	0.0038
	Ver	0.9909	0.0002	0.0009	0.0016
	Dia	0.9878	0.0017	0.0008	0.0038

12.6.1 Correlation Analysis

The correlation coefficient can assess the relationship between adjacent pixels in an image. For a cipher, the correlation coefficient should be close to zero. Tables 12.1–12.3 present the horizontally, vertically, and diagonally correlate γ_h, γ_v, γ_d.

TABLE 12.3
Correlations for the FOHCLU system

Image	Correlation	Input image	Rate of measurement		
			0.5	0.3	0.1
Image CT 1	Hor	0.9943	0.0014	0.00009	0.0054
	Ver	0.9848	0.0004	0.00014	0.00007
	Dia	0.9805	0.0026	0.0038	0.0008
Image CT 2	Hor	0.9959	0.0002	0.0026	0.0009
	Ver	0.9909	0.0018	0.0032	0.0019
	Dia	0.9878	0.0033	0.0009	0.0007

TABLE 12.4
Reconstruction performance PSNR in (dB) (FOHC Chen measurement matrix)

Image	Rate of measurement		
	0.5	0.3	0.1
	PSNR in dB		
Image CT 1	26.4922	20.792	12.1216
Image CT 2	27.3439	22.7488	14.3623

TABLE 12.5
Reconstruction performance PSNR in (dB) (FOHC Lorenz measurement matrix)

Image	Rate of measurement		
	0.5	0.3	0.1
	PSNR in dB		
Image CT 1	26.1976	20.6649	11.9852
Image CT 2	27.3325	22.7427	14.4321

The correlation coefficients for each of the input images are obviously quite near to unity. On the other hand, the correlation is nearly zero for the cipher images produced with the three FOHC measurement matrices. The study findings in the tables show that there is almost no difference in the correlation between the chaotic sensing matrices.

TABLE 12.6
Reconstruction performance PSNR in (dB) (FOHC Lü measurement matrix)

Image	Rate of measurement		
	0.5	0.3	0.1
	PSNR in dB		
Image CT 1	26.2778	20.5662	11.987
Image CT 2	27.3682	22.6226	14.4179

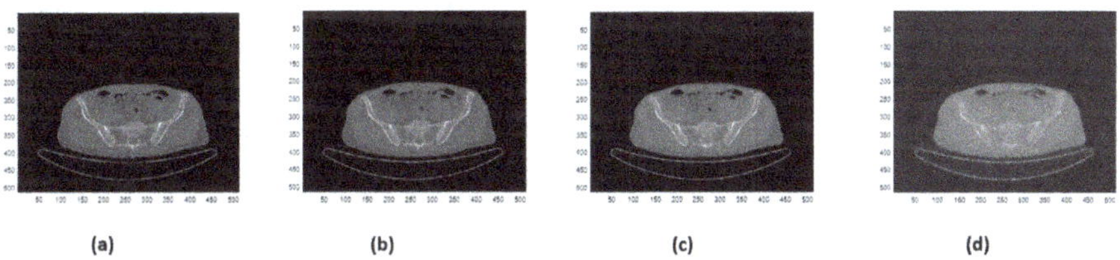

FIGURE 12.4 Image CT 1(FOHC Chen measurement matrix).

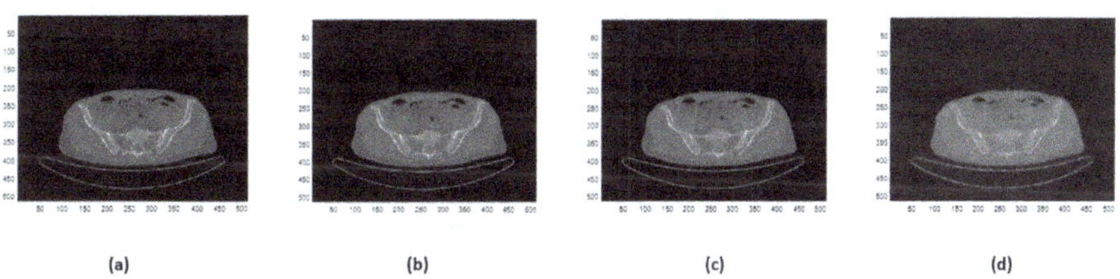

FIGURE 12.5 Image CT 1 (FOHC Lü measurement matrix).

12.6.2 Reconstruction Performance

With the PSNR, the restoration efficiency is evaluated. Various hyperchaotic sequences show that the higher the PSNR value, the greater the reconstruction accuracy. The findings in Tables 12.4–12.6, as well as Figures 12.4–12.9, show that the PSNR is nearly equal across different chaotic sensing matrices, with only minimal variation.

12.7 CONCLUSION

In this chapter, we used three distinct 4D fractional hyperchaotic sequences to generate measurement matrices. We evaluated the effectiveness of both encryption quality and image reconstruction. According to experimental findings, matrices

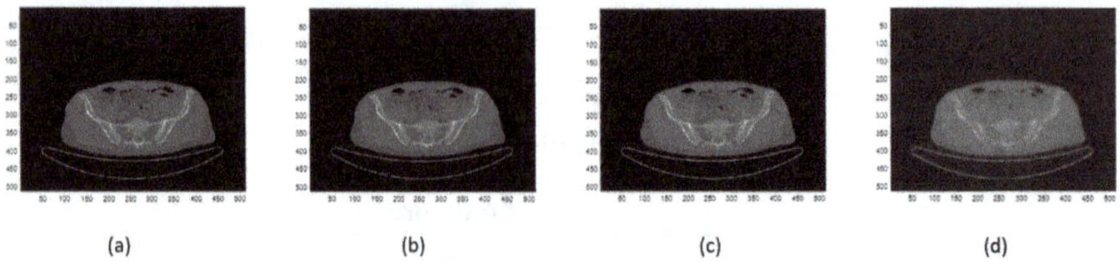

FIGURE 12.6 Image CT 1 (FOHC Lorenz measurement matrix).

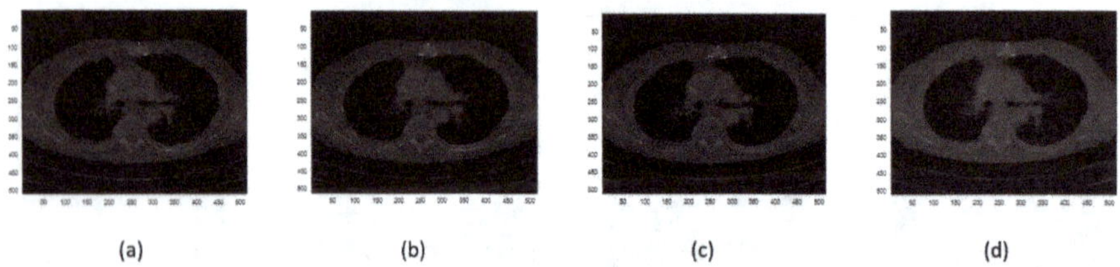

FIGURE 12.7 Image CT 2 (FOHC Chen measurement matrix).

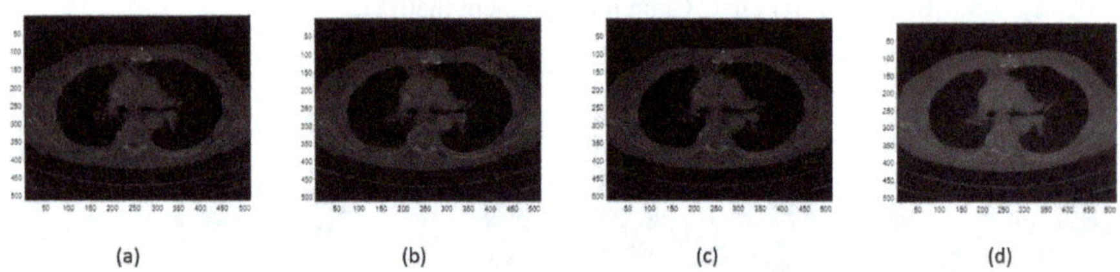

FIGURE 12.8 Image CT 2 (FOHC Lü measurement matrix).

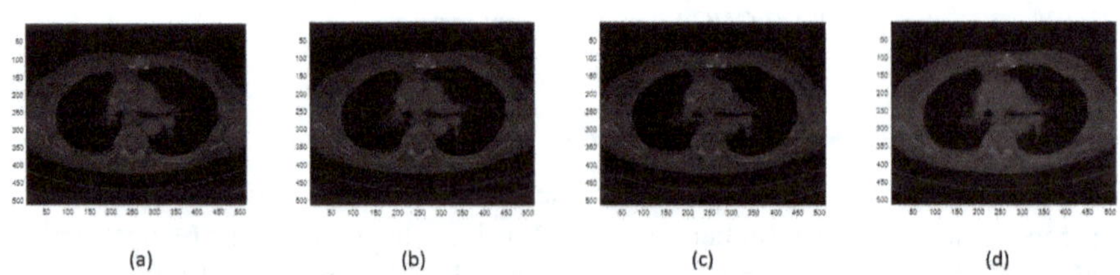

FIGURE 12.9 Image CT 2 (FOHC Lorenz measurement matrix).

produced by FOHC sequences have substantial randomness and extended dynamics, which makes them perfect for producing safe measurement matrices with excellent reconstruction. Furthermore, the three distinct FOHC sensing matrices operate almost identically.

REFERENCES

[1] D. L. Donoho, "Compressed sensing," *IEEE Transaction of Information Theory*, vol. 52, no. 4, pp. 1289–1306, 2006.

[2] R. Baraniuk, "Compressive sensing [lecture notes]," *IEEE Signal Proceeding Magazine*, vol. 24, no. 4, pp. 118–121, 2007.

[3] Y. Wu, G. Yang, H. Jin, and J. P. Noonan, "Image encryption using the two-dimensional logistic chaotic map," *Journal of Electronic Imaging*, vol. 21, no.1, Article ID 013014, 2012.

[4] M. Frunzete, Y. Lei, J. Barbot, and A.Vlad, "Compressive sensing matrix designed by tent map, for secure data transmission," *Signal Processing Algorithms, Architectures, Arrangements, and Applications Conference Proceedings, Vol 1,* pp.1–6, 2011.

[5] Y. Lei, J. P. Barbot, Z. Gang, and S. Hong,"Compressive sensing with chaotic sequence," *IEEE Signal Processing Letters*, vol. 17, no. 8, pp. 731734, 2010.

[6] V. Kafedziski, and T. Stojanovski," Compressive sampling with chaotic dynamical systems," *Telecommunications Forum*, pp. 695–698, 2011.

[7] C. Zhu, "A novel image encryption scheme based on improved hyperchaotic sequences," *Optics Communications*, vol. 285, no. 1, pp. 29–37, 2012.

[8] B. Norouzi, S. Mirzakuchaki, S. M. Seyedzadeh, and M. R. Mosavi, "A simple, sensitive and secure image encryption algorithm based on hyperchaotic system with only one round diffusion process," *Multimedia Tools and Applications,* vol. 71, no. 3, pp. 1469–1497, 2014.

[9] X. Wang and H. Zhang, "A novel image encryption algorithm based on genetic recombination and hyper-chaotic systems," *Nonlinear Dynamics*, vol. 1, pp. 333–346, 2016.

[10] T. Li, Y. Wang, and Y. Yang "Synchronization of fractional-order hyperchaotic systems via fractional-order controllers" *Discrete Dynamics in Nature and Society*, 2014, 408972, 14 pages, 2014.

[11] I. Podlubny, I. Petras, B. M. Vinagre, and L. Dorcak, "Analogue realizations of fractional-order controllers," *Nonlinear Dynamics*, vol. 29, no. 1–4, pp. 281–296, 2002.

[12] Z. Wang, X. Huang, Y.-X. Li, and X.-N. Song, "A new image encryption algorithm based on the fractional-order hyperchaotic Lorenz system," *Chinese Physics B*, vol. 22, no. 1, Article ID010504, 2013.

[13] Z. Wang, X. Huang, Y.-X. Li, and X.-N. Song, "A new image encryption algorithm based on the fractional-order hyperchaotic Lorenz system," *Chinese Physics B*, vol. 22, no. 1, Article ID010504, 2013.

[14] J. Zhao, S. Wang, Y. Chang, and X. Li, "A novel image encryption scheme based on an improper fractional-order chaotic system," *Nonlinear Dynamics*, vol. 80, no. 4, pp. 1721–1729, 2015.

[15] Y. Li, W. K. S. Tang, and G. R. Chen, "Generating hyperchaos via state feedback control," International *Journal of Bifurcation and Chaos in Applied Sciences and Engineering*, vol. 15, no. 10, pp. 3367 3375, 2005.

[16] X. Y.Wang and M. J. Wang, "A hyperchaos generated from Lorenz system," *Physica A*, vol. 387, no. 14, pp. 3751–3758, 2008.

[17] X. Y. Wang and J. M. Song, "Synchronization of the fractional order hyperchaos Lorenz systems with activation feedback control," *Communications in Nonlinear Science and Numerical Simulation*, vol. 14, no. 8, pp. 3351–3357, 2009.

[18] M. Chen, J. A. Lu, J. H. L¨u, and S. M. Yu, "Generating hyperchaotic L¨uattractorvia state feed backcontrol," *Physica A, Elsevier,* vol. 364, pp. 103–110, 2006.

[19] Gan, L. "Block compressed sensing of natural images," *15th International Conference on Digital Signal Processing, IEEE Xplore* , pp. 403–406, 2007.

[20] J. Haupt and R. Nowak, "Signal reconstruction from noisy random projections," *IEEE Transactions on Information Theory*, vol. 52, no. 9, pp. 4036–4048, September 2006.

[21] S. Mun, and J. Fowler, "Block compressed sensing of images using directional transforms," *16th IEEE International Conference on Image Processing (ICIP), 2009*, IEEE, pp. 3021–3024, 2009.

[22] M. N. Do, and M. Vetterli, "The contourlet transform: An efficient directional multiresolution image representation," *IEEE Transactions on Image Processing*, vol. 14, no. 12, pp. 2091–2106, 2005.

13 Early-Stage Lung Cancer Classification Using Spatial FusionNet

Meghna Vaddadi, Netaliya Ahmed, Nimmy B. Mathew, and A. Anilet Bala

13.1 INTRODUCTION

Lung cancer is a variation of cancer that affects the lungs, whereby cells in the lung transform and form a malignant tumor. Lung cancer exists in two main types: non-small-cell lung cancer (NSCLC) and small-cell lung cancer (SCLC). Globally, lung cancer is an important public health concern due to its high prevalence, association with smoking, and often delayed diagnosis. Lung cancer is one of the most common cancers globally, both in new cases and deaths. It is one of the major causes of death from any disease. The primary cause of lung cancer is tobacco smoke [1]. Smoking is the leading risk factor for lung cancer, and the risk doubles with each 20-pack-year increase. Despite smoking being a key risk factor, some non-smokers suffer from this condition too. Non-smokers get it through passive smoke inhalation or factors like environmental pollution and genetic predisposition.

Every year, there are over 2.2 million new cases of lung cancer. It causes a significant number of cancer-related mortalities, estimated at more than 1.8 million each year [2]. While most countries with high smoking rates have the highest incidence levels, lung cancer also affects non-smokers. Early diagnostics are essential for better outcomes, as the prognosis of lung cancer often depends on the stage of diagnosis. This is because the symptoms develop as the condition progresses, making it difficult to detect during the early stages. Such individuals may be asked by their doctors to take tests such as low-dose computed tomography (CT) scans or any other screening modality specifically designed for those considered at risk [3]. Regarding early lung cancer detection, CT scans are thought to be among the best tools available [4]. Surgical intervention, chemotherapy, radiotherapy, targeted therapy, and immune-based therapy are some of the ways to treat the disease. Its type and stage determine how best to manage it.

Quitting smoking is essential for preventing lung cancer. Health educators recommend quitting smoking so that the chances of getting lung cancer can be minimized. Current ongoing research explores the genetic and molecular basis of lung cancer in an attempt to develop targeted therapies, as well as personalized treatment options.

DOI: 10.1201/9781003484233-13

Lung cancer is a worldwide public health burden that has major implications [5]. To be able to minimize the impact of this disease, prevention and early detection are important. The most important way of preventing lung cancer is by quitting smoking, which consequently points out public health programs and personal lifestyles as means to lessen the burden of this infection, among other intervention measures. The early identification of lung cancer is essential for effective treatments and better patient results. Recent breakthroughs in deep learning approaches have demonstrated significant improvements in the precision and speed of classifying lung cancer from medical imaging data.

13.2 RELATED WORK

Several studies have delved into the realm of lung cancer segmentation, and classification utilizing deep learning algorithms. Rathod et al. developed the Spatial FusionNet framework to create and assess a new method for categorizing early-stage lung cancer in the study paper [6].

Spatial FusionNet is a model that merges the capabilities of the Inception v3 and ResNet-50 models to develop DLCTLungDetectNet, a model tailored for detecting lung cancer. DLCTLungDetectNet combines various deep learning architectures to utilize spatial information in medical imaging data for enhanced accuracy in early-stage lung cancer classification. Multiple studies in the literature have emphasized the importance of detecting early-stage lung cancer. Gu et al. [7] proposed an optimization technique for convolutional neural networks (CNNs) that improved accuracy and decreased false positives in lung cancer detection. Blanc et al. [8] suggested an artificial intelligence (AI) method that combines three-dimensional (3D) U-Net, 3D Retina-UNET, and support vector machine (SVM) algorithms, showing impressive results on various datasets.

Furthermore, Wankhade et al. [9] proposed a hybrid architecture that integrates 3D CNN with RNN, demonstrating exceptional performance in the initial stage prediction of lung cancer. The article highlights the increasing interest in and efforts to improve lung cancer diagnosis and classification through AI and deep learning techniques. This work evaluates the effectiveness of Spatial FusionNet, specifically DLCTLungDetectNet, in accurately categorizing early-stage lung cancer using medical imaging data.

Rajasekar et al. [10] presented a predictive approach using feature analysis and deep learning models, stressing the significance of early lung cancer detection. Thong et al. [11] conducted a systematic review highlighting the promising efficacy of AI-based imaging in lung cancer screening and advocating for further high-quality studies. Jin et al. [12] conducted a systematic review that compared the effectiveness of machine learning (ML) algorithms in pulmonary lump computer-aided diagnosis (CAD), emphasizing tailored algorithm choices for different stages of diagnosis. Similarly, several ML approaches are employed for a variety of applications, including forest cover classification [13].

Chaunzwa et al. [14] introduced a deep neural network approach to classify lung cancer histology, employing transfer learning and model interpretability techniques. Teramoto et al. [15] proposed a rapid lung nodule identification method by combining cylindrical nodule enhancement filters with SVMs for false-positive reduction. Cao et al. [16] suggested a multi-scale approach for nodule detection, incorporating attention mechanisms and a ResSCBlock module for enhanced feature extraction. Sheriff et al. [17] developed a web application utilizing the VGGNet-16 architecture for early lung cancer detection. Sravani et al. [18] employed VGG16 and Inception v3 models for precise lung cancer diagnosis, utilizing data augmentation and supercomputing resources for efficient training and evaluation.

Swaminathan et al. [19] introduced an approach that optimizes complexity for lung cancer classification by employing dense and sparse neural networks, highlighting Inception v3's reduced computational overhead, showing promise for accurate classification. Raju et al. [20] utilized Wiener filtering, generative adversarial network (GAN)-based segmentation (SSSOA optimization), and VGG16 CNN. This approach achieves a 97% prediction rate for early-stage lung cancer detection, emphasizing VGG16's impressive accuracy in deep learning methodologies.

In [21], the smaller VGGNet CNN innovatively classifies interstitial lung diseases from HRCT images, with a remarkable 95% average accuracy across 17 interstitial lung disease (ILD) categories, showcasing its potential for early detection. The modified version of the VGG network is beneficial for various applications, in addition to disease detection [22].

Wang et al. [23] proposed a medical image denoising approach that integrates adaptive deep CNN with adaptive watershed segmentation, achieves superior performance on magnetic resonance imaging (MRI) and CT images (Jaccard index of 0.95 and peak signal-to-noise ratio (PSNR) of 43.76 dB), and enhances denoising with marker-based watershed segmentation. Ma et al. [24] introduced a novel histogram equalization algorithm in CIE LCH color space. They enhanced color image contrast with competitive performance across diverse testing images. Pawar et al. [25] created MedSAM, a basic model for universal medical image segmentation that is more flexible, works better than specialist models, and takes less time to annotate, which is a big step forward. Makaju et al. [26] suggested an ML model for detecting lung cancer. It uses a fine-tuned ResNet-50 with 88.89% accuracy, putting recall first in medical settings. This could assist doctors in resolving a major healthcare problem.

Bhatt et al. [27] proposed a CAD system with watershed segmentation and SVM classification for early lung cancer detection. This research achieved an improved 92% accuracy compared to current models, marking a significant step in precise lung cancer diagnosis. Gugulothu et al. [28] focused on early lung cancer detection by employing computer vision and SVM algorithms for effective bi-classification of inpatient CT lung scans, crucial for improved survival rates. Achanta et al. [29] introduced LNDC-HDL, a hybrid deep learning approach. This study employs optimization techniques for lung nodule feature extraction, and classification from CT scans, highlighting increased sensitivity and reduced false positives. Durgesh et al. [30] introduced a lung cancer detection method based on a modified Faster R-CNN called the HFRCNN approach. They achieved a 97% detection accuracy on the LUNA16 dataset.

Underscoring the importance of Matplotlib and Seaborn in data visualization, Gupta et al. [31] recognized them as foundational tools for transforming raw data into impactful visual representations using Python. The knowledge gathered from several research projects that have tackled similar obstacles includes improving CNN structures, introducing innovative segmentation methods, and applying ML models for lung cancer identification. The capabilities of visualization libraries like Matplotlib and Seaborn are investigated as highlighted in recent research [31] to provide relevant visualizations that help in understanding categorization outcomes. Our research aims to enhance early-stage lung cancer classification by incorporating findings from various studies and utilizing advancements in AI techniques.

More precise techniques will be developed as a result, enabling timely intervention and enhancing patient outcomes. Highlighting Matplotlib and Seaborn's proficiency, this chapter emphasizes their role as foundational tools in Python for creating impactful and clear data-driven visuals, facilitating effective communication.

13.3 METHODOLOGY

The process begins with the acquisition of a lung cancer dataset, sourced from Kaggle and comprising 1080 CT scan images. Following dataset retrieval, pre-processing methods are employed to improve image quality, extract relevant features, and facilitate accurate diagnoses by healthcare professionals. After pre-processing, several deep learning (DL) models, including VGG16, VGG19, Inception v3, and the newly introduced FusionNet called 'TriadNet', are applied to the CT scan dataset using standard hold-out validation, along with the proposed model. The proposed system model is illustrated in Figure 13.1. The dataset is divided into 70% for training, 20% for testing, and 10% for validation. Following this, CT images are classified into normal, benign, or malignant categories. An in-depth analysis of the results is then performed for each DL model and the proposed model to derive meaningful insights.

13.3.1 Main Objective

The following is a concise summary of the main goals of "TriadNet: Deep Learning for Lung Tumor Detection in CT Scans":

- **Lung Tumor Detection:** To precisely identify lung tumors in CT scans, construct the specialized deep learning model TriadNet.
- **Improved Precision and Dependability:** Elevate the reliability and accuracy of detection beyond traditional methods, with a focus on reducing both false positives and false negatives.
- **Early-Stage Disease Prediction:** Automatically analyzing medical images can aid in the early diagnosis of lung tumors, potentially improving patient outcomes by detecting tumors at an early stage.
- **Streamlined Operations:** Automated analysis can improve tumor identification efficiency, which in turn reduces radiologists' burden and speeds up the diagnosis process.

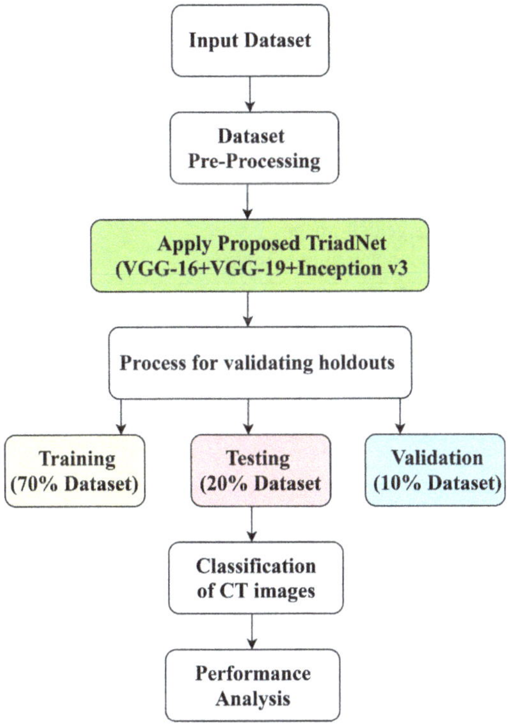

FIGURE 13.1 Proposed system model.

- **Practical Applicability in Clinical Settings:** Assure the applicability and clinical significance of TriadNet for medical practitioners, supporting the field of lung cancer diagnosis and medical imaging.
- **Adaptability and Scalability:** As it may be integrated into larger healthcare facilities and systems, the deep learning model should be designed to be both adaptable and scalable.
- **Advancement in Medical AI:** It advances the field of deep learning in medical imaging by developing advanced methods to recognize lung tumors.
- **Improved Patient Outcomes:** In the end, it uses cutting-edge AI algorithms to help with early and more accurate lung tumor diagnosis to improve patient treatment and outcomes.

13.4 DATASET COLLECTION

The dataset collected from DLCTLungDetectNet – Lung Tumor Dataset includes a wide array of data essential for training and evaluating the proposed model. The dataset includes three different forms of malignancies and a group for normal imaging. The dataset image split is given in Table 13.1.

TABLE 13.1
Split of dataset images

Total no. of images	1080
No. of non-cancerous images	235
No. of squamous cell images	265
No. of large cell images	212
No. of adenocarcinoma images	368

Our dataset includes three major forms of chest cancer:

a) Lung adenocarcinoma is the common type of lung cancer, representing about 30% of all lung cancer cases and over 40% of NSCLC. Nodules typically appear in the outer regions of the lung, mainly within mucus-producing glands. Symptoms may include coughing, hoarseness, unexpected weight loss, and weakness.
b) Large-cell undifferentiated carcinoma, known for its rapid growth and widespread dissemination in the lung, is classified as large cell carcinoma. It usually accounts for 10–15% of all cases of NSCLC and is known for its extremely aggressive nature.
c) Squamous cell lung cancer typically occurs in the lung's middle region, most frequently in or around the bigger bronchi with the trachea or in major respiratory branches. Smoking strongly links it to over 30% of NSCLC.
d) Our dataset contains normal chest CT-scan images for comparison analysis, in addition to malignant samples.

This organized dataset helped us to build an efficient and accurate chest cancer detection system using the proposed TriadNet.

13.4.1 Dataset Pre-Processing

Pre-processing methods are essential for identifying lung cancer from X-rays and CT scans. These methods improve image quality, extract pertinent information, and aid radiologists and healthcare professionals in making precise diagnoses. Figure 13.2 displays raw input image with noise. Post-pre-processing, we acquire histogram-equalized pictures. Figure 13.2 shows a few typical image pre-processing methods used for lung cancer prediction.

13.4.1.1 Enhancement Techniques

i. Contrast Enhancement: Increasing the contrast of the image helps to enhance the details and lesions. The contrast-enhanced image can be calculated using a contrast stretching function, as follows, where $I(x, y)$ is the original image:

$$I_{enhanced}(x,y) = a * I(x,y) + b \tag{1}$$

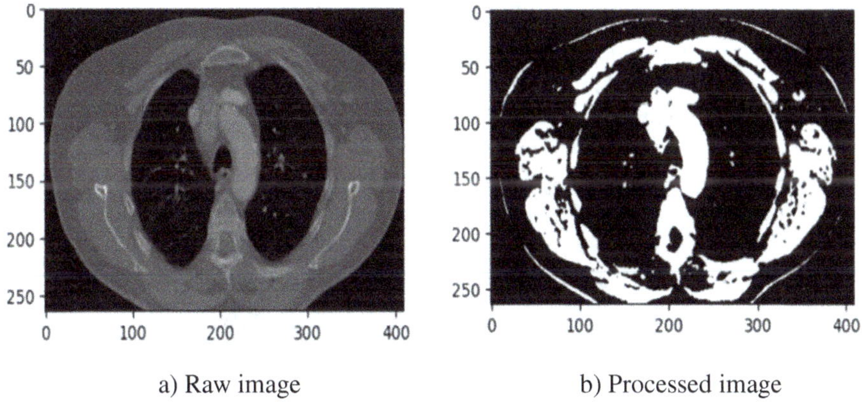

FIGURE 13.2 Unprocessed and processed lung cancer image.

ii. Noise Reduction: The Gaussian blur approach removes image noise from equipment constraints or patient movement. This technique eliminates noise while preserving information regarding the details. The Gaussian blur operation can be expressed as follows:

$$I_{blurred}(x, y) = \frac{1}{K} \sum_{i=1}^{M} \sum_{j=1}^{N} G(i, j) I(x + i, y + j) \tag{2}$$

where $M \times N$ is the size of the image, $G(i, j)$ is the Gaussian kernel, and K is the normalization constant given by

$$K = \sum_{i=1}^{M} \sum_{j=1}^{N} G(i, j) \tag{3}$$

Gaussian kernel G is applied to the equalized image to generate a denoised image:

$$I_{denoised}(x, y) = I_{equalized}(x, y) * G \tag{4}$$

iii. Histogram Equalization (HE): HE changes the intensity distribution to enhance clarity. The histogram equalized image is given by

$$I_{equalized}(x, y) = L * \frac{CDF(I(x, y))}{M \times N} \tag{5}$$

where L is the number of intensity levels, $M \times N$ is the size of the image, and CDF is the cumulative distribution function.

13.4.1.2 Adaptive Histogram Equalization (AHE)

The HE output undergoes further processing to obtain the AHE [32]. After the denoised image is divided into distinct tiles $T(x, y)$, the HE for each tile is determined, and then the $CDF(T)$ is computed. AHE is mainly useful for medical images [33]:

$$I_{adaptive\ equalised} = I_{equalized}\left(x, y\right) - CDF(T\left(x, y\right) \quad (6)$$

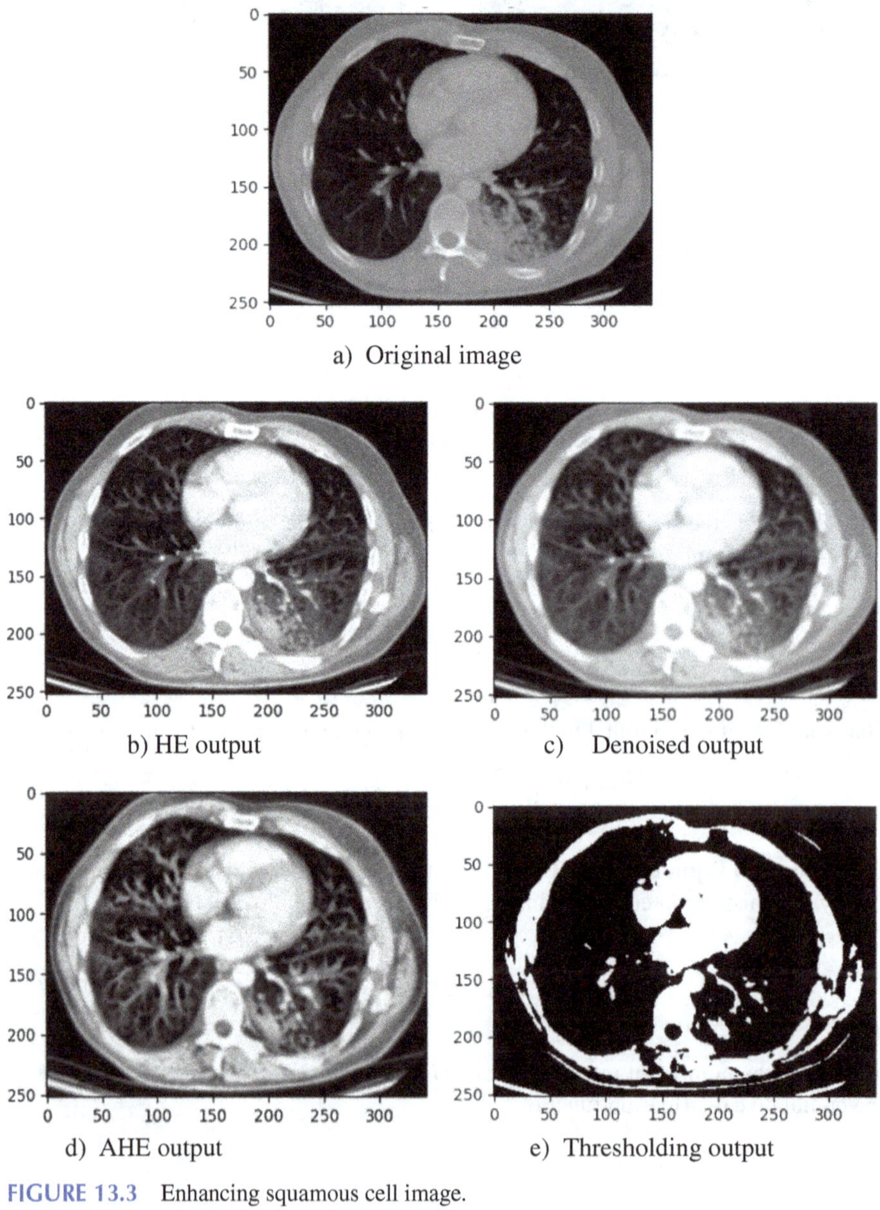

a) Original image

b) HE output

c) Denoised output

d) AHE output

e) Thresholding output

FIGURE 13.3 Enhancing squamous cell image.

13.4.1.3 Binary Thresholding

A segmented image is generated by applying the thresholding technique. The intensity levels of 180 or above are assigned a value of 255 (white), while the rest are assigned a value of 0 (black). The lung region is isolated from the background through this method. Figures 13.3 and 13.4 display the original images with histogram conversion, noise reduction, adaptive processing, and thresholding applied.

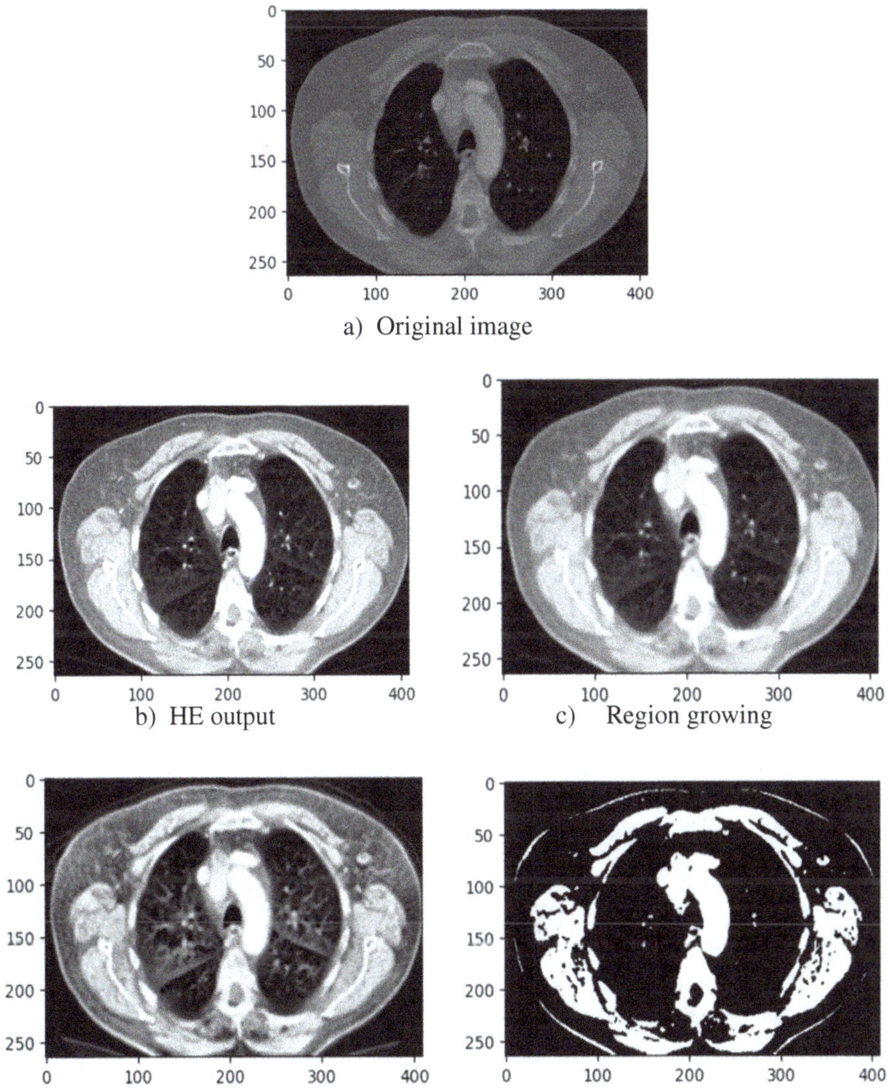

a) Original image

b) HE output

c) Region growing

d) Gradient output

e) Watershed transform output

FIGURE 13.4 Enhancing an adenocarcinoma image.

13.5 IMAGE SEGMENTATION

13.5.1 Region Growing

Region growing is a segmentation method that groups pixels with similar features. Region growth begins with a seed point. The coordinates in the image are set to (100, 100). The process starts with the initial point and the method grows a region by adding neighbouring pixels whose intensity levels are within a certain range.

13.5.2 Watershed Transform

The watershed transform isolates objects based on their topographical properties for image segmentation. It is commonly utilized to separate intersecting objects. The image gradient is computed by applying a morphological operation with a kernel size of (3, 3). This gradient graphic emphasizes the borders between things then the watershed transform is implemented. The watershed transform output is shown in Figures 13.5 and 13.6.

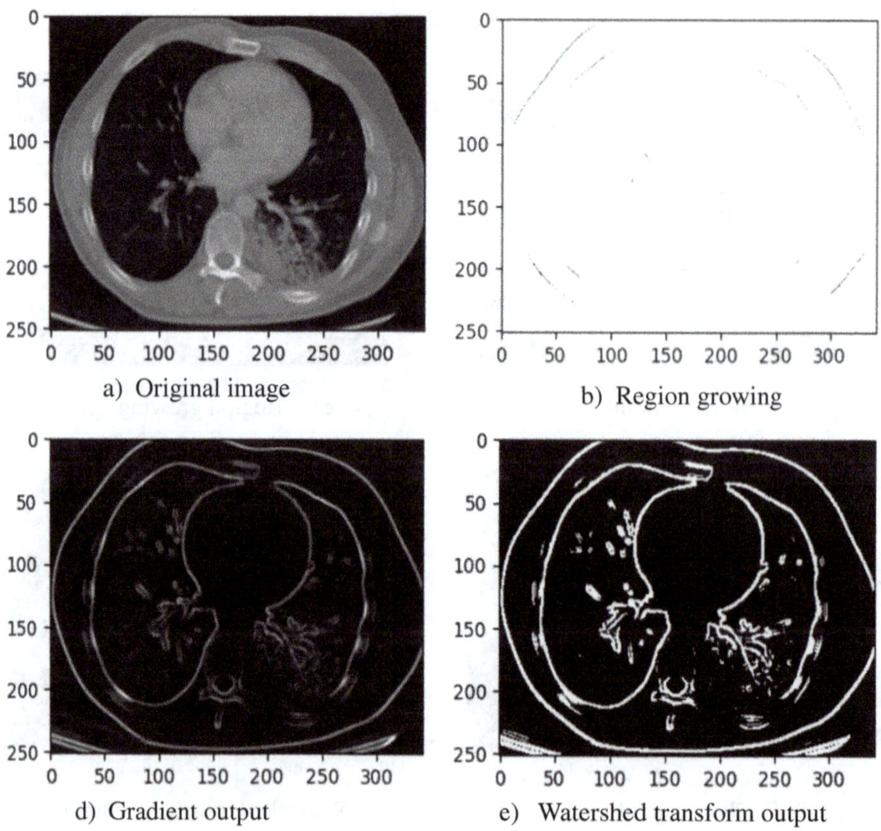

FIGURE 13.5 Segmenting a squamous cell cancerous image.

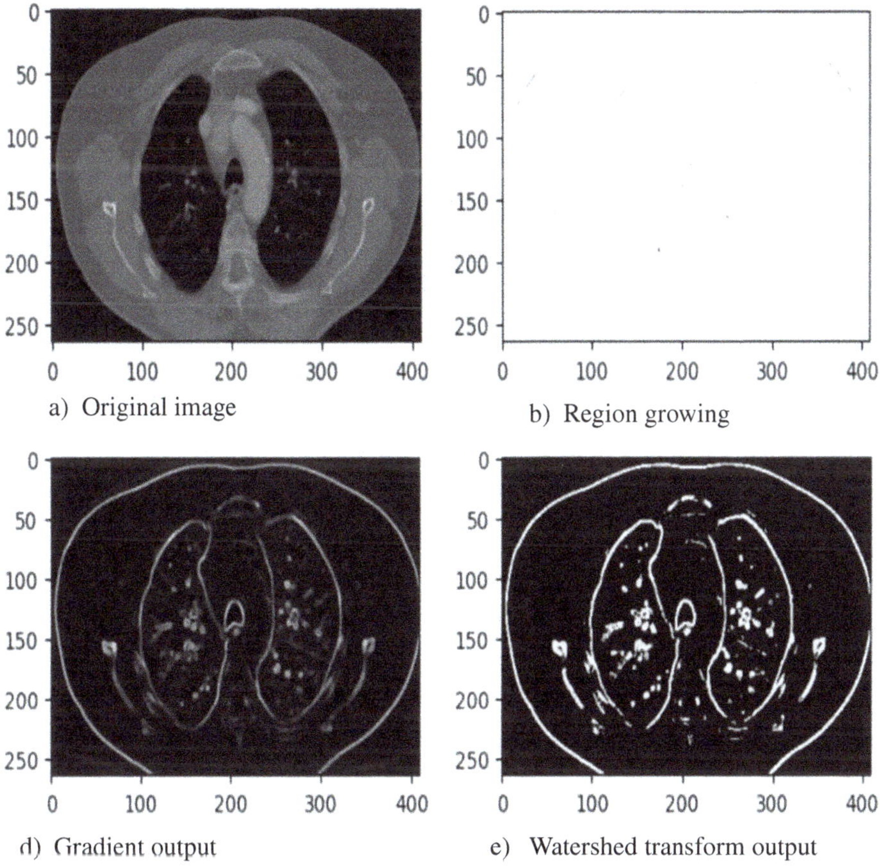

FIGURE 13.6 Segmenting an adenocarcinoma cancerous image.

13.5.2.1 Pre-Processing Algorithm

Step 1. Load Lung Image: Load the CT scan image of the lungs, which serves as the input for subsequent processing steps.

Step 2. Apply HE: Perform histogram equalization to increase the overall contrast, improving the visibility of structures and details.

Step 3. Enhance Image Contrast: Apply contrast enhancement techniques to further improve the visibility of features within the lung image, aiding in better analysis and interpretation.

Step 4. Reduce Noise using Gaussian Blur: Employ Gaussian blur to reduce noise in the image, promoting a smoother and more refined representation of the lung structures.

Step 5. Apply AHE: Implement adaptive histogram equalization to locally enhance the contrast in different regions of the lung image, ensuring optimal visibility across various intensity levels.

Step 6. Lung Region Extraction using Thresholding: Utilize thresholding techniques to segment and extract the lung region from the pre-processed image, isolating it from the surrounding tissues.

Step 7. Segmented lung region (S): Using thresholding, segment the lung area (S).

The algorithm successfully pre-processed and extracted the lung region from the CT scan for further analysis or medical interpretation.

13.6 LAYER ARCHITECTURES OF THE PROPOSED TRIADNET

The proposed architecture in Figure 13.7 begins with a pre-trained base model loaded with weights from ImageNet and includes additional layers for fine-tuning and customization to suit the specific requirements of the chest cancer detection task.

First, the VGG16 base model is used and then a dropout layer is used for regularization. Next, the 3D output is flattened to make it a one-dimensional (1D) vector. Finally, three dense layers contain batch normalization (BN) and rectified linear unit (ReLU) functions. The final dense layer has a sigmoid activation function, indicating binary classification output. Similarly, the VGG19 model follows the same structure as VGG16, using the VGG19 base model instead. The added layers include dropout, flattening, BN, and three dense layers with ReLU, culminating in the last sigmoid

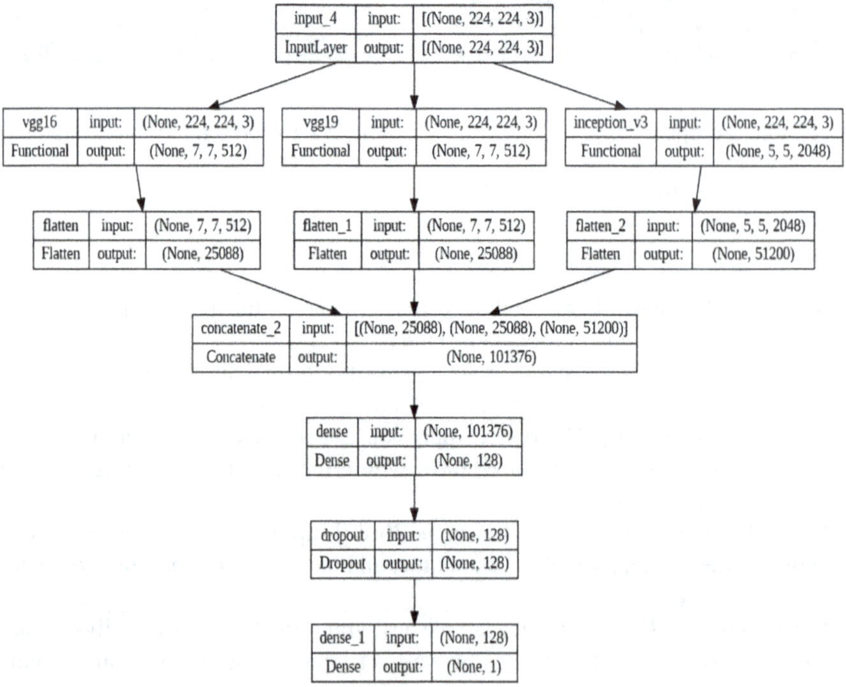

FIGURE 13.7 Layer architecture diagram of the proposed TriadNet model.

activation layer. The Inception v3 model integrates the Inception v3 base model with additional layers, including dropout, flattening, BN, and three dense layers with ReLU activation functions. The final dense layer has a sigmoid activation, reflecting the binary nature of the classification task.

To create the hybrid model, features are extracted from each of the base models (VGG16, VGG19, and Inception v3) using their respective pre-trained weights. These features are then concatenated into a single vector, which serves as input for subsequent dense layers in the hybrid model. Putting these different features together is meant to take advantage of the unique representations that each base model has learned. This could make the overall model better at finding complex patterns in the chest cancer dataset.

The chosen layers for the hybrid model include the flattened features from each base model and three subsequent dense layers for further processing. The goal of concatenating these features is to make use of the complementary data that each base model has collected, potentially improving the model's performance in detecting chest cancer. It was decided to freeze the layers of the pre-trained models during training. This keeps the hierarchical representations that were learned before, and the trainable dense layers let the models adapt to the task at hand. The hybrid model that is made is put together, trained, and tested using a binary cross-entropy loss function and different metrics. This gives us a complete and effective way to find chest cancer.

Feature Extraction:

$$F_{VGG16}(I),\ F_{VGG19}(I),\ F_{InceptionV3}(I) \tag{7}$$

Concatenation of Features:
Let *Concatenated*(*I*) represent the concatenated feature vector:

$$Concatenated(I) = [F_{VGG16}(I),\ F_{VGG19}(I),\ F_{InceptionV3}(I) \tag{8}$$

Dense Layers:
Let $W1$, $b1$, $W2$, and $b2$ be the weights and biases of the dense layers.
Let *ReLU*(*x*) represent the ReLU activation function:

$$Output(I) = Sigmoid(W_2 \cdot ReLU\left(W_1 \cdot Concatenated(I) + b_1\right) + b_2 \tag{9}$$

where $\cdot$ represents matrix multiplication, and *Sigmoid* and *ReLU* are activation functions applied element-wise to the vectors.

13.7 PROPOSED ARCHITECTURE

The proposed TriadNet is used to enhance the categorization of lung tumors in the field of medical imaging. This novel method is based on combining three powerful pre-trained frameworks, VGG16, VGG19, and Inception v3, to incorporate their unique characteristics and knowledge into a single architecture. The TriadNet model effectively utilizes VGG16, VGG19, and Inception v3 as feature extractors to analyze input photos. By combining and compressing these collected characteristics, a comprehensive representation is obtained, enhancing the feature set necessary for accurate lung tumor categorization. The model is improved by dense layers and dropout regularization. It is finished off with a sigmoid-activated output layer for binary classification, which accurately finds lung cancers when they are present or not. The model detects tumors in a CT scan and categorizes them based on phases using the proposed CNN model.

Several crucial factors demonstrate the significance of TriadNet in lung tumor categorization. TriadNet utilizes a tri-model feature fusion approach to combine the feature representation capabilities of VGG16, VGG19, and Inception v3. This strategic integration enables a wide range of features to be included, capturing the detailed patterns necessary for precise lung tumor categorization.

An innovative approach to learning and regularization is required when integrating different pre-trained DL models. TriadNet effectively combines learning from both DL models by using shared dense layers and dropout regularization to stop overfitting. This balance guarantees the model's ability to generalize and remain strong. TriadNet outperforms standalone VGG16, VGG19, and Inception v3 deep learning models in lung tumor classification based on comparative studies.

The performance metric values demonstrate the enhanced performance of the hybrid model in terms of improving classification outcomes. TriadNet remains computationally efficient despite combining three intricate DL models, focusing on resource optimization. By stopping pre-trained layers and speeding up the fusion process, computing power is used more efficiently. The success of TriadNet in accurately categorizing lung tumors suggests its potential for broader applications in medical imaging.

Additionally, compressive sensing [34] is useful for reducing the size of CT image datasets while preserving crucial diagnostic features. This leads to enhanced storage efficiency and accelerated processing speeds.

The algorithm presents a standard architectural framework for a deep learning model commonly used in picture classification applications. Let's thoroughly examine each stage in detail:

1. **Loading Pre-Trained Models:** This stage includes importing pre-trained DL models such as VGG16, VGG19, and Inception v3. The models have undergone prior training on large datasets for broad image recognition tasks, featuring convolutional layers that are highly proficient at extracting features from images.
2. **Image Input (*X*):** *X* represents the input images intended for processing by the model. The photos may vary in size, but are usually adjusted to match the input dimensions required by the pre-trained models, such as 224 × 224 pixels.
3. **Feature Extraction:** During this stage, pre-trained models such as VGG16, VGG19, and Inception v3 are utilized to extract features from the input images. The models utilize a series of convolutional layers and transformations to

detect patterns and high-level representations in the images. The output feature maps produced by VGG16, VGG19, and Inception v3 are referred to as FVGG16, FVGG19, and FInception v3, respectively. The feature maps are matrices of numerical values that encode the discovered visual features.

4. **Post-Feature Extraction:** The feature maps are usually multi-dimensional, for example, in terms of height, width, and depth. These features are flattened into 1D vectors for use in the following layers. FflatVGG16, FflatVGG19, and FflatInception v3 are the flattened feature vectors obtained from FResNet-50 and FInception v3, respectively. FConcat is the result of combining the flattened feature vectors. This fusion combines the retrieved features from VGG16, VGG19, and Inception v3 into a unified vector.
5. **Dense Layers:** The flattened feature vector, FConcat, passes through a series of dense (completely linked) layers. The layers consist of neurons (nodes) that are fully linked. H1 represents the output of the first dense layer, while H2 represents the output of the following dense layer. The layers utilize the ReLU activation function to help the model learn complex patterns.
6. **Output Layer:** The last layer in the architectural design is labeled Y and is in charge of providing the model's predictions. The sigmoid activation function (σ) is typically used for binary classification tasks with two classes. The sigmoid activation function is applied at the last dense layer (H2), along with weights (Wout) and biases (bout) that are linked to the output layer.

This building system uses models that have already been trained (VGG16, VGG19, and Inception v3) to pull out features and fully linked dense layers to make predictions based on those features. The output layer plays a crucial role in deciding the final classification or prediction results.

This architectural design serves as the foundational framework for classifying CT scan pictures into two categories: tumor and non-tumor. If the scans detect tumors, a deep learning model is utilized to classify the tumors into different stages: Stage 1, Stage 2, Stage 3, and Stage 4.

13.8 RESULTS AND DISCUSSION

The performance metrics provide a detailed assessment of the models' effectiveness in classification tasks. The outcomes of extensive testing and analysis of several frameworks for the categorization of lung tumors have produced insightful findings that validate TriadNet's dominance as the best model in this field. The comparison analysis's main conclusions are summarized in Table 13.2. TriadNet is an inventive hybrid model that demonstrates remarkable performance in the training, validation, and testing stages. It combines features from VGG16, VGG19, and Inception v3. This data are also compared with DLCTLungDetectNet, a spatial FusionNet consisting of ResNet-50 and Inception v3.

For randomly selected images, the Prediction vs. Truth Analysis comparison for all the different deep learning models is shown in Figure 13.8.

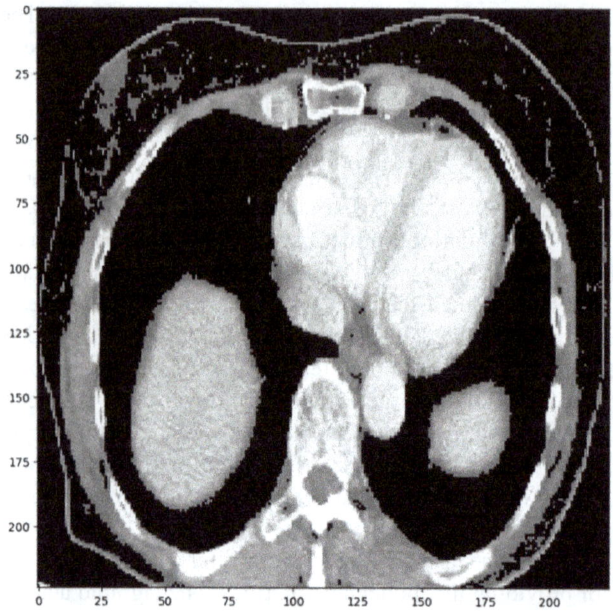

a) **VGG16:** Non-cancerous, **VGG19:** Cancerous, **Inception v3:** Cancerous, **TriadNet:** Cancerous, **Truth:** Cancerous

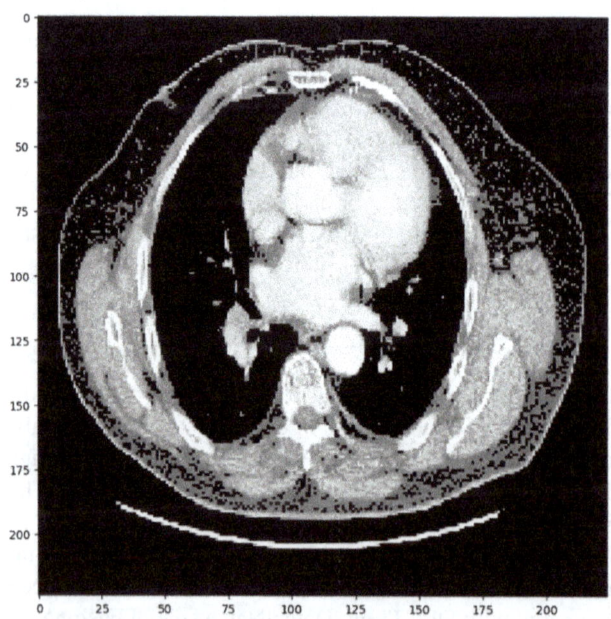

b) **VGG16:** Cancerous, **VGG19:** Cancerous, **Inception v3:** Cancerous, **TriadNet:** Cancerous, **Truth:** Cancerous

FIGURE 13.8 Label prediction of randomly selected dataset images.

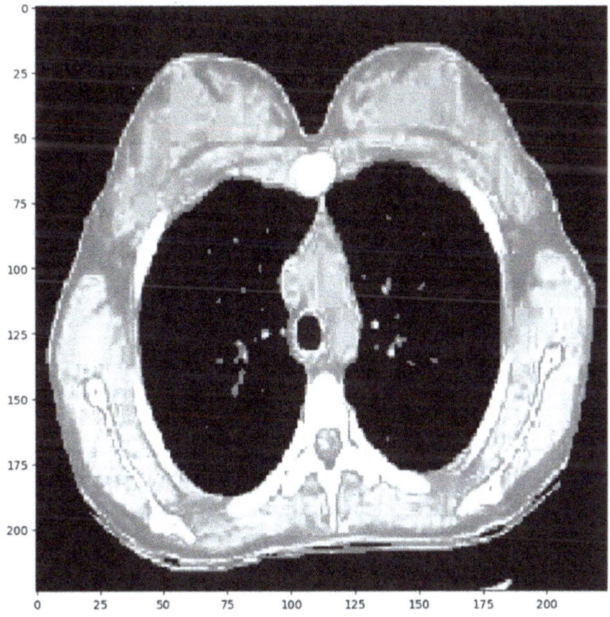

c) **VGG16:** Non-cancerous, **VGG19:** Non-cancerous, **Inception v3:** Non-cancerous, **TriadNet:** Non-cancerous, **Truth:** Non-cancerous

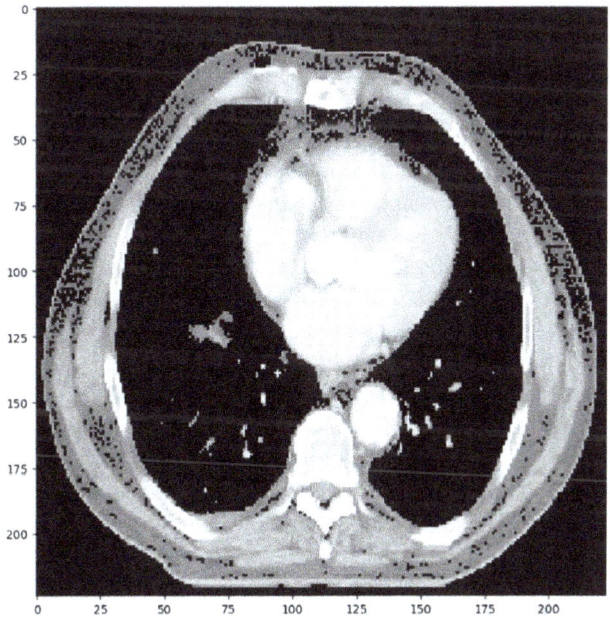

d) **VGG16:** Cancerous, **VGG19:** Non-cancerous, **Inception v3:** Cancerous, **TriadNet:** Cancerous, **Truth:** Cancerous

FIGURE 13.8 (Continued)

TABLE 13.2
Performance metric comparison of various models

Framework	Accuracy	Precision	Recall	Loss	F1
VGG16	0.9703	0.8800	0.9653	0.0600	0.9402
VGG19	0.9703	0.8916	0.8636	0.1000	0.9302
Inception v3	0.9802	0.9521	0.9091	0.1000	0.9452
DLCTLungDetectNet	0.9653	0.9111	0.9318	0.0900	0.8832
TriadNet Model (proposed model)	**0.9901**	**0.9773**	**0.9773**	**0.0500**	**0.9746**

The performance metrics for different DL models in a classification task are summarized in Table 13.2. With an accuracy of 0.9901, the proposed TriadNet model successfully classified 99.01% of the cases. With a precision of 0.9773, the "TriadNet Model" has the highest accuracy, meaning that almost all of its positive predictions came true. With the highest F1 score of 0.9746, the "TriadNet Model" exhibits a strong balance between recall and precision. It is observed that the TriadNet model improves accuracy by 1%, precision by 2.64%, recall by 1.24%, F1 score by 3.11, and loss by 16.66% over existing models. A graphical representation of the model comparison is shown in Figure 13.9.

13.9 CONCLUSION

TriadNet stands out as the top-performing model, outperforming others in accuracy, recall, precision, and loss measures. The feature fusion method enhances feature sets, which are essential for precise tumor classification, while also maintaining computational efficiency, a vital component for practical medical imaging applications. After a thorough examination of the outcomes in all stages, TriadNet continually proves to be the top-performing model. FusionNet combines features from VGG16, VGG19 and Inception v3 to enhance the feature set, collecting detailed patterns essential for accurate lung tumor classification. The proposed TriadNet model outperforms other models, achieving 1% improvements in accuracy, 2.64 percent improvements in precision, 1.24 percent improvements in recall, 3.11 percent improvements in F1 score, and a 16.66 percent reduction in loss.

The TriadNet model outperforms the other models based on the specified performance metrics. The TriadNet model earns a top accuracy score of 0.9901. It accurately classifies 99.01% of the data points. This strongly suggests that the model is producing precise predictions, surpassing all other models in this regard.

The FusionNet model has a precision score of 0.9773, meaning it accurately predicts most of the positive classes every time. It has the lowest false positive rate among all the models, which makes it very dependable for categorizing positive events. The TriadNet model achieves a flawless recall score of 97.73%. This indicates that it accurately recognizes all good situations. The FusionNet model had the highest F1 score of 0.9746 compared to all other models. The F1 score considers

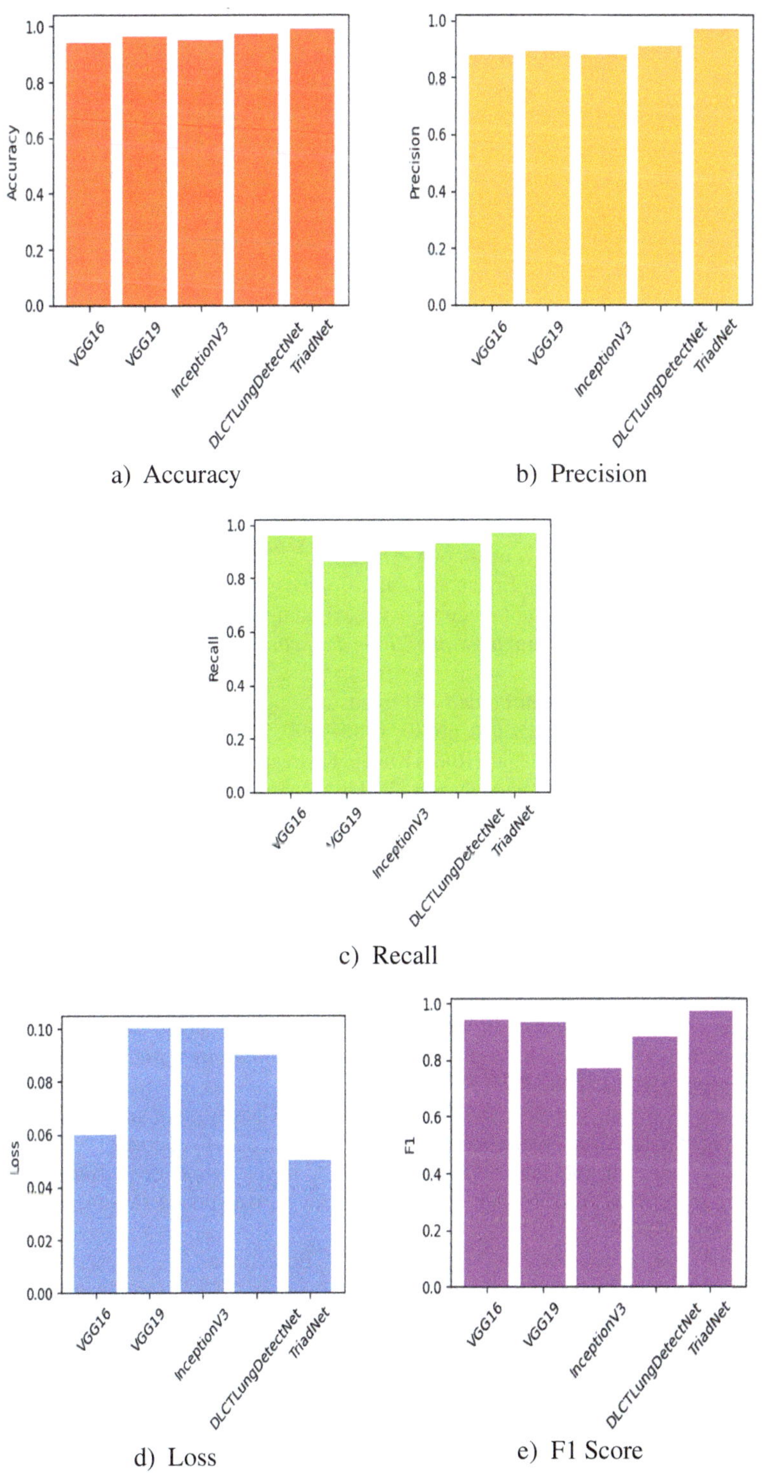

FIGURE 13.9 Graphs for the comparison of deep learning models for various metrics.

precision and recall offering a balanced evaluation of performance. A 0.99% score indicates a great ability to accurately identify positive cases while reducing FP. The demonstration showcases the ideal equilibrium between precision and recall, especially beneficial in applications wherein achieving high accuracy and reducing FP is crucial. The FusionNet model outperforms all other models in this comparison and is the optimal choice for the specified task or problem. In the future, this work can be further developed to accommodate newer pre-processing techniques. The proposed model is currently being used for binary classification, however, there exists future scope to further develop the model for multi-stage classification. This work can also be accommodated to employ an unsupervised dataset. As new algorithms come into light with new research, this model can be further improved to fit newly arising requirements.

REFERENCES

1. Sharma, Rajesh. "Mapping of global, regional and national incidence, mortality and mortality-to-incidence ratio of lung cancer in 2020 and 2050." *International Journal of Clinical Oncology* 27, no. 4: 665–675, 2022.
2. Toğaçar, Mesut, Burhan Ergen, and Zafer Cömert. "Detection of lung cancer on chest CT images using minimum redundancy maximum relevance feature selection method with convolutional neural networks." *Biocybernetics and Biomedical Engineering* 40, no. 1: 23–39, 2020.
3. Li, Chao, et al. "Global burden and trends of lung cancer incidence and mortality." *Chinese Medical Journal* 136, no. 13: 1583–1590, 2023.
4. Ramana, Kadiyala, Madapuri Rudra Kumar, K. Sreenivasulu, Thippa Reddy Gadekallu, Surbhi Bhatia, Parul Agarwal, and Sheikh Mohammad Idrees. "Early prediction of lung cancers using deep saliency capsule and pre-trained deep learning frameworks." *Frontiers in Oncology* 12: 886739, 2022.
5. Yousefi, Mahmood, et al. "Cost of lung cancer: A systematic review." *Value in Health Regional Issues* 33: 17–26, 2023.
6. Rathod, Seema B., and Lata L. Ragha. "DLCT LUNG Detect Net: Leveraging Deep Learning for Lung Tumor Detection in CT scans." *Journal of Electrical Systems* 20, no.2s:1290-1308,2024..
7. Gu, Dongdong, Guocai Liu, and Zhong Xue. "On the performance of lung nodule detection, segmentation and classification." *Computerized Medical Imaging and Graphics* 89: 101886, 2021.
8. Blanc, D., et al. "Artificial intelligence solution to classify pulmonary nodules on CT." *Diagnostic and Interventional Imaging* 101, no. 12: 803–810, 2020.
9. Wankhade, Shalini, and S. Vigneshwari. "A novel hybrid deep learning method for early detection of lung cancer using neural networks." *Healthcare Analytics* 3: 100195, 2023.
10. Rajasekar, Vani, M. P. Vaishnnave, S. Premkumar, V. Sarveshwaran, and V. Rangaraaj. "Lung cancer disease prediction with CT scan and histopathological images feature analysis using deep learning techniques." *Results in Engineering* 18: 101111, 2023.
11. Thong, Lay Teng, Hui Shan Chou, Han Shi Jocelyn Chew, and L. A. U. Ying. "Diagnostic test accuracy of artificial intelligence-based imaging for lung cancer screening: A systematic review and meta-analysis." *Lung Cancer* 176: 4–13, 2023.

12. Jin, Haizhe, Cheng Yu, Zibo Gong, Renjie Zheng, Yinan Zhao, and Quanwei Fu. "Machine learning techniques for pulmonary nodule computer-aided diagnosis using CT images: A systematic review." *Biomedical Signal Processing and Control* 79: 104104, 2023.
13. Nagaesvara, E. B. R., M. Aadhithya, and A. Malini. "An analysis of machine learning techniques for forest cover type classification." In *2023 6th International Conference on Contemporary Computing and Informatics (IC3I)*, vol. 6, pp. 489–494. IEEE, 2023.
14. Chaunzwa, Tafadzwa L., Ahmed Hosny, Yiwen Xu, Andrea Shafer, Nancy Diao, Michael Lanuti, David C. Christiani, Raymond H. Mak, and H. J. W. L. Aerts. "Deep learning classification of lung cancer histology using CT images." *Scientific Reports* 11, no. 1: 5471, 2021.
15. Teramoto, Atsushi, and Hiroshi Fujita. "Fast lung nodule detection in chest CT images using cylindrical nodule-enhancement filter." *International Journal of Computer Assisted Radiology and Surgery* 8: 193–205, 2013.
16. Cao, Zhenguan, Rui Li, Xun Yang, Liao Fang, Zhuoqin Li, and Jinbiao Li. "Multi-scale detection of pulmonary nodules by integrating attention mechanism." *Scientific Reports* 13, no. 1: 5517, 2023.
17. Sheriff, S. Thanzeem Mohamed, J. Venkat Kumar, S. Vigneshwaran, Aida Jones, and Jose Anand. "Lung cancer detection using vgg net 16 architecture." In *Journal of Physics: Conference Series* (vol. 2040, no. 1, p. 012001). IOP Publishing, 2021.
18. Sravani, Meesala, Meesala Krishna Murthy, and Satish Muppidi. "Utilizing Visual Geometry Group (VGG16) and InceptionV3 convolutional Neural Network (CNN) models for accurate diagnosis of lung cancer: An Artificial Intelligence (AI)-based approach." *Multimedia Tools and Applications 83,* no.19: 57477-57494, 2024.
19. Swaminathan, Vishnu Priyan, Ramesh Balasubramani, S. Parvathavarthini, Vidhya Gopal, Kanagaselvam Raju, Tamil Selvan Sivalingam, and Sounder Rajan Thennarasu. "GAN based image segmentation and classification using Vgg16 for prediction of lung cancer." *Journal of Advanced Research in Applied Sciences and Engineering Technology* 35, no. 1: 45–61, 2024.
20. Raju, Nidhin, D. Peter Augustine, and J. Chandra. "A novel artificial intelligence system for the prediction of interstitial lung diseases." *SN Computer Science* 5, no. 1: 143, 2024.
21. Annavarapu, Ambika, and Surekha Borra. "An adaptive watershed segmentation based medical image denoising using deep convolutional neural networks." *Biomedical Signal Processing and Control* 93: 106119, 2024.
22. Malini, A., P. Priyadharshini, and S. Sabeena. "An automatic assessment of road condition from aerial imagery using modified VGG architecture in faster-RCNN framework." *Journal of Intelligent & Fuzzy Systems* 40, no. 6: 11411–11422, 2021.
23. Wang, Wei, and Yuming Yang. "A histogram equalization model for color image contrast enhancement." *Signal, Image and Video Processing* 18, no. 2: 1725–1732, 2024.
24. Ma, Jun, Yuting He, Feifei Li, Lin Han, Chenyu You, and Bo Wang. "Segment anything in medical images." *Nature Communications* 15, no. 1: 654, 2024.
25. Pawar, Shreya. "Deep learning for lung cancer detection and classification in CT scans." *Journal of High School Science* 8, no. 1: 60–73, 2024.
26. Makaju, Suren, P. W. C. Prasad, Abeer Alsadoon, A. K. Singh, and A. Elchouemi. "Lung cancer detection using CT scan images." *Procedia Computer Science* 125: 107–114, 2018.
27. Bhatt, Sanjeev Kumar, and S. Srinivasan. "Lung cancer detection using AI and different techniques of machine learning." *International Journal of Intelligent Systems and Applications in Engineering* 12, no. 8s: 630–638, 2024.

28. Gugulothu, Vijay Kumar, and Savadam Balaji. "An early prediction and classification of lung nodule diagnosis on CT images based on hybrid deep learning techniques." *Multimedia Tools and Applications* 83, no. 1: 1041–1061, 2024.
29. Achanta, Alekhya, and Roja Boina. "Advanced techniques in Python for effective data visualization." *International Journal of Science and Research (IJSR)* 12: 1–8, 2023.
30. Srivastava, Durgesh, Santosh Kumar Srivastava, Surbhi Bhatia Khan, Hare Ram Singh, Sunil K. Maakar, Ambuj Kumar Agarwal, Areej A. Malibari, and Eid Albalawi. "Early detection of lung nodules using a revolutionized deep learning model." *Diagnostics* 13, no. 22: 3485, 2023.
31. Gupta, P., and A. Bagchi. "Data visualization with Python." In *Essentials of Python for Artificial Intelligence and Machine Learning James E. Hetrick,Ed. Synthesis Lectures on Engineering, Science, and Technology*. Cham: Springer, 2024.
32. Pizer, Stephen M., E. Philip Amburn, John D. Austin, Robert Cromartie, Ari Geselowitz, Trey Greer, Bartter Haar Romeny, John B. Zimmerman, and Karel Zuiderveld. "Adaptive histogram equalization and its variations." *Computer Vision, Graphics, and Image Processing*, 39, no. 3, 355–368,1987.
33. Setiawan, Agung W., et al. "Color retinal image enhancement using CLAHE." In *International Conference on ICT for Smart Society*. IEEE, 2013.
34. Kayalvizhi, S., and S. Malarvizhi. "A novel encrypted compressive sensing of images based on fractional order hyper chaotic Chen system and DNA operations." *Multimedia Tools and Applications* 79, no. 5: 3957–3974, 2020.

14 Practical Applications: Specific Diseases or Conditions Where AI Has Made a Significant Impact

A Review

Saranya J., Selvakumar V. S., Suganthi S., and Dinesh K.

14.1 INTRODUCTION

Healthcare is one of the sectors that has benefited the most from the introduction of artificial intelligence (AI). The field of patient care, diagnosis, and treatment may change as a result of AI, which is described as technology, particularly computer systems, imitating human intellectual processes. This chapter explores the practical applications of AI in diagnosing and managing specific diseases and conditions, highlighting the significant impact it has made in the healthcare industry. The development of complex algorithms, increases in computer power, and the exponential rise of data have all contributed to the integration of AI in healthcare. AI technologies have been used to extract insights from complicated medical data, enabling more precise diagnosis, individualized therapies, and better patient outcomes. These technologies include machine learning (ML), deep learning, computer vision, and natural language processing (NLP) [1].

Medical imaging has been one of the first and largest areas where AI has had an impact on healthcare. AI algorithms have been developed to evaluate pictures from magnetic resonance imaging (MRI), computed tomography (CT) scans, and X-rays, with surprising precision. This technology can help diagnose diseases like cancer, cardiovascular issues, and neurological disorders early on. For instance, AI-powered tools can now identify malignant tumors in mammograms with precision comparable to, or even surpassing, that of human radiologists. Beyond diagnostics, AI has shown promise in predicting disease progression and treatment outcomes. ML models are trained to examine patient data and find trends that might point to a higher risk of

DOI: 10.1201/9781003484233-14

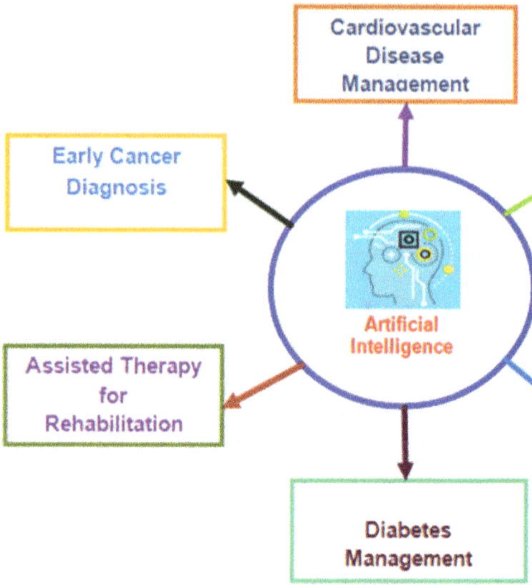

FIGURE 14.1 Graphical abstract.

developing specific diseases, like diabetes or Alzheimer's. This predictive capability is invaluable for early intervention and preventive healthcare strategies [2].

The relevance of AI in healthcare cannot be overstated, as it represents a paradigm shift in how medical data is analyzed, diagnoses are made, and treatments are administered. The medical community faces several urgent difficulties, and the incorporation of AI technology has significantly improved the efficiency, accuracy, and personalized nature of healthcare services. AI's ability to overcome human limitations in the diagnosis of complicated diseases is one of the main areas in which it proves its usefulness. For healthcare practitioners, the sheer amount of medical data–including genetic data, imaging data, and electronic health records–can be excessive to handle manually [3]. The issue can be solved by AI algorithms, which can quickly process and interpret enormous volumes of data, allowing for more precise and timely diagnosis.

AI has played a key role in the creation of personalized medicine in the field of treatment. AI algorithms are able to provide individualized treatment regimens that are more successful and cause fewer negative effects by examining a patient's genetic composition, medical background, and other pertinent data. This approach has had a particularly significant effect in oncology, where targeted medicines for various cancer types have been developed as a result of AI-driven insights. Furthermore, a large investment in infrastructure and healthcare professional training is needed for the integration of AI technologies into healthcare systems.

AI has enormous potential in the healthcare industry, despite these challenges. AI is anticipated to become more and more important in patient care, treatment planning, and illness diagnosis as technology advances [4]. The current investigations and advancements in this domain have the potential to reveal novel uses and augment the potential of AI in the healthcare sector.

14.2 AI IN CANCER DIAGNOSIS AND THERAPY

A ground-breaking development in oncology, the use of AI in cancer diagnosis and therapy holds the promise of improving the accuracy, efficacy, and personalization of cancer care. AI technologies–in particular, ML and deep learning algorithms–have been exceptionally good at interpreting medical imaging, including CT, MRI, and mammograms, in the field of cancer diagnosis. This has made it possible to diagnose a variety of tumors early on. For instance, in breast cancer detection, AI algorithms have been developed to scrutinize mammograms with high accuracy, identifying subtle indications of cancer that might be overlooked by human radiologists. This has the potential to reduce false positives and false negatives, leading to more accurate diagnoses. Similar to this, AI is used to evaluate low-dose CT scans in order to find nodules and patterns that might point to the presence of lung cancer in order to diagnose the disease in its early stages. These AI-driven diagnostic tools not only aid in early detection but also help in reducing the workload of radiologists and improving the overall efficiency of the diagnostic process. In the realm of skin cancer, AI-driven dermatology tools are being developed to analyze images of skin lesions and moles. These methods use ML to distinguish between benign lesions and skin cancers, including melanoma, the most deadly kind of the disease [5]. By providing an initial assessment, AI can help prioritize cases that require further examination by a dermatologist, thus streamlining the diagnostic process and potentially saving lives through early detection. The use of AI in prostate cancer detection is changing the diagnosis process by providing a more precise and effective method of spotting the illness early on. Prostate cancer is one of the most prevalent cancers in males and requires early detection in order to effectively treat it. Multiparametric MRI (mpMRI) is being used more and more to analyze the presence of prostate cancer utilizing AI techniques, especially those based on deep learning. These sophisticated AI models are capable of the detection of suspicious areas that may signify the presence of cancer, thereby assisting radiologists in making more precise diagnoses. AI-enabled MRI image analysis automation increases cancer detection accuracy while also saving a great deal of time and effort compared to manual interpretation. This results in earlier diagnosis and immediate action. As AI technology continues to advance, its application in prostate cancer detection is expected to further improve this disease.

AI is essential to the development of tailored therapy regimens for cancer patients. AI systems are able to provide individualized therapy recommendations that are less likely to cause adverse effects and more successful by examining a patient's genetic information, medical history, and other pertinent data. AI, for instance, can forecast how several medications would interact with the tumor and the patient's body throughout chemotherapy, enabling physicians to select the most effective drug combination. AI is also being utilized in radiation therapy to improve treatment plans, making sure that the tumor receives the maximal dose while the surrounding healthy tissues receive the least amount of exposure [6]. In the area of immunotherapy, AI is also making progress in identifying biomarkers that indicate a patient's prognosis for a given course of treatment. This aids in recognizing individuals who would most likely benefit from immunotherapy, enhancing the results of treatment. AI-powered technologies are also being created to monitor patients while they are receiving therapy. These systems use data from electronic health records and wearable devices to identify early indicators of treatment resistance or adverse responses. To guarantee the safe and efficient application of AI in oncology, a number of obstacles must be overcome, including ethical questions, data privacy concerns, and the requirement for strong regulatory frameworks. Furthermore, in order to guarantee that AI tools are created and applied in a way that complies with clinical requirements and standards, cooperation between AI specialists, oncologists, and other healthcare professionals is necessary for the effective application of AI in clinical settings [7].

14.3 AI IN CARDIOVASCULAR DISEASE MANAGEMENT

The application of AI in the treatment of cardiovascular illnesses is growing, as these conditions are among the world's top causes of death. AI is transforming the diagnosis, treatment, and monitoring of heart disorders by utilizing cutting-edge algorithms and ML approaches. This section explores the application of AI in detecting arrhythmias and heart failure, as well as its role in predicting cardiovascular risks and outcomes. If not detected and addressed right away, arrhythmias, also known as irregular heartbeats, are a common cardiovascular ailment that can cause major health problems. AI has become a potent instrument for identifying and categorizing arrhythmias [8], providing more accuracy and efficiency than conventional techniques. One of the most common applications of AI in arrhythmia detection is the analysis of electrocardiogram (ECG) data. Deep learning models in particular, ML algorithms, have been developed to identify patterns in ECG signals that signify the presence of different kinds of arrhythmias, including bradycardia, ventricular tachycardia, and atrial fibrillation [9]. Large volumes of ECG data may be processed in real-time by these AI models, which enable quick and precise diagnosis–a crucial component of prompt intervention [10].

Moreover, AI-powered wearable devices have become increasingly popular for the continuous monitoring of heart rhythms. Even in the absence of symptoms, these gadgets' sensors and AI algorithms can identify minute variations in heartbeats and notify users of possible arrhythmias. This proactive approach in monitoring enables the early detection and management of arrhythmias, reducing the risk of complications such as stroke and heart failure. AI is also enhancing the interpretation of ambulatory ECG monitoring, such as Holter monitors, by automating the analysis of long-term ECG recordings. This automation reduces the workload of healthcare professionals and minimizes the likelihood of human error in identifying arrhythmias [11].

AI is being used not just for detection but also for arrhythmia onset prediction. Utilizing a variety of patient data, such as heart rate variability, ECG characteristics, and clinical indicators, predictive models are able to identify patients who are at an increased risk of experiencing arrhythmias. Predictive insights have the potential to enhance patient outcomes by informing tailored treatment regimens and preventive interventions. The ability to accurately predict cardiovascular risks and outcomes is crucial for the prevention and management of heart diseases. AI is making a significant contribution in the healthcare domain through the prediction and evaluation of a variety of datasets that are specific to the detection of a particular disease after seeing current trends in false diagnostic estimation by professional doctors. Based on a variety of variables, such as genetic markers, lifestyle decisions, blood pressure, cholesterol levels, and other clinical indicators, ML models are being used to forecast the risk of acquiring cardiovascular illnesses. These models provide personalized risk assessments, enabling targeted interventions and lifestyle modifications to prevent the onset of heart diseases [12–14].

AI is also being employed to predict outcomes in patients with existing cardiovascular conditions. AI systems, for instance, may evaluate cardiac imaging data, including cardiac MRI and echocardiograms, to determine how heart disorders are progressing and to forecast the possibility of unfavorable outcomes like heart attacks or heart failure. This information is invaluable for guiding treatment decisions and optimizing patient care. In the realm of heart failure management, AI is being used to predict hospital readmissions and mortality rates. AI models are able to identify high-risk patients who may need more comprehensive monitoring and aggressive treatment by evaluating patient data, including medical history, medication adherence, and physiological markers [15].

Furthermore, AI is contributing to the development of precision medicine in cardiovascular care. AI algorithms can forecast a patient's unique response to a given treatment by combining genetic and clinical data. This enables medical professionals to customize therapy to meet the unique needs of each patient. AI is transforming the management of cardiovascular diseases by providing advanced tools for detecting arrhythmias and predicting cardiovascular risks and outcomes. The use of AI in therapeutic settings includes enhancing diagnosis efficiency and accuracy, facilitating early intervention, and customizing treatment plans. It is anticipated that if AI technology develops further, it will have a greater influence on the management of cardiovascular disease and present new chances to improve patient outcomes [16].

14.4 AI IN NEUROLOGICAL DISORDERS

The diagnosis, monitoring, and treatment of neurological illnesses are being revolutionized by the use of AI in neurology. AI is gaining new insights into diseases like epilepsy, Parkinson's, and Alzheimer's and improving the efficacy of treatments and rehabilitation for these conditions thanks to its capacity to analyze complex data and spot patterns. Early and accurate diagnosis of neurological disorders is crucial for effective management and treatment. In this context, AI is crucial, especially for the diagnosis of epilepsy, Parkinson's disease, and Alzheimer's disease. AI systems are being used to evaluate brain imaging data, such as MRI and PET scans, in order to identify early indications of Alzheimer's disease. These algorithms can identify subtle changes in brain structure and function that may not be visible to the human eye, enabling earlier diagnosis and intervention [17]. Additionally, AI is being used to analyze cognitive test results and other clinical data to differentiate between Alzheimer's and other forms of dementia. AI is being used to evaluate movement data for Parkinson's disease that is gathered from smartphone apps and wearable sensors. ML models can detect patterns such as tremors, rigidity, and bradykinesia using this data that are indicators of Parkinson's disease. With the use of this technology, we can continuously monitor symptoms and gather important data that can be used to modify treatment regimens and enhance patient outcomes. AI is being utilized to analyze electroencephalogram (EEG) recordings in epilepsy patients in order to identify and anticipate events [18]. AI algorithms can identify specific patterns in brain activity that precede a seizure, offering the potential for early intervention and better seizure management. This is particularly beneficial for patients with drug-resistant epilepsy, where traditional treatment options are limited.

AI is not only transforming the diagnosis and monitoring of neurological disorders but also revolutionizing the way therapies and rehabilitation are delivered. AI-assisted therapies and rehabilitation programs are becoming increasingly personalized and effective, thanks to the insights provided by ML algorithms. AI-powered solutions are being employed in the field of stroke rehabilitation to offer patients individualized exercise regimens that change based on their progress. These systems can analyze data from sensors and wearable devices to assess the patient's motor abilities and adjust the difficulty of exercises accordingly. For individuals with Parkinson's disease [19], AI is being used to develop tailored physical therapy programs that address specific symptoms such as tremors and gait disturbances. By continuously monitoring the patient's movements, AI algorithms can adjust the therapy regimen in real-time, ensuring that it remains effective as the disease progresses. In the treatment of epilepsy, AI is being applied to develop personalized medication regimens. By analyzing data from EEG recordings, genetic information, and patient history, AI models can predict how an individual will respond to different antiepileptic drugs. This allows for the selection of the most effective medication with the fewest side effects, improving the patient's quality of life [20].

AI is also being explored in the development of brain-computer interfaces (BCIs) for patients with severe neurological impairments. These interfaces use AI algorithms to interpret brain signals and translate them into commands for assistive devices, enabling individuals with conditions like amyotrophic lateral sclerosis (ALS) to communicate and interact with their environment. In the discipline of neurology, AI has transformed the diagnostic, monitoring, and treatment of neurological illnesses by opening up new avenues. The precise classification and adequate processing of natural and perceptual emotions are necessary for the accurate prediction of the onset of neurological diseases [21]. AI is enhancing the efficacy of rehabilitation programs and improving the quality of life for people suffering from diseases like epilepsy, Parkinson's disease, and Alzheimer's by offering tailored and adaptable therapy.AI technology is predicted to have a greater influence on neurological treatment as it develops, providing patients with better prospects and care [22].

14.5 AI IN DIABETES MANAGEMENT

The management of diabetes, a chronic and complex disease affecting millions worldwide, is being revolutionized by the integration of AI. AI is transforming the way diabetes is diagnosed, monitored, and treated, offering personalized care and improved outcomes for patients. The early detection and management of diabetes are crucial for preventing complications. AI algorithms are being used to analyze a variety of data, including genetic data, lifestyle factors, and biomarkers, in order to forecast the onset of diabetes. Preventive and early intervention are made possible by

ML models that are able to identify those who are at a high risk of getting diabetes. AI is also being used to personalize diabetes management plans. AI systems can offer real-time recommendations for insulin dose, dietary modifications, and physical exercise by evaluating data from continuous glucose monitoring(CGM) devices, insulin pumps, and other wearable devices. This personalized approach helps patients maintain optimal blood glucose levels, and reduces the risk of hypoglycemia and hyperglycemia [23,24]. People who have acute diabetes are significantly more likely to develop diabetic retinopathy (DR). Although DR doesn't often cause symptoms, if it isn't treated, it can cause low vision and visual impairment [25].

The continuous monitoring of glucose levels is essential for effective diabetes management. AI-powered CGMs are becoming increasingly sophisticated, providing accurate and real-time glucose readings. These devices use advanced algorithms to predict glucose trends and alert patients to potential episodes of high or low blood sugar, allowing for timely intervention. AI is also being applied to non-invasive glucose monitoring technologies. Researchers are developing AI-driven devices that can measure glucose levels through the skin or in tears, offering a painless alternative to traditional finger-prick tests. Since glucose monitoring is now more convenient and less intrusive thanks to these developments, people with diabetes may live longer and have better quality of life.

Diabetes therapy is very customized, and AI is helping to customize medications to meet the specific needs of each patient. AI algorithms are able to assess data from multiple sources, such as genetic profiles, electronic health records, and patient-reported results, in order to suggest the best drugs and dosages. This precision medicine approach ensures that patients receive the treatment that is most likely to be effective for their specific condition. AI is also being used to optimize insulin therapy. ML models can predict how different factors, such as food intake, physical activity, and stress, will affect a patient's blood glucose levels. This information can be used to adjust insulin doses in real-time, helping patients achieve better glycemic control.

The prevention of long-term consequences, such as cardiovascular disease, kidney failure, and neuropathy, is one of the main concerns in managing diabetes. By examining trends in patient data, AI algorithms are being created to forecast the likelihood of these issues. Because of its ability for prediction, early intervention and focused management techniques can be used to lower the risk of problems. Additionally, DR, a major condition that can result in blindness, is being better detected with the assistance of AI. Early detection and treatment of retinopathy are made possible by deep learning algorithms that analyze retinal pictures to identify symptoms of the condition [26].

Although AI has made great strides in managing diabetes, there are still issues that need to be resolved, such as data privacy issues, the requirement for strong regulatory frameworks, and guaranteeing that AI-driven technologies are available to everybody. AI is predicted to become more and more important in the treatment of diabetes as it develops, providing new avenues for individualized care, enhanced monitoring, and enhanced problem avoidance. In conclusion, AI is transforming diabetes management by providing personalized care, improving glucose monitoring, optimizing treatment, and preventing complications. The potential of AI in the treatment of diabetes is anticipated to increase as technology develops, providing patients with this chronic

TABLE 14.1
AI applications in diabetes management

Aspect of diabetes management	Description	AI applications
Early detection and risk prediction	Identifying individuals at high risk of developing diabetes for early intervention.	AI algorithms analyze genetic, lifestyle, and biomarker data to predict diabetes onset.
Personalized management plans	Tailoring diabetes management to individual needs, including insulin dosing and lifestyle adjustments.	AI systems evaluate information from wearables, insulin pumps, and CGMs to offer suggestions in real time.
Continuous glucose monitoring (CGM)	Monitoring glucose levels in real-time to manage diabetes effectively.	AI-powered CGMs provide accurate and real-time glucose readings, predicting trends and alerting patients to potential episodes of high or low blood sugar.
Non-invasive glucose monitoring	Developing painless alternatives to traditional finger-prick tests for glucose monitoring.	Researchers are using AI to develop devices that measure glucose levels through the skin or in tears.
Treatment personalization	Tailoring diabetes treatment to individual patient needs, including medication and insulin therapy.	AI algorithms analyse various data sources to recommend effective medications and dosages. AI models predict how different factors affect blood glucose levels to adjust insulin doses in real-time.
Prevention of long-term complications	Predicting and managing complications such as cardiovascular disease, kidney failure, and neuropathy.	AI algorithms analyse patterns in patient data to predict the risk of complications and improve detection of diabetic retinopathy.

illness with hope for improved results and a higher quality of life [27]. Table 14.1 presents applications of AI in various aspects of diabetes management which includes early detection of diabetes, CGM, personalization treatments, and prevention of long-term complications.

14.6 AI IN INFECTIOUS DISEASES

The detection, monitoring, and treatment of infectious diseases are being revolutionized by the use of AI. AI algorithms, particularly those based on ML and deep learning, are being used to analyze clinical data, laboratory results, and imaging studies to identify patterns indicative of specific infections. It makes it possible for early identification and precise diagnosis, both of which are essential for efficient containment and treatment.AI also plays a significant role in epidemiological modeling and prediction. In order to forecast outbreaks and their possible effects, ML algorithms can evaluate data from a variety of sources, such as social media, travel trends, and climatic conditions. These predictive models are essential for public health planning and response, enabling authorities to allocate resources effectively and implement timely interventions.

In the realm of genomics, AI algorithms are being used to analyze genomic data from pathogens, identifying mutations and tracking the emergence of new strains. This genomic analysis is particularly important in the context of antimicrobial resistance, as it helps in identifying resistant genes and informing the development of new treatments.AI is also accelerating the process of drug discovery and vaccine development for infectious diseases. ML models can analyze vast chemical libraries to identify potential compounds with antimicrobial activity, while AI algorithms can predict the immune response to different vaccine candidates, aiding in the design of effective vaccines. Table 14.2 presents AI-powered instruments for early infectious disease detection.

TABLE 14.2
AI-driven tools for the early detection of infectious disease

Problem in infectious disease management	AI application	Description
Early detection and diagnosis	AI-driven diagnostic tools	AI algorithms analyze clinical data, laboratory results, and imaging studies to identify patterns indicating specific infections, enabling early detection and accurate diagnosis.
Epidemiological modeling and prediction	MLmodels	AI models are used to predict outbreaks and their possible effects by analyzing data from multiple sources, such as social media, travel patterns, and climate conditions. This helps with public health response and preparation.
Genomic analysis of pathogens	AI in genomics	AI algorithms are used to analyze genomic data from pathogens, identifying mutations and tracking the emergence of new strains, which is crucial for understanding antimicrobial resistance and informing treatment development.
Drug discovery and vaccine development	AI in drug and vaccine research	ML models analyze vast chemical libraries to identify potential compounds with antimicrobial activity, and AI algorithms predict the immune response to different vaccine candidates, speeding up the development process.
Public health surveillance and contact tracing	AI-powered surveillance systems	Natural language processing algorithms analyze news reports and social media posts for early signals of disease outbreaks, and AI-powered contact tracing apps automate the process of identifying and notifying individuals who have been in contact with infected persons.

Moreover, AI technologies are being used to enhance public health surveillance and contact tracing efforts. NLP algorithms can analyze news reports and social media posts to detect early signals of disease outbreaks, while AI-powered contact tracing apps can automate the process of identifying and notifying individuals who have been in contact with infected persons, helping to control the spread of infections. Even though AI has great promise to manage infectious diseases, there are still issues and moral questions that need to be resolved, like data security, privacy, and the possibility of algorithmic bias. Ensuring the transparency and interpretability of AI models is also crucial for building trust and acceptance among the public and healthcare professionals [28].

AI is predicted to become more and more significant in global health as it develops, providing new avenues for the prevention and management of infectious diseases. It is anticipated that the combination of AI and other technologies, such as wearables and the Internet of Things (IoT), would improve illness monitoring and management even further, providing hope for improved results and a healthier future.

14.7 AI IN REHABILITATION

Rehabilitation is a critical aspect of healthcare aimed at helping individuals recover from injuries, surgeries, or chronic conditions. AI is causing a revolutionary change in the rehabilitation industry by providing new avenues for individualized and efficient care. AI-driven technologies are being integrated into rehabilitation programs to provide real-time feedback, adapt therapies to individual needs, and predict patient outcomes, thereby enhancing the overall effectiveness of rehabilitation services. One of the key applications of AI in rehabilitation is in physical therapy. AI-powered systems can analyze patients' movements and provide instant feedback, helping therapists to tailor exercises and track progress more accurately. Wearable sensors equipped with AI algorithms can monitor patients' activities and provide insights into their mobility and biomechanics. This data-driven approach enables therapists to design personalized rehabilitation programs that address specific deficits and goals.

AI is also making significant strides in neurorehabilitation, where it is used to assist patients recovering from neurological conditions such as stroke or spinal cord injuries. BCIs powered by AI can interpret neural signals and translate them into commands for assistive devices, enabling patients to regain control over their movements. Virtual reality (VR) combined with AI provides immersive environments for patients to practice motor skills, with adaptive algorithms adjusting the difficulty level based on the patient's performance [29]. In speech and language therapy, AI-driven tools are being developed to assess and treat communication disorders. These tools use NLP to analyze speech patterns and provide targeted exercises for improving language skills. They can also offer real-time feedback and track progress over time, making therapy more interactive and engaging. In the realm of occupational therapy, AI is being used to create adaptive environments that respond to the needs of patients. Smart home technologies, powered by AI, can adjust lighting, temperature, and other environmental factors to accommodate the physical limitations of individuals undergoing rehabilitation. These intelligent systems can also remind patients to perform

TABLE 14.3
AI – assisted therapy for rehabilitation

Aspect of Rehabilitation	Description	AI Applications
Physical therapy	Tailoring exercises to a patient's specific needs and tracking progress.	AI-powered systems analyze movements and provide real-time feedback. Wearable sensors monitor mobility and biomechanics.
Neurorehabilitation	Assisting patients recovering from neurological conditions like stroke or spinal cord injuries.	BCIs interpret neural signals for assistive devices. VR with AI provides adaptive environments for practicing motor skills.
Speech and language therapy	Assessing and treating communication disorders.	AI-driven tools use natural language processing to analyze speech patterns and provide targeted exercises.
Occupational therapy	Creating adaptive environments for patients with physical limitations.	Smart home technologies adjust environmental factors like lighting and temperature. Systems remind patients to perform exercises and follow treatment plans.
Clinic efficiency	Optimizing scheduling, resource allocation, and patient management.	Predictive analytics forecast patient outcomes and identify individuals at risk of slow recovery.

exercises, take medications, and follow other aspects of their treatment plans, thereby promoting adherence and improving outcomes.

AI is also enhancing the efficiency of rehabilitation clinics by optimizing scheduling, resource allocation, and patient management. Clinicians can intervene early and modify treatment strategies by using predictive analytics to forecast patient outcomes and identify patients who may recover slowly. Despite the potential benefits, the integration of AI into rehabilitation poses several challenges. AI system correctness and dependability must be guaranteed since mistakes might have a serious negative impact on patient care. Privacy and security concerns must be addressed, as AI systems often require access to sensitive health data. Furthermore, as Table 14.3 illustrates, strong clinical trials are required to confirm the efficacy of AI-based therapies in rehabilitation.

14.8 CHALLENGES AND LIMITATIONS

AI has significantly improved healthcare, particularly in the fields of specific illness and ailment diagnosis and treatment, but it is not without challenges and limitations. Security and privacy of data are two main issues. Large volumes of private health data must be accessed by AI systems, which raises questions regarding patient confidentiality and the possibility of data breaches. The absence of standards in healthcare data is another difficulty. AI algorithms require consistent and standardized data to function effectively, but healthcare data are often fragmented and inconsistent, making them difficult for AI systems to interpret and analyze.

Fairness and bias in AI systems are equally significant issues. Since AI systems can only be as objective as the data they are trained on, biased data will probably cause the system to reinforce its own biases and produce incorrect diagnosis or treatment suggestions. The complexity of medical conditions also poses a challenge for AI. Many diseases are complex and multifactorial, making it difficult for AI algorithms to accurately diagnose or predict outcomes. Additionally, AI systems may struggle to adapt to new and emerging diseases, as they rely on historical data for training. The integration of AI into clinical workflows is another challenge. Healthcare workers may be reluctant to use AI technologies because they don't believe the recommendations made by the technology or they fear losing their jobs. Additionally, there may be technical and logistical barriers in integrating AI systems into existing healthcare infrastructure.

The application of AI in healthcare is likewise fraught with ethical and legal issues. The complicated web of legal requirements and moral standards that AI systems must abide by may impede the advancement and application of AI technology. The cost of developing and implementing AI systems can be prohibitive for many healthcare organizations, particularly in low-resource settings. This can exacerbate existing health disparities, as only well-resourced healthcare systems may be able to afford the latest AI technologies [30].

Despite the obstacles and restrictions, there are a number of possible paths for the future and ways to solve these problems that could assist optimize the advantages of AI in healthcare. Enhancing data privacy and security is paramount, and healthcare organizations and AI developers can implement advanced encryption techniques, secure data-sharing protocols, and robust access controls. Developing and enforcing strict data governance policies will also be crucial to ensure that patient data is handled responsibly and securely. Efforts to standardize healthcare data can significantly improve the effectiveness of AI algorithms. Initiatives such as the development of common data models and interoperability standards can facilitate the consistent and accurate exchange of health information across different systems and platforms. Addressing bias in AI requires a multifaceted approach. This entails incorporating a varied range of stakeholders in the creation and assessment of AI systems, implementing bias detection and correction algorithms, and diversifying training datasets. Regular auditing and monitoring of AI algorithms can also help identify and mitigate biases over time.

AI algorithms can be built to integrate multi-modal data, such as genetic, clinical, and environmental information, to address the complexity of medical diseases. More advanced models that better capture the subtleties of complicated diseases can be developed through collaborative efforts between physicians, data scientists, and domain specialists. Seamless integration into clinical workflows is essential for the successful adoption of AI in healthcare. This can be achieved through user-centered design, ongoing training and support for healthcare professionals, and the development of intuitive interfaces that facilitate the use of AI tools in clinical decision-making.

Regulatory frameworks and ethical guidelines must evolve to keep pace with advancements in AI. A transparent, accountable, and socially conscious approach to the development and application of AI technology can be achieved by collaborating with ethicists, regulatory agencies, and patient advocacy groups. Addressing the cost barrier is crucial to ensure the equitable distribution of AI benefits across different healthcare settings. This may involve developing cost-effective AI solutions, exploring innovative financing models, and advocating for policies that support the widespread adoption of AI in healthcare [31].

In summary, AI in healthcare has a bright future, but its viability will depend on our capacity to overcome the obstacles and constraints that currently exist. By fostering collaboration, innovation, and ethical practices, we can harness the full potential of AI to transform healthcare and improve patient outcomes [32].

14.9 FUTURE DIRECTIONS

AI has enormous potential to change healthcare as it develops further. The future directions of AI in healthcare are shaped by technological advancements, interdisciplinary collaboration, and a commitment towards addressing current limitations. Deep learning techniques and bio-inspired AI algorithms have produced encouraging results in a variety of disciplines [33].

One of the key areas of focus is the advancement in deep learning and neural networks. With the advancement of these technologies, complex medical data may now be interpreted with greater accuracy and subtlety. This can lead to improved diagnostic accuracy and personalized treatment plans. Another significant direction is the integration of AI with other emerging technologies such as genomics, wearable devices, and the Internet of Medical Things (IoMT) [34]. This convergence can lead to a more holistic approach to healthcare, where AI not only assists in diagnosis and treatment but also in preventive care and continuous monitoring of patients' health. For instance, wearable device data can be analyzed by AI algorithms to track the development of a chronic illness or identify early warning indicators of sickness. The expansion of AI applications in telemedicine and remote patient monitoring is also a promising direction. With the COVID-19 pandemic highlighting the importance of remote healthcare services, AI can play a crucial role in making telemedicine more effective and accessible. AI-powered chatbots and virtual health assistants can provide preliminary consultations, triage, and follow-up care, reducing the burden on healthcare professionals and improving patient engagement. Furthermore, the development of explainable AI (XAI) is gaining traction. As AI systems become more involved in healthcare decision-making, the need for transparency and interpretability increases. XAI aims to make AI algorithms more understandable to human users, which is crucial for building trust among healthcare professionals and patients. This transparency is essential for the ethical and responsible use of AI in healthcare.

For AI to be successfully implemented in healthcare, cooperation between researchers, practitioners, and policymakers is essential. Interdisciplinary teams can ensure that AI solutions are clinically relevant, ethically sound, and aligned with healthcare goals. Additionally, policies and regulations need to be updated to keep pace with technological advancements, ensuring that AI is used safely and effectively in healthcare settings. The journey of AI in healthcare is fraught with challenges, from data privacy concerns to the complexity of medical conditions. However, the road ahead is paved with potential solutions and innovative strategies that promise to overcome these obstacles. Protecting patient data is paramount in the era of AI, and advanced cryptographic techniques such as homomorphic encryption offer a promising solution by allowing data to be processed in an encrypted form. Moreover, blockchain technology can be leveraged to create secure and immutable records of patient data. The lack of standardization in healthcare data hampers AI's potential, but initiatives aimed at harmonizing health data through universal coding systems and interoperable formats are crucial. To mitigate bias in AI, the development and training of algorithms must prioritize diversity and inclusivity, involving gathering and utilizing datasets that reflect the demographic variety of the global population. Addressing the complexity of medical conditions requires AI systems that can learn and adapt over time, integrating continuous learning algorithms and incorporating multi-disciplinary data. For AI to be truly effective, it must be seamlessly integrated into existing clinical workflows, calling for the development of user-friendly AI tools that complement healthcare professionals' work [35].

For the development, testing, and application of AI in healthcare, precise standards and guidelines must be established, and these frameworks must advance in tandem with AI technology. The high cost of AI development and deployment poses a significant barrier, especially in under-resourced settings, but investing in open-source AI projects and public-private partnerships can reduce costs and promote the democratization of AI technology. Fostering partnerships between AI technologists, healthcare professionals, patients, and policymakers is essential to develop AI solutions that are not only technologically advanced but also clinically relevant and patient-centered. Preparing the healthcare workforce for the AI revolution is critical, with educational initiatives and training programs equipping healthcare professionals with the necessary knowledge and skills to effectively utilize AI tools. The path to fully realize AI's potential in healthcare is complex and filled with challenges. Yet, with innovative solutions and a commitment to collaboration, transparency, and ethical practice, these obstacles can be overcome. The future of healthcare, augmented by AI, promises to be one of enhanced diagnosis, personalized treatment, and improved patient outcomes. As we move forward, it is imperative that we navigate this path with a focus on equity, ensuring that the benefits of AI in healthcare are accessible to all [36]. The findings of analysis on the pharmaceutical sector showcase that the random forest algorithm exhibits superior performance in comparison to the decision tree algorithm [37]. Deep learning algorithms have been found to perform better than ML algorithms; however, their computing needs have been challenged [38].

14.10 CONCLUSION

AI in healthcare is a paradigm shift that has the potential to completely transform all facets of medical treatment. AI is revolutionizing healthcare by providing never-before-seen possibilities for enhancing patient outcomes and streamlining healthcare delivery, from early detection and diagnosis to customized therapy and continuous management. The journey of AI in healthcare, however, is not without its challenges. Data privacy and security remain paramount concerns, as the reliance on vast amounts of personal health data raises critical questions about patient confidentiality and the potential for breaches. Moreover, the lack of standardization in healthcare data poses a significant hurdle, as AI algorithms require consistent and standardized data to function effectively. Addressing these challenges requires a concerted effort from all stakeholders in the healthcare ecosystem, including policymakers, healthcare providers, and technology developers, to establish robust data governance frameworks and interoperable data standards.

Bias and fairness in AI algorithms also demand attention. The risk of perpetuating existing biases through AI systems highlights the need for diverse and representative training datasets, as well as transparent and accountable algorithmic processes. Ensuring that AI technologies are equitable and just is essential for their ethical application in healthcare. The complexity of medical conditions adds another layer of difficulty. Many diseases are multifactorial, requiring AI algorithms to navigate a labyrinth of factors to provide accurate diagnoses and predictions. This necessitates the development of sophisticated models that can handle the intricacies of medical data and evolve with the emergence of new diseases and treatments.

AI use in healthcare will not be successful unless it is successfully integrated into clinical workflows. Healthcare professionals' resistance, motivated by worries about losing their jobs or a lack of confidence in recommendations made by AI, needs to be overcome via cooperation and education. Developing user-friendly AI tools that seamlessly fit into existing healthcare infrastructures will be key to ensuring their widespread acceptance and use.

The proper application of AI in healthcare requires careful attention to ethical and legal issues. To ensure responsibility and trust as AI systems participate in decision-making processes more, it is imperative to create clear norms and ethical standards. Engaging with regulatory bodies, ethicists, and patient advocacy groups will be essential to navigate the complex ethical landscape of AI in healthcare. The cost of developing and implementing AI systems poses a significant barrier, particularly in low-resource settings. This financial challenge can exacerbate health disparities, as only well-resourced healthcare systems may be able to afford the latest AI technologies. Addressing this issue requires innovative financing models and policies that support the equitable distribution of AI benefits across different healthcare settings. Looking into the future, the potential of AI in healthcare is large. AI is anticipated to become more and more important in patient care, treatment planning, and illness diagnosis as technology develops. Ongoing research and development promise to uncover new applications and further enhance the capabilities of AI in healthcare.

In conclusion, there are a lot of opportunities and significant challenges ahead for AI in healthcare. It takes a cooperative, moral approach to navigate this route, with an emphasis on equity and patient-centered treatment. We have the ability to make healthcare more streamlined, precise, and customized if we solve the existing obstacles and fully utilize AI.

REFERENCES

[1] Gandhi, Z., Gurram, P., Amgai, B., Lekkala, S.P., Lokhandwala, A., Manne, S., Mohammed, A., Koshiya, H., Dewaswala, N., Desai, R. and Bhopalwala, H., 2023. Artificial intelligence and lung cancer: Impact on improving patient outcomes. *Cancers*, *15*(21), p.5236.

[2] Lee, D. and Yoon, S.N., 2021. Application of artificial intelligence-based technologies in the healthcare industry: Opportunities and challenges. *International Journal of Environmental Research and Public Health*, *18*(1), p.271.

[3] Jiang, F., Jiang, Y., Zhi, H., Dong, Y., Li, H., Ma, S., Wang, Y., Dong, Q., Shen, H. and Wang, Y., 2017. Artificial intelligence in healthcare: Past, present and future. *Stroke and Vascular Neurology*, *2*(4) ; e000101. doi:10.1136/svn-2017-000101; pp. (230 – 243).

[4] Kasula, B.Y., 2021. AI-driven innovations in healthcare: Improving diagnostics and patient care. *International Journal of Machine Learning and Artificial Intelligence*, *2*(2), pp.1–8.

[5] Das, K., Cockerell, C.J., Patil, A., Pietkiewicz, P., Giulini, M., Grabbe, S. and Goldust, M., 2021. Machine learning and its application in skin cancer. *International Journal of Environmental Research and Public Health*, *18*(24), p.13409.

[6] Banerjee, A., Chakraborty, C. and RathiSr, M., 2020. Medical imaging, artificial intelligence, internet of things, wearable devices in terahertz healthcare technologies. In*Terahertz biomedical and healthcare technologies*(pp. 145–165). Elsevier, Materials to Devices 2020, Pages 145-165.

[7] Hernandez-Boussard, T., Bozkurt, S., Ioannidis, J.P. and Shah, N.H., 2020. MINIMAR (MINimum Information for Medical AI Reporting): Developing reporting standards for artificial intelligence in health care. *Journal of the American Medical Informatics Association*, *27*(12), pp.2011–2015.

[8] Asatryan, B., Bleijendaal, H. and Wilde, A.A., 2023. Towards advanced diagnosis and management of inherited arrhythmia syndromes: Harnessing the capabilities of artificial intelligence and machine learning. *Heart Rhythm, Volume 20, Issue 10, Pages 1399-1407.*

[9] Arvinti, B., Iacob, E.R., Isar, A., Iacob, D. and Costache, M., 2021. Automated medical care: Bradycardia detection and cardiac monitoring of preterm infants. *Medicina*, *57*(11), p.1199.

[10] Nadarzynski, T., Miles, O., Cowie, A. and Ridge, D., 2019. Acceptability of artificial intelligence (AI)-led chatbot services in healthcare: A mixed-methods study. *Digital Health*, *5*, p.2055207619871808.

[11] Hazari, M.S., Haykal-Coates, N., Winsett, D.W., Krantz, Q.T., King, C., Costa, D.L. and Farraj, A.K., 2011. TRPA1 and sympathetic activation contribute to increased risk of triggered cardiac arrhythmias in hypertensive rats exposed to diesel exhaust. *Environmental Health Perspectives*, *119*(7), pp.951–957.

[12] Mohsin, S.N., Gapizov, A., Ekhator, C., Ain, N.U., Ahmad, S., Khan, M., Barker, C., Hussain, M., Malineni, J., Ramadhan, A. and Nagaraj, R.H., 2023. The role of artificial intelligence in prediction, risk stratification, and personalized treatment planning for congenital heart diseases. *Cureus*, *15*(8) :e44374. doi: 10.7759/cureus.44374. PMID: 37664359; PMCID: PMC10469091

[13] Mansour, R.F., El Amraoui, A., Nouaouri, I., Díaz, V.G., Gupta, D. and Kumar, S., 2021. Artificial intelligence and internet of things enabled disease diagnosis model for smart healthcare systems. *IEEE Access*, *9*, pp.45137–45146.

[14] Golec, M., Gill, S.S., Parlikad, A.K. and Uhlig, S., 2023. HealthFaaS: AI based smart healthcare system for heart patients using serverlesscomputing. *IEEE Internet of Things Journal*, vol. 10, Issue no. 21, pp. 18469-18476, 2023, doi: 10.1109/JIOT.2023.3277500.

[15] Tay, J.L., Li, Z. and Sim, K., 2022. Effectiveness of artificial intelligence methods in personalized aggression risk prediction within inpatient psychiatric treatment settings—A systematic review. *Journal of Personalized Medicine*, *12*(9), p.1470.

[16] Choudhury, A. and Asan, O., 2020. Role of artificial intelligence in patient safety outcomes: Systematic literature review. *JMIR Medical Informatics*, *8*(7), p.e18599.

[17] Jones, O.T., Calanzani, N., Saji, S., Duffy, S.W., Emery, J., Hamilton, W., Singh, H., de Wit, N.J. and Walter, F.M., 2021. Artificial intelligence techniques that may be applied to primary care data to facilitate earlier diagnosis of cancer: Systematic review. *Journal of Medical Internet Research*, *23*(3), p.e23483.

[18] Rong, G., Mendez, A., Assi, E.B., Zhao, B. and Sawan, M., 2020. Artificial intelligence in healthcare: Review and prediction case studies. *Engineering*, *6*(3), pp.291–301.

[19] Perju-Dumbrava, L., Barsan, M., Leucuta, D.C., Popa, L.C., Pop, C., Tohanean, N. and Popa, S.L., 2022. Artificial intelligence applications and robotic systems in Parkinson's disease. *Experimental and Therapeutic Medicine*, *23*(2), pp.1–11.

[20] Padhan, S., Mohapatra, A., Ramasamy, S.K., Agrawal, S. and Ramasamy, S., 2023. Artificial Intelligence (AI) and robotics in elderly healthcare: Enabling independence and quality of life. *Cureus*, *15*(8):e42905. doi: 10.7759/cureus.42905. PMID: 37664381; PMCID: PMC10474924.

[21] Pravin, S.C., Sivaraman, V.B. and Saranya, J.,2023.Deep ensemble models for speech emotion classification.*Microprocessors and Microsystems*, *98*, 104790.

[22] Poalelungi, D.G., Musat, C.L., Fulga, A., Neagu, M., Neagu, A.I., Piraianu, A.I. and Fulga, I., 2023. Advancing patient care: How artificial intelligence is transforming healthcare. *Journal of Personalized Medicine*, *13*(8), p.1214.

[23] Mujahid, O., Contreras, I. and Vehi, J., 2021. Machine learning techniques for hypoglycemia prediction: Trends and challenges. *Sensors*, *21*(2), p.546.

[24] Hsu, C.C., Kao, Y., Hsu, C.C., Chen, C.J., Hsu, S.L., Liu, T.L., Lin, H.J., Wang, J.J., Liu, C.F. and Huang, C.C., 2023. Using artificial intelligence to predict adverse outcomes in emergency department patients with hyperglycemic crises in real time. *BMC Endocrine Disorders*, *23*(1), p.234.

[25] Pravin, S.C., Sindhu Priya, K., Suganthi, S., Saranya, J.andSelva Kumar, V.S.,2023. LabVIEW based anomaly detection for screening diabetic retinopathy. In *IoT Based Control Networks and Intelligent Systems,* . Lecture Notes in Networks and Systems, vol 528. Springer, Singapore. https://doi.org/10.1007/978-981-19-5845-8_1

[26] Khanna, N.N., Maindarkar, M.A., Viswanathan, V., Fernandes, J.F.E., Paul, S., Bhagawati, M., Ahluwalia, P., Ruzsa, Z., Sharma, A., Kolluri, R. and Singh, I.M., 2022, December. Economics of artificial intelligence in healthcare: Diagnosis vs. treatment. *Healthcare*, *10*(12), p. 2493.

[27] Bin Sawad, A., Narayan, B., Alnefaie, A., Maqbool, A., Mckie, I., Smith, J., Yuksel, B., Puthal, D., Prasad, M. and Kocaballi, A.B., 2022. A systematic review on healthcare artificial intelligent conversational agents for chronic conditions. *Sensors*, *22*(7), p.2625.

[28] Sun, T.Q. and Medaglia, R., 2019. Mapping the challenges of Artificial Intelligence in the public sector: Evidence from public healthcare. *Government Information Quarterly*, *36*(2), pp.368–383.

[29] Meng, W., Liu, Q., Zhou, Z., Ai, Q., Sheng, B. and Xie, S.S., 2015. Recent development of mechanisms and control strategies for robot-assisted lower limb rehabilitation. *Mechatronics*, *31*, pp.132–145.

[30] Kasula, B.Y., 2023. AI applications in healthcare a comprehensive review of advancements and challenges,, IJISCS (International Journal of Information System and Computer Science, *6*(6) pp. (1-9).

[31] Lee, D. and Yoon, S.N., 2021. Application of artificial intelligence-based technologies in the healthcare industry: Opportunities and challenges. *International Journal of Environmental Research and Public Health, 18*(1), p.271.

[32] Lee, D. and Yoon, S.N., 2021. Application of artificial intelligence-based technologies in the healthcare industry: Opportunities and challenges. *International Journal of Environmental Research and Public Health, 18*(1), p.271.

[33] Dev,K., Khowaja, S.A., Bist,A.S.,Saini,V.,andBhatia, S., 2023. Triage of potential COVID-19 patients from chest X-ray images using hierarchical convolutional networks.*Neural Computing and Applications*, *35*, pp. 23861–23876.

[34] Manickam, P., Mariappan, S.A., Murugesan, S.M., Hansda, S., Kaushik, A., Shinde, R. and Thipperudraswamy, S.P., 2022. Artificial intelligence (AI) and internet of medical things (IoMT) assisted biomedical systems for intelligent healthcare. *Biosensors*, *12*(8), p.562.

[35] Nguyen, D.C., Pham, Q.V., Pathirana, P.N., Ding, M., Seneviratne, A., Lin, Z., Dobre, O. and Hwang, W.J., 2022. Federated learning for smart healthcare: A survey. *ACM Computing Surveys (CSUR)*, *55*(3), pp.1–37.

[36] Patil, S. and Shankar, H., 2023. Transforming healthcare: Harnessing the power of AI in the modern era. *International Journal of Multidisciplinary Sciences and Arts*, *2*(1), pp.60–70.

[37] Sakthi Ganesh Dharani, R., Lokheshram, S.V., and Malini, A.,2023.Seasonal disease based demand forecasting for pharmaceutical medications using random forest.), Lecture Notes in Computer Science(), vol 13924. Springer, Cham. https://doi.org/10.1007/978-3-031-44084-7_25Springer pp. 261–268.

[38] Rajasekaran, U., Sriram, G.K., Ramyavarshini, P., andMalini, A.,2023.XAI-based light-weight CNN-HAR model using random sampling. In*Lecture Notes in Networks and Systems, 730 LNNS*, pp. 377–388.

15 Medical Impact Assessment of Industrial Emissions

Predicting the Air Quality Index

Eshaan Abbas Jafri, Raj Tetarwal, Udhaya Kumar, and Kasthuri Bha J. K.

15.1 INTRODUCTION

Air pollution poses a ubiquitous environmental challenge, with profound impacts on human health, ecosystems, and global climate trends. Ensuring the effective monitoring and prediction of air quality is imperative for public health management and environmental preservation efforts. Notably, industrial activities emerge as significant contributors to air pollution, releasing various gases and particulate matter into the atmosphere. This study aims to unravel the complexities of air pollution by harnessing data analysis and predictive modeling techniques to discern the Air Quality Index (AQI).

Through a meticulous analysis of key pollutants, including sulfur dioxide (SO_2), nitrogen oxides (NO_x), respirable suspended particulate matter (RSPM), and suspended particulate matter (SPM), their influence on air quality levels was comprehensively explored. Several regression techniques, spanning random forest regression, linear regression, AdaBoost regression, support vector machine (SVM), gradient boosting, boosting regression, ridge regression, and stacking regression, are employed to construct the predictive model. Moreover, beyond the model development phase, the project expanded its scope to encompass the creation of a user-friendly web interface for AQI forecasting. This interface enables users to input gas concentrations and promptly obtain the AQI computation. To enhance user engagement, educational components such as a detailed table elucidating various AQI levels and their corresponding health impacts were integrated into the website.

This project was implemented to promote public awareness about the detrimental impacts of air pollution on human health and the environment.

The *x*-axis depicts concentration and the *y*-axis depicts frequency.

DOI: 10.1201/9781003484233-15

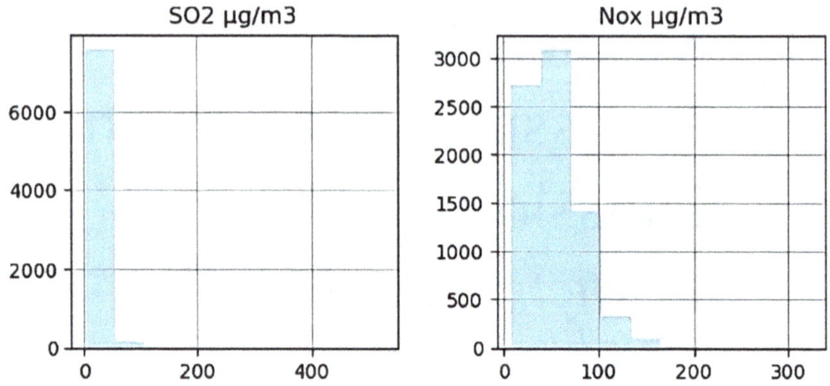

FIGURE 15.1 Distribution of the SO_2 and NO_x concentration data values.

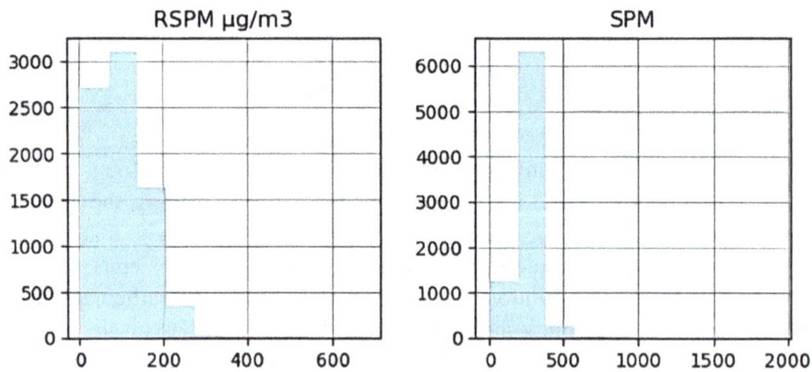

FIGURE 15.2 Distribution of the RSPM and SPM concentration data values.

15.2 METHODOLOGY

15.2.1 Data Preprocessing and Collection

The process of data collecting and preprocessing entails the acquisition of information pertaining to various industrial gases and particulate matter. The data are meticulously acquired from dependable sources or monitoring stations. Once acquired, rigorous preparation procedures are implemented to uphold the quality and uniformity of the data. The tasks entail managing null values, transforming data types into suitable formats, and eliminating duplicate entries from the dataset.

15.2.2 Exploratory Data Analysis (EDA)

Once the data pretreatment stage is over, the next step is to begin exploratory data analysis (EDA). Data exploration is a crucial procedure that involves thoroughly

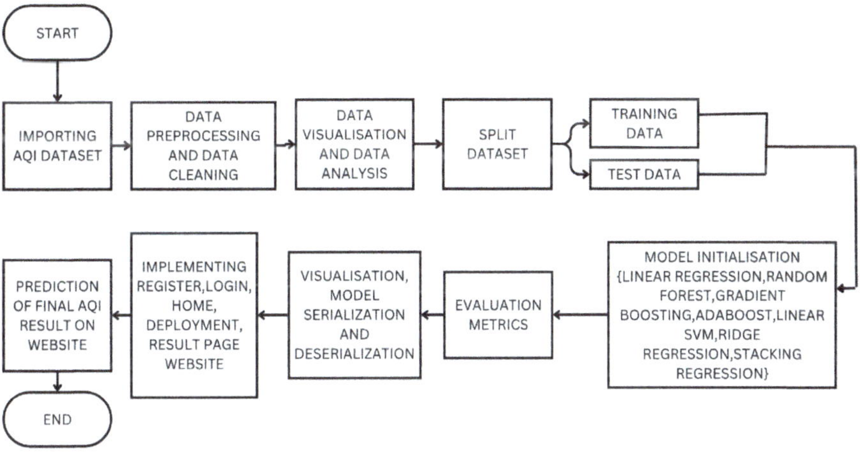

FIGURE 15.3 AQI prediction block diagram.

	SO_2 µg/m3	NO_x µg/m3	RSPM µg/m3	SPM	AQI
SO_2 µg/m3	1.000000	0.240843	0.117720	0.093823	0.186419
NO_x µg/m3	0.240843	1.000000	0.371171	0.259338	0.557226
RSPM µg/m3	0.117720	0.371171	1.000000	0.487040	0.930327
SPM	0.093823	0.259338	0.487040	1.000000	0.466647
AQI	0.186419	0.557226	0.930327	0.466647	1.000000

FIGURE 15.4 Correlation matrix of air pollutants.

examining the information to acquire a comprehensive understanding of its properties and uncover any inherent patterns or trends. Descriptive statistics, measures such as the median, mean, and standard deviation, are calculated to give a brief assessment of the core tendencies and dispersion of the dataset. Moreover, visual depictions such as histograms, scatter plots, and box plots are generated to visually analyze the relationships between variables and detect any atypical or anomalous data points in the dataset.

15.2.3 Regression Model Development

Through the process of conducting EDA, we are able to gain a comprehensive and detailed understanding of the dataset. Subsequently, we construct regression models with the objective of forecasting the AQI using the given attributes. The scope of our inquiry includes a range of regression approaches such as support vector regression (SVR), AdaBoost regression, linear regression, gradient boosting regression, ridge regression, random forest regression, and stacking regression. Typically, these models are trained using a portion of the data and then assessed for their performance using important criteria.

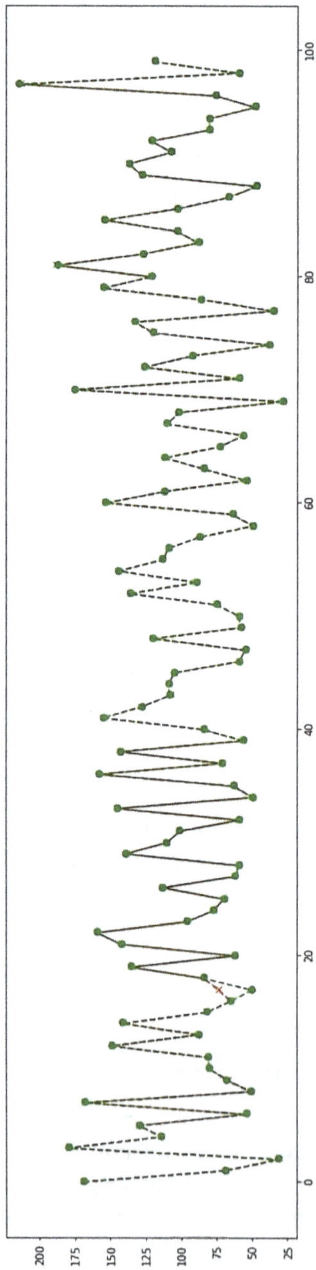

FIGURE 15.5 Random forest line graph.

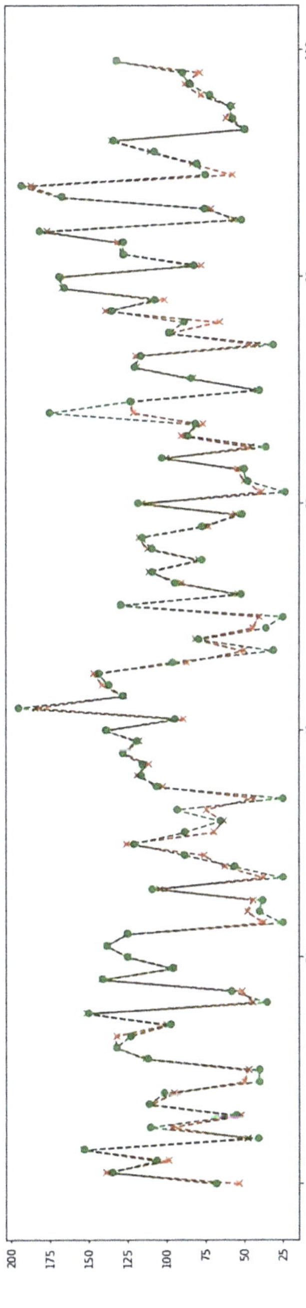

FIGURE 15.6 SVR line graph.

15.2.4 Linear Regression

Linear regression is a statistical method used to create a linear equation that models the relationship between a dependent variable and many independent variables based on observed data [1]. Linear regression is a statistical method used to determine the linear relationship between industrial gases (SO_2, NO_2, RSPM, and SPM) and the AQI in the context of prediction. The model calculates the coefficients for each gas, which indicate the effect of changes in gas concentrations on AQI. Linear regression offers a direct method for estimating air quality by minimizing the total of squared differences between projected and actual AQI values, using industrial gas concentrations as the basis.

The mathematical expression for the model is extended to

$$y = m1x + c \tag{1}$$

$$m1 = \frac{n\sum(x_i y_i) - \sum x_i \sum y_i}{n\sum(x_i^2) - (\sum x_i)^2} \tag{2}$$

$$C = \frac{\sum y_i - m1\sum x_i}{n} \tag{3}$$

where n is equal to the number of data points.

For multiple linear regression with multiple independent variables:

$$y = b_0 + b_1x_1 + b_2x_2 + \ldots + x_nx_n \tag{4}$$

a) The dependent variable is represented by the symbol y.
b) The variable x is considered to be the independent variable.
c) The variable "m" represents the slope of the line.
d) The y-intercept, denoted by c, represents the value of y when x is equal to 0.

The project utilizes linear regression to model the linear correlation between industrial gases (SO_2, NO_x, RSPM, and SPM) and AQI. It aids in assessing the linear correlation between gases and AQI, offering insights into the impact of changes in gas concentrations on air quality.

15.2.5 Ridge Regression

Ridge regression is a form of linear regression that deals with the problem of multicollinearity among independent variables and avoids overfitting by incorporating a penalty term into the regression coefficients [2]. The project utilizes ridge regression to enhance the resilience of the linear regression model by reducing the coefficients towards zero, while still permitting a certain level of adaptability in the model. Ridge regression improves the stability and reliability of predicting the AQI by punishing large coefficients and lowering the influence of multicollinearity caused

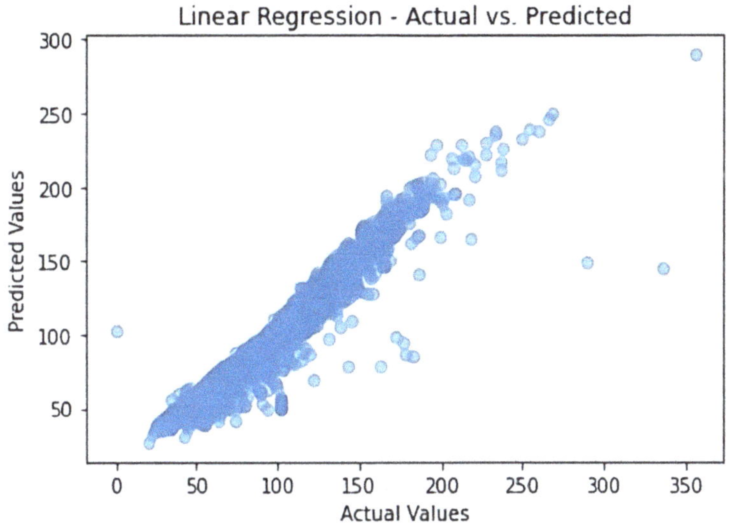

FIGURE 15.7 Linear regression (actual vs. predicted value).

by industrial gas concentrations. Ridge regression incorporates a regularization component into the linear regression equation:

$$\sum_{i=1}^{n}\left(y_i - \beta_0 - \beta_1 x_{i1} - \beta_2 x_{i2} - \ldots - \beta_n x_{in}\right)^2 + \lambda\sum_{j=1}^{n}\beta_j^2 \quad (5)$$

where λ is the regularization parameter.

$$\lambda\sum_{j=1}^{n}\beta_j^2 \quad (6)$$

The regularization term imposes a penalty on coefficients with large values, thus limiting overfitting and diminishing the influence of multicollinearity. Ridge regression is utilized to enhance the resilience of the linear regression model by tackling multicollinearity among the independent variables. When multicollinearity is present, the coefficient estimates obtained from ordinary linear regression can be incorrect. Ridge regression addresses this problem by incorporating a regularization term into the regression coefficients, which enhances the stability and dependability of the predictions.

15.2.6 Support Vector Regression (SVR)

SVR is a regression technique that utilizes SVMs to perform regression problems [3]. The SVM algorithm functions by converting input variables into a feature space characterized by a large number of dimensions. It then determines the hyperplane that efficiently divides the data points while maximizing the margin. When forecasting the AQI, SVMs aim to minimize the difference between the predicted and actual values, while simultaneously optimizing the separation margin.

SVM is a reliable approach for predicting air quality using industrial gas concentrations since it efficiently deals with nonlinear connections and outliers.

Mathematical expression:

$$min_{\omega.b,\xi,\xi^*} \frac{1}{2}\|\omega\|^2 + C\sum_{i=1}^{n}(\xi_i + \xi_i^*) \tag{7}$$

Assistance vector regression seeks to identify a hyperplane, denoted by $\omega.x + b = 0$, that closely approximates the connection among the input variables x, the output variable y, while minimizing the amount of error.

Subject to the constraints:

$$y_i - \omega.x_i - b \leq \in + \xi_i \tag{8}$$

$$\omega.x_i + b - y_i \leq + \xi_i^* \tag{9}$$

$$\xi_i, \xi_i^* \geq 0 \tag{10}$$

where:

a) ω is the weight vector
b) b is the bias term
c) ξ_i and ξ_i^* are slack variables
d) C is the regularization parameter.

The SVM technique is employed to predict the AQI by accurately capturing the intricate and nonlinear relationships between industrial gases and AQI.

SVMs are adept at capturing intricate correlations and managing nonlinearities within the data. The modeling approach used is very adaptable to different patterns found in air quality data, resulting in improved accuracy

15.2.7 Random Forest Regression

Random forest regression is a technique that builds numerous decision trees during training and produces the average forecast of each tree [3]. The model is designed to be resistant to overfitting and able to capture intricate relationships in the data By training each tree on a randomly selected fraction of the data and a randomly chosen subset of the features [3]. The study uses random forest regression to describe the complex connections between industrial gases and AQI, applying ensemble learning techniques to improve the accuracy and reliability of predictions[4].

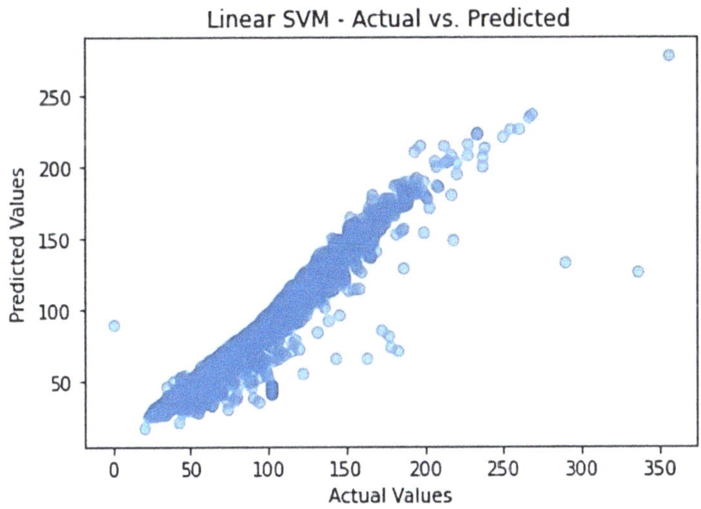

FIGURE 15.8 SVR (actual vs. predicted value).

Mathematical expression:

$$\hat{y} = \frac{i}{N}\sum_{i=1}^{N} h_i(x) \tag{11}$$

where:

a) variable $\hat{y}$ represents the projected output
b) N is the numerical value that corresponds to the quantity of decision trees
c) $h_i(x)$ is the forecast of the decision tree denoted by x.

The application of random forest regression is used to represent the complex connections between industrial gases and the AQI. Random forest regression utilizes ensemble learning to effectively capture intricate relationships between variables and generate reliable predictions. It is especially beneficial when working with data that have several dimensions and nonlinear connections, leading to enhanced accuracy in predictions [5].

15.2.8 Gradient Boosting Regression

Gradient boosting regression is a technique that constructs learners, where each subsequent learner aims to minimize the errors generated by the prior ones. The process involves constructing a sequence of decision trees based on the discrepancies between the expected and actual values. These trees are then utilized to generate the ultimate output by aggregating their predictions. Gradient boosting regression is a powerful method for capturing intricate relationships and is more resistant to overfitting than

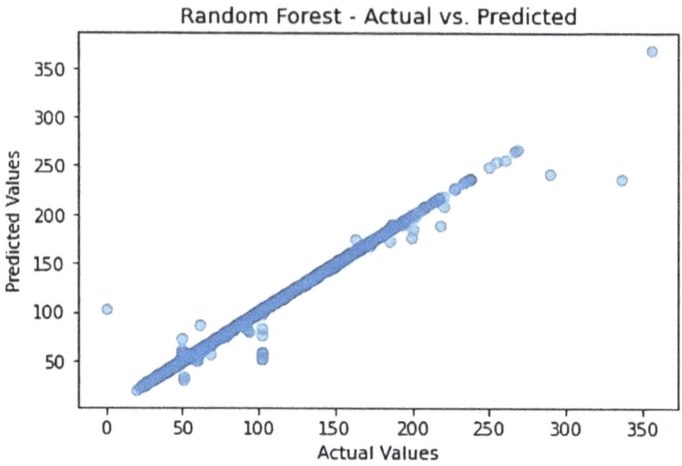

FIGURE 15.9 Random forest (actual vs. predicted value).

conventional decision trees [3,4]. The study utilizes gradient boosting regression to forecast the AQI by iteratively enhancing prediction accuracy through learning from the residuals of the prior models:

Mathematical expression:

$$F_o(x) = arg_{\gamma} min \sum_{i=1}^{n} L(y_i, \gamma) \tag{12}$$

The loss function L and the projected value γ are crucial elements. The goal is to minimize the loss function by identifying the anticipated value that results in the lowest loss function. Gradient boosting regression improves prediction accuracy by iteratively learning from the residuals of previous models [3,4]. It efficiently captures complex relationships and minimizes errors with every iteration. By sequentially adding weak learners, it is possible to improve the accuracy of predictions, resulting in more precise forecasts of AQI.

15.2.9 AdaBoost Regression

AdaBoost regression, also known as adaptive boosting regression, is a technique that utilizes numerous weak learners to construct a powerful learner [1]. The algorithm provides weights to data points based on their performance in prior rounds, with a greater emphasis on misclassified data points in following iterations. AdaBoost regression is highly advantageous when working with noisy data and can adjust to intricate correlations within the data. The project utilizes AdaBoost regression as an ensemble method to enhance the prediction accuracy and robustness of the AQI by

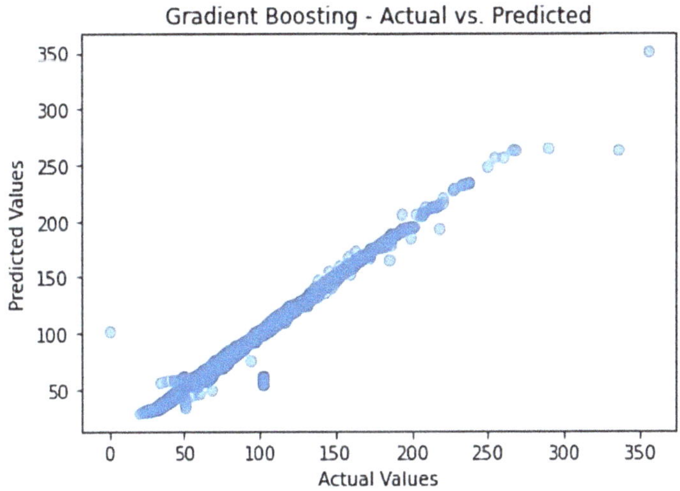

FIGURE 15.10 Gradient boosting (actual vs. predicted value).

exploiting the advantages of boosting. AdaBoost regression is an ensemble method used to predict AQI. It places more emphasis on the misclassified data points in each iteration. AdaBoost is proficient at managing noisy data and adjusting to intricate relationships. By increasing the weights of incorrectly identified data points, it is possible to enhance the accuracy and resilience of predictions, particularly in difficult conditions.

15.2.10 Stacking Regression

Stacking regression, or stacked generalization, is a technique that combines multiple regression models as base estimators. It then employs another model as a final estimator to create predictions based on the outputs of the base models [3,4]. It utilizes a variety of several models to capture a broad spectrum of patterns in the data and frequently results in enhanced predictive performance in comparison to individual models. The research utilizes stacking regression to improve the accuracy of predicting the AQI by leveraging the capabilities of several regression algorithms. This approach offers a more dependable forecast of air quality by considering the concentrations of industrial gases. Stacking regression is used to amalgamate the forecasts of various regression models and offer a more dependable prediction of AQI. Stacking regression utilizes the variety of distinct models to effectively capture a broad spectrum of patterns present in the data [1]. By amalgamating the merits of diverse regression methods, it might enhance the precision and resilience of predictions, ultimately yielding more dependable forecasts of air quality based on industrial gas concentrations.

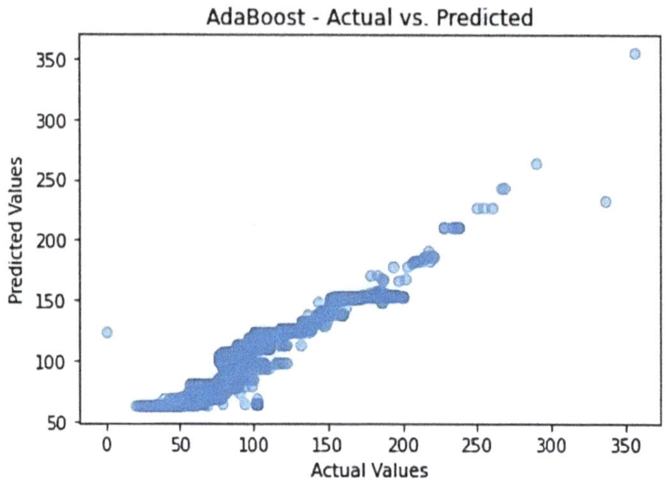

FIGURE 15.11 AdaBoost (actual vs. predicted value).

15.2.11 Evaluation Metrics

During this stage, the regression models' performance is assessed by employing several metrics to evaluate their capacity to predict the AQI using input features. The term "quantifies" refers to the process of measuring or determining the amount of anything. In this case, it is used to describe the action of determining the proportion of variation that is accounted for by the model. Conversely, the root mean squared error (RMSE), mean square error (MSE), and mean absolute error (MAE) are used to evaluate the average differences between the predicted and actual values. The Explained Volatility Score assesses the level of volatility present in the target variable [6].

These metrics offer valuable information about the models' appropriateness for predicting the AQI and help in identifying areas for improvement.

15.2.12 Mean Absolute Error (MAE)

The MAE is calculated by taking the average of the absolute discrepancies between each predicted value $\hat{y}_i$ and its corresponding actual value y_i for all n data points [2,4]. This is the procedure by which it is computed:

$$\text{MAE} = \frac{1}{n}\sum_{i=1}^{n}\left|y_i - \hat{y}_i\right| \tag{13}$$

The absolute difference $|y_i - \hat{y}_i|$ represents the magnitude of the error and is the difference between the predicted value ($\hat{y}_i$) and the actual value (y_i) for each data point (i). The MAE is computed by accumulating the absolute deviations between

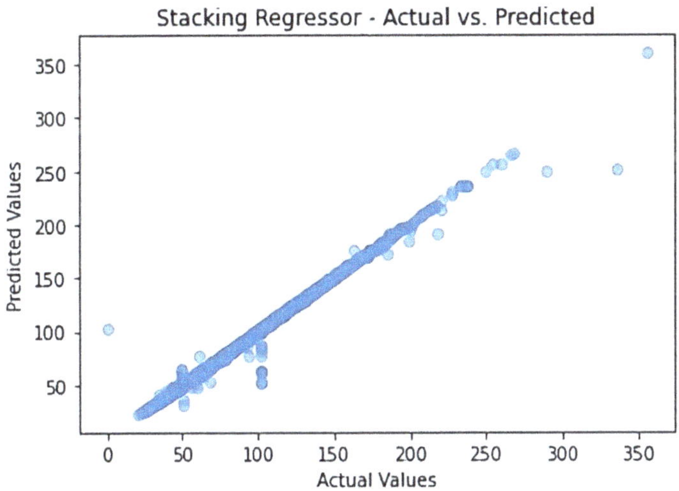

FIGURE 15.12 Stacking regression (actual vs. predicted value).

each data point and the mean, and thereafter dividing by the total number of data points, denoted by n.

15.2.13 Mean Square Error (MSE)

The MSE is computed by averaging the squared differences between each predicted value $\hat{y}_i$ and its corresponding actual value y_i across all data points n:

$$MSE = \frac{1}{n}\sum_{i=1}^{n}\left(y_i - \hat{y}_i\right)^2 \tag{14}$$

The squared difference $\left(y_i - \hat{y}_i\right)^2$ is computed for each data point i, which amplifies the impact of greater mistakes as a result of the squaring process [6]. The squared discrepancies between each data point and their respective values are summed and then divided by the number of data points, n, to calculate the MSE.

15.2.14 Root Mean Squared Error (RMSE)

The RMSE is the root square of MSE and is calculated as follows:

$$\text{RMSE} = \sqrt{MSE} \tag{15}$$

RMSE measures the average deviation between the predicted and actual values. RMSE is derived by taking the square root of the MSE. An advantage of using RMSE is that it is expressed in the same unit as the target variable, which improves its clarity.

The lower the RMSE number, the greater the superiority of prediction performance, as it signifies smaller disparities between the predicted and actual values [3].

15.2.15 Web Interface Development

The research explores the complexities of the website interface, specifically focusing on its design and functionality. The text provides detailed information on how to successfully manage personal information, such as usernames, email addresses, and localities, in order to customize air quality insights. This information may be found in references [7,8].

The deployment processes give priority to scalability, reliability, and performance optimization in order to ensure smooth user access. Integrating with a backend database enables the secure storage and retrieval of air quality data and user preferences. User authentication procedures guarantee secure access to crucial functions and data. Furthermore, the inclusion of mechanisms for user feedback and support channels highlights the dedication to actively engage with users and constantly enhance the interface.

An intuitive web interface enhances the prediction of the AQI and offers valuable insights into the state of air quality. Through the interface, users can input values for industrial gases, and the website utilizes trained regression models to dynamically compute the AQI. Furthermore, the inclusion of a table that outlines the various ranges of the AQI and their corresponding health impacts serves to enhance knowledge regarding the potential health hazards posed by air pollution. This web interface functions as a significant instrument for making informed decisions and increasing public knowledge about air quality problems [4,9].

15.3 RESULTS

In the final phase, a visual illustration delineates the concentrations of SO_2, NO_x, RSPM, and SPM gases, offering a succinct overview of the analyzed air quality

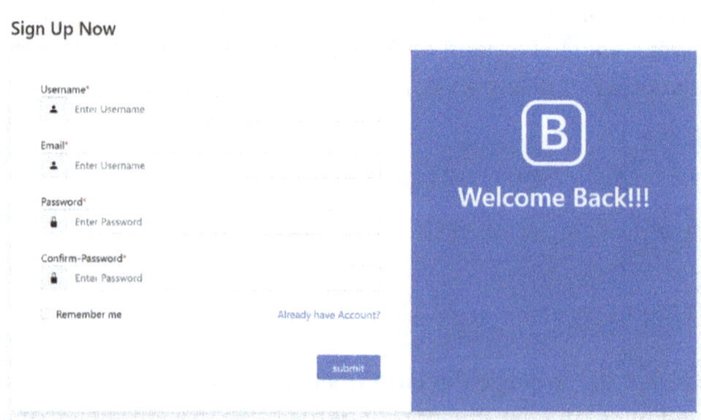

FIGURE 15.13 User information page.

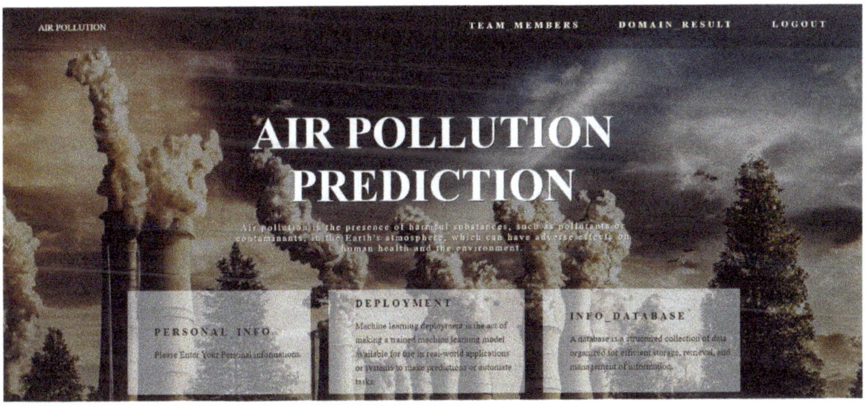

FIGURE 15.14 Main menu of the website.

TABLE 15.1
AQI reference table

AQI range	Category	Health effects
0–50	Good	Good air quality
51–100	Satisfactory	Low air pollution and no ill effects on health.
101–200	Moderate	Moderate pollution, breathing discomfort for people with lung, asthma and heart diseases
201–300	Poor	Mild aggravation of symptoms among high-risk persons, like those with heart or lung disease.
301–400	Very poor	Significant aggravation of symptoms and decreased exercise tolerance in persons with heart or lung disease
401–500 or more	Severe	Severe aggravation of symptoms and danger to health

parameters through a medical lens. This graphical representation serves as a vital tool in comprehending the health implications associated with varying levels of these pollutants. Users are encouraged to actively engage with the interface by inputting their gas concentration values, thereby fostering a collaborative approach towards addressing public health concerns related to air pollution. This interactive component not only increases user engagement but also assists in making well-informed decisions, especially when applying medical measures to reduce the negative impact of air pollution on human health.

The calculated AQI value was determined to be 96.3734, based on the input concentrations of SO_2, NO_x, RSPM, and SPM gases. This numerical representation of the AQI is pivotal in gauging the current air quality status, thereby providing essential insights into potential health risks posed by atmospheric pollutants.

Additionally, we expound on the significance of this AQI value by offering a detailed exposition of the corresponding air quality category. This description encompasses

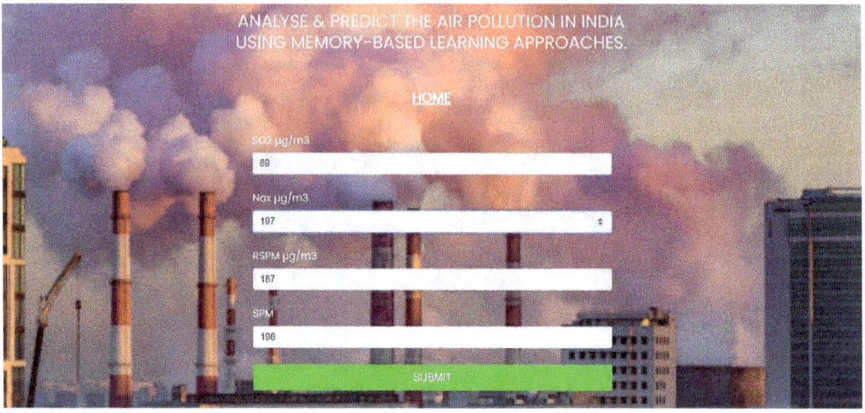

FIGURE 15.15 Data entry of values for prediction.

API range	Category	Health effects
0-50	Good	Good air quality
51-100	Satisfactory	Low air pollution and no ill effects on health.
101-200	Moderate	Moderate pollution, Breathing discomfort to the people with lungs, asthma and heart diseases
201-300	Poor	Mild aggravation of symptoms among high-risk persons, like those with heart or lung disease.
301-400	Very poor	Significant aggravation of symptoms and decreased exercise tolerance in persons with heart or lung disease.
401-500 or more	Severe	Severe aggravation of symptoms and endangers health

FIGURE 15.16 Predicted result of the website.

critical factors such as pollutant concentrations, associated health implications, and recommended precautionary measures. By presenting both the numerical AQI value and its contextual interpretation, our findings empower users with a comprehensive understanding of the prevailing air quality conditions, thereby facilitating informed decision-making processes regarding public health interventions.

15.4 CONCLUSION AND FUTURE WORK

This project has achieved the successful development and evaluation of regression models tailored for predicting the AQI, which is determined by measuring the levels of industrial gases present in the air. Notably, SO_2, NO_x, RSPM, and SPM were considered. Through the utilization of a diverse array of algorithms, comprehensive insights into air quality dynamics have been attained. The user-friendly web interface enhances engagement by enabling users to input gas concentrations and view corresponding AQI values. Future endeavors will focus on refining existing models,

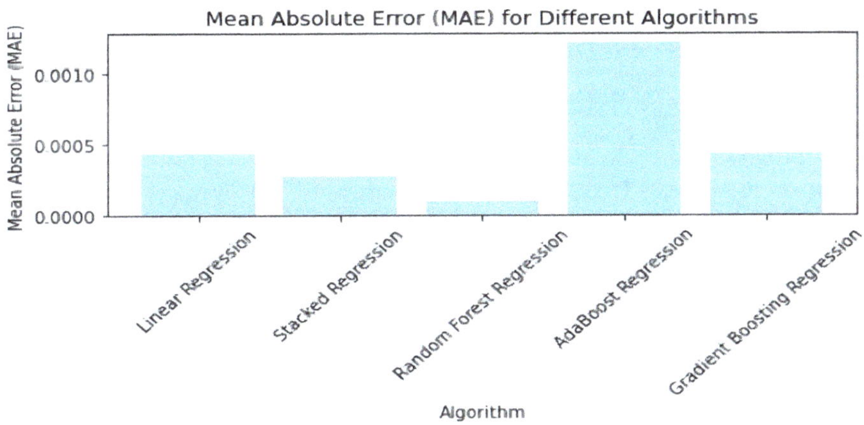

FIGURE 15.17 Comparison of the MAE of different algorithms.

integrating additional data sources to augment predictive accuracy, and enhancing the user experience to foster more efficient air quality management strategies.

REFERENCES

[1] A.-S. Chowdhury, M. S. Uddin, M. R. Tanjim, F. Noor, and R. M. Rahman, "Application of data mining techniques on air pollution of Dhaka City," in *Proceedings of the 2020 IEEE 10th International Conference on Intelligent Systems (IS)*, Varna, Bulgaria, August 2020, pp. 562–567.

[2] M. Castelli, F. M. Clemente, A. Popovic, S. Silva, and L. Vanneschi, "A machine learning approach to predict air quality in California," Hindawi *Complexity*, vol. 2020, Article ID 8049504, p. 23, 2020.

[3] R. W. Gore and D. S. Deshpande, "An approach for classification of health risks based on air quality levels," IEEE in *Proceedings of the 2017 1st International Conference on Intelligent Systems and Information Management (ICISIM)*, Aurangabad, India, October 2017, pp. 58–61.

[4] S.Y. Muhammad, M. Makhtar, A. Rozaimee, A. Abdul, and A. A. Jamal, "Classification model for air quality using machine learning techniques," *International Journal of Software Engineering and Its Applications*,vol. 7 pp. 45–52, 2015.

[5] R. Janarthanan, P. Partheeban, K. Somasundaram, and P. Navin Elamparithi, "A deep learning approach for prediction of air quality index in a metropolitan city," *Sustainable Cities and Society*, vol. 67, pp 1-11, Article ID 102720, 2021.

[6] W. F. Ip, C. M. Vong, J. Y. Yang, and P. K. Wong, "Least squares support vector prediction for daily atmospheric pollutant level," IEEE in *Proceedings of 2010 IEEE/ACIS 9th International Conference on Computer and Information Science (ICIS)*, IEEE, August 2010, pp. 23–28.

[7] P. Sai Swetha, M. A. Chiranjath Shakthi, S. Hrushikesh, and A. Malini, "Prediction of column average carbon dioxide emission using random forest regression," Springer, Singapore, in *International Conference on Data Analytics & Management, ICDAM*, vol. 1, pp. 377–388, 2023.

[8] E. Haque, S. Tabassum and E. Hossain, "A Comparative Analysis of Deep Neural Networks for Hourly Temperature Forecasting," IEEE Access, in R*ecent Advances in Computer Science and Communications*, vol. 9, pp. 160646-160660 2021.

[9] S. Kayalvizhi, K. Ferents Koni Jiavana, K. Suganthi, and S. Malarvizhi, "Prediction of ground water quality in western regions of Tamil Nadu using deep auto encoders," *Urban Climate*, vol. 49, Febuary 2023.

[10] C. R. Aditya, C. R. Deshmukh, D. K. Nayana, and P. G. Vidyavastu, "Detection and prediction of air pollution using machine learning models," *International Journal of Engineering Trends and Technology (IJETT)*, vol. 59, no. 4, May 2018.

[11] P. Shah, A. Yashwant, U. Khaitan and S. Kayalvizhi, "Weather management system using machine learning algorithm and IOT," in *IEEE xplore – 2023 International Conference on Recent Advances in Electrical, Electronics, Ubiquitous Communication, and Computational Intelligence (RAEEUCCI)*, Chennai, India, 2023, pp. 1–4.

Index

A

Abstraction, 115
Access attack, 118
Access layer, 116
Accuracy, 13, 17–18
AI, 11–12
AI applications in diabetes management, 250
AI-assisted therapy for rehabilitation, 253
AI-driven tools for the early detection of infectious disease, 251
AI in cancer diagnosis, 245
AI in drug and vaccine research, 251
AI in genomics, 251
AI in healthcare, 256
AI into clinical workflows, 254
AI-powered continuous glucose monitors, 249
AI-powered wearable devices, 246
Algorithms, 11–13
Application programming interfaces, 111
Architecture, 14, 17
Artificial neural network (ANN), 202
Association rule learning (ARL), 199–200
Attack on data transition, 119
Attacks by routing, 119
Attention mechanism, 162, 163
Augmentation, 159
Automatic ischemia detection, 135

B

Bagging techniques, 203
BigIoT, 115
Blockchain interoperability, 123
Blockchain technology, 106, 116
Boosting, 198
Brain, 13–14, 17–18
Brain-computer interfaces using AI, 248
Breast, 12, 18
Breast cancer classification (BCC), 194
Breast cancer classification using machine learning, 193
Bridge, 112
Byzantine consensus method, 122

C

Calinski–Harabasz index, 99
Cancer, 11–12, 18
Cardiac imaging using AI systems, 247
Cardiomyopathy, 134
Cerebral, 18
Classification, 13, 15
Cluster approach, 95, 97, 98
Compose layer, 116
Computed tomography, 55, 64, 66–7
Conclusion 167
Constrained application protocol (CoaP) 116
Convolutional neural networks (CNNs), 13–14, 54–6, 58–9, 61–8, 70–1
CT, 12–13
Customization of diabetes therapy using AI, 249

D

Data, 11–15
Data adapter, 111
Data mapping, 111
Data processing, 107, 110
Dataset description, 159
Datasets, 11–12
Davies–Bouldin index, 101
Decision-making, 12
Decision tree (DT), 195
Deep learning, 53–5, 61–4, 67–71, 159, 161
Deep learning algorithms, 256
Deep neural networks, 13
Detection, 11–13
Diagnosis, 54, 57–9, 62–71
Diagnostics, 11–12
Dictionary, 112
Distributed denial of service, 118
Distributed intelligent digital archive, 113
Drugs, 18
Dyspepsia, 137
Dyspnea, 132

E

Eavesdropping and interference, 118
Electronic health records, 123
Employs, 11, 14
Encryption, 109
Ensemble learning, 13
Evaluation of cognitive test results using AI systems, 247
Explainable AI (XAI), 255
Extensible markup language, 111
Extensible messaging, 116

F

Face feature extraction, 85, 86
Face statistical features, 95, 96, 98

Find layer, 116
Fireware, 113
Forecast, 11
Foundational level, 114
Frequent, 18
Full-service operator, 115

G

Gastro esophageal reflux disease (GERD), 137
Gastrointestinal, 18
Gateway, 108
GoogLeNet, 14–16
Gradient descent, 13
GreenIoT framework, 115

H

Healthcare, 11
Heterogeneity, 110, 111
Hidden layers, 13
Horizontal communication, 108
Hyperparameters, 15
Hypertext transfer protocol, 116

I

Information, 11, 13–14, 16
Injection of false data, 117
Integrated development environment, 116
Internet of Medical Things (IoMT), 255
Internet of Things, 106
Interoperability, 106–11
Interoperability platforms, 115
InterSensor, 112
Introduction, 156, 193
IoT development stages, 108
IoT ecosystem, 114, 116
IoT hierarchy, 108
Isotonic separation, 200

J

JavaScript Object Notation, 111
Jobs, 17

K

K-Means, 202
K-nearest neighbor (KNN), 16, 201

L

Layer, 13–17
Least squares support vector machine (LS-SVM), 198
Levels of interoperability, 108
LIME, 165
Linear discriminant analysis (LDA), 203
Linear PCA, 83, 84
Logistic regression (LR), 196–7

M

Machine learning (ML), 11
Machine learning, 53, 55, 61, 64, 67, 194
Machine learning techniques, 195
Magnetic resonance imaging, 55–6, 63, 65
Malicious code injection attack, 117
Malignancy, 18
Mapping, 111
MATLAB, 14
Merkle tree, 120
Message exchange, 112
Message Queuing Telemetry Transport (MQTT) protocol, 111
Metastases, 18
Methodology, 159
Middleware, 111
ML algorithms, 251
ML and deep learning, 250
Model, 15–16
Model interpretability, 165, 166
Molecular, 12
MRI, 12–13

N

Naive Bayes (NB), 199
Negative, 13, 17–18
Network things, 116
Neurological treatment and rehabilitation programs using AI technology, 248
NLP algorithms, 252
Node capture, 117
Non-interoperability, 106

O

Ontology, 112, 113
Open data, 109–10, 114
Open information, 115
OpenSensors, 113
Optimization, 13, 15

P

Patients, 13, 18
Performance metrics, 95, 97, 98
Period, 13
PET, 12–13
Phishing site attack, 118
Photoplethysmography (PPG), 136
Planning, 11
Platform for development, 115

Positive, 13, 17–18
Practical Byzantine Fault Tolerance, 122
Precision medicine in cardiovascular care, 247
Prediction, 11, 13, 18
Pre-processing, 53, 58, 62, 71
Prognosis, 11
Proof of elapsed time, 121
Proof of importance, 120
Proof of stake, 120
Proof of work, 120
Proposed model, 162
Publishing and marketplace system, 115
Publish-subscribe system, 111

Q

Quality, 14, 18

R

Radio-frequency identifications, 116
Radiography, 12
Random forest, 13, 200–201
Real-time information, 109
Related work, 157
Reprogram attack 119
Research, 11–12, 18
ResNet101 15–17
Resource description framework, 113
Restricted Boltzmann Machines (RBM), 203
Results and discussion, 163
Robot operating system (ROS), 111

S

Second epidemic, 133
Security threats, 117
Seizure, 18
Self-care, 114
Semantic level, 108, 114
Semantics, 113
Sensitivity, 13, 17
Sensors, 107, 110
Sequential, 13
Service-oriented architecture, 112
SHAP, 165, 166
Share layer, 116
Side-channel attacks, 118
Signatures, 12
Silhouette score, 98
Sleep deprivation attacks, 118
Slurred speech, 132
Smart buildings, 107
Smart city, 109
Smart healthcare, 110
Smart transports, 113
Sniffing out attacks, 119
Software framework, 112
SOM, 202
Specificity, 17
Standardized protocols, 115
Standardizing, 113
Structural level, 108, 114
Supervised machine learning, 86
Support vector machine (SVM), 197–198

T

TabDoc, 113
Technique, 12–14, 16
Theft of data, 119
ThinkSpeak, 113
Three-level hybrid, 114
Toolbox, 14
Translator, 111
Treatment, 11–12, 18
Triglyceride-glucose (TyG), 137
t-Stochastic Neighbour Embedding, 94
Tumor, 11–14, 16–17

U

Unsupervised machine learning, 93
Utilization, 18

V

Value, 17–18
Vector machine, 16
Vertical communication, 108
VGG19, 161, 162

W

Web of Things (WoT), 115
Wrapper, 111

Z

Zero, 17

www.ingramcontent.com/pod-product-compliance
Lightning Source LLC
LaVergne TN
LVHW011117300926
849160LV00008B/417
* 9 7 8 1 0 3 2 7 7 6 5 8 3 *